T0362439

Diversity, Equity, and Inclusion in Obstetrics and Gynecology

Editor

VERSHA PLEASANT

OBSTETRICS AND GYNECOLOGY CLINICS OF NORTH AMERICA

www.obgyn.theclinics.com

Consulting Editor
WILLIAM F. RAYBURN

March 2024 • Volume 51 • Number 1

ELSEVIER

1600 John F. Kennedy Boulevard • Suite 1800 • Philadelphia, Pennsylvania, 19103-2899

http://www.theclinics.com

OBSTETRICS AND GYNECOLOGY CLINICS OF NORTH AMERICA Volume 51 Number 1
March 2024 ISSN 0889-8545, ISBN-13: 978-0-443-13149-3

Editor: Kerry Holland
Developmental Editor: Saswoti Nath

© **2024 Elsevier Inc. All rights are reserved, including those for text and data mining, AI training, and similar technologies.**

This periodical and the individual contributions contained in it are protected under copyright by Elsevier, and the following terms and conditions apply to their use:

Photocopying
Single photocopies of single articles may be made for personal use as allowed by national copyright laws. Permission of the Publisher and payment of a fee is required for all other photocopying, including multiple or systematic copying, copying for advertising or promotional purposes, resale, and all forms of document delivery. Special rates are available for educational institutions that wish to make photocopies for non-profit educational classroom use. For information on how to seek permission visit www.elsevier.com/permissions or call: (+44) 1865 843830 (UK)/(+1) 215 239 3804 (USA).

Derivative Works
Subscribers may reproduce tables of contents or prepare lists of articles including abstracts for internal circulation within their institutions. Permission of the Publisher is required for resale or distribution outside the institution. Permission of the Publisher is required for all other derivative works, including compilations and translations (please consult www.elsevier.com/permissions).

Electronic Storage or Usage
Permission of the Publisher is required to store or use electronically any material contained in this periodical, including any article or part of an article (please consult www.elsevier.com/permissions). Except as outlined above, no part of this publication may be reproduced, stored in a retrieval system or transmitted in any form or by any means, electronic, mechanical, photocopying, recording or otherwise, without prior written permission of the Publisher.

Notice
No responsibility is assumed by the Publisher for any injury and/or damage to persons or property as a matter of products liability, negligence or otherwise, or from any use or operation of any methods, products, instructions or ideas contained in the material herein. Because of rapid advances in the medical sciences, in particular, independent verification of diagnoses and drug dosages should be made.

Although all advertising material is expected to conform to ethical (medical) standards, inclusion in this publication does not constitute a guarantee or endorsement of the quality or value of such product or of the claims made of it by its manufacturer.

Obstetrics and Gynecology Clinics (ISSN 0889-8545) is published quarterly by Elsevier Inc., 360 Park Avenue South, New York, NY 10010-1710. Months of issue are March, June, September, and December. Periodicals postage paid at New York, NY, and additional mailing offices. Subscription price per year is $355.00 (US individuals), $100.00 (US students), $428.00 (Canadian individuals), $100.00 (Canadian students), $497.00 (international individuals), $956.00 (international institutions), and $225.00 (international students). For institutional access pricing please contact Customer Service via the contact information below. To receive student/resident rate, orders must be accompanied by name of affiliated institution, date of term, and the signature of program/residency coordinator on institution letterhead. Orders will be billed at individual rate until proof of status is received. Foreign air speed delivery is included in all *Clinics* subscription prices. All prices are subject to change without notice. POSTMASTER: Send address changes to *Obstetrics and Gynecology Clinics*, Elsevier Health Sciences Division, Subscription Customer Service, 3251 Riverport Lane, Maryland Heights, MO 63043. **Customer Service: Telephone: 1-800-654-2452 (U.S. and Canada); 314-447-8871 (outside U.S. and Canada). Fax: 314-447-8029. E-mail: journalscustomerservice-usa@elsevier.com (for print support); journalsonlinesupport-usa@elsevier.com (for online support).**

Reprints. For copies of 100 or more of articles in this publication, please contact the Commercial Reprints Department, Elsevier Inc., 360 Park Avenue South, New York, New York 10010-1710. Tel.: 212-633-3874; Fax: 212-633-3820; E-mail: reprints@elsevier.com.

Obstetrics and Gynecology Clinics of North America is also published in Spanish by McGraw-Hill Interamericana Editores S.A., P.O. Box 5-237, 06500, Mexico; in Portuguese by Reichmann and Affonso Editores, Rio de Janeiro, Brazil; and in Greek by Paschalidis Medical Publications, Athens, Greece.

Obstetrics and Gynecology Clinics of North America is covered in MEDLINE/PubMed (Index Medicus), Excerpta Medica, Current Concepts/Clinical Medicine, Science Citation Index, BIOSIS, CINAHL, and ISI/BIOMED.

Contributors

CONSULTING EDITOR

WILLIAM F. RAYBURN, MD, MBA
Affiliate Professor, Department of Obstetrics and Gynecology and College of Graduate Studies, Medical University of South Carolina Charleston, South Carolina; Emeritus Distinguished Professor, Department of Obstetrics and Gynecology, University of New Mexico School of Medicine, Albuquerque, New Mexico

EDITOR

VERSHA PLEASANT, MD, MPH
Clinical Assistant Professor, Director, Cancer Genetics and Breast Health Clinic, Department of Obstetrics and Gynecology, University of Michigan, Ann Arbor, Michigan

AUTHORS

MARY F. ACKENBOM, MD, MSc
Assistant Professor, Obstetrics and Gynecology, Magee-Womens Research Institute, University of Pittsburgh, Pittsburgh, Pennsylvania

LEEN AL KASSAB, MD
Department of Obstetrics and Gynecology, Harvard Medical School, Brigham and Women's Hospital, Boston, Massachusetts

IMAN K. BERRAHOU, MD
Department of Obstetrics, Gynecology and Reproductive Sciences, Yale School of Medicine, New Haven, Connecticut

OLUWATENIOLA E. BROWN, MD
Assistant Professor, Obstetrics and Gynecology, Northwestern University Feinberg School of Medicine, Chicago, Illinois

AMANDA S. BRUEGL, MD, MCR (ONEIDA, STOCKBRIDGE-MUNSEE NATIONS)
Associate Professor, Division of Gynecologic Oncology, Oregon Health and Science University, Portland, Oregon

CHARELLE M. CARTER-BROOKS, MD, MSc
Assistant Professor OB/GYN & Urology, The George Washington School of Medicine and Health Sciences, Washington, DC

AGENA R. DAVENPORT-NICHOLSON, MD, FACOG
Department of Gynecology and Obstetrics, Emory University School of Medicine, Atlanta, Georgia

JESSICA BUCK DISILVESTRO, MD (CADDO NATION OF OKLAHOMA)
Gynecologic Oncology Fellow, Brown University, Women & Infants Hospital, Providence, Rhode Island

SUSAN DWYER ERNST, MD
Clinical Associate Professor of Obstetrics and Gynecology, University of Michigan Medical School, and Chief of Gynecology at the University Health Service, Michigan Medicine, Ann Arbor, Michigan

JASMIN A. EATMAN, MS
Emory University School of Medicine, Rollins School of Public Health, Emory University, Atlanta, Georgia

JOSHUA GEORGE, MD, MPH
Maternal Fetal Medicine Fellow, Department of Obstetrics and Gynecology, University of Michigan, Ann Arbor, Michigan

LEAH HABERSHAM, MD
Assistant Professor, Department of Obstetrics, Gynecology, and Reproductive Science, Icahn School of Medicine at Mount Sinai, New York, New York

FELICIA L. HAMILTON, MD, FACOG
OB/Gyn Residency Program Director, Chair, OB/Gyn Practice Committee, Department of Obstetrics and Gynecology, MedStar Washington Hospital Center; Associate Clinical Professor, Georgetown University Medical Center, Washington, DC

MADELINE HEDGES
Undergraduate Student, University of Arizona, Tucson, Arizona

CHERIE C. HILL, MD, FACOG
Assistant Professor, Department of Gynecology and Obstetrics, Emory University School of Medicine, Atlanta, Georgia

JASMINE D. JOHNSON, MD
Assistant Professor of Clinical Obstetrics and Gynecology, Division of Maternal-Fetal Medicine, Indiana University School of Medicine, Indianapolis, Indiana

KIMBERLY KARDONSKY, MD (JAMESTOWN S'KLALLAM TRIBE)
Assistant Professor, Department of Family Medicine, University of Washington School of Medicine, Health Sciences Center, Seattle, Washington

CHARISSE LODER, MD, MSc
Assistant Professor, Department of Obstetrics and Gynecology, University of Michigan, Ann Arbor, Michigan

BLAIR McNAMARA, MD
Instructor, Department of Obstetrics, Gynecology and Reproductive Sciences, Yale School of Medicine, New Haven, Connecticut

KATHLEEN E. O'BRIEN, MD
Clinical Instructor, Michigan Medicine, Ann Arbor, Michigan

RIEHAM OWDA, MD
Assistant Professor, Department of Obstetrics and Gynecology, University of Michigan, Ann Arbor, Michigan

VERSHA PLEASANT, MD, MPH
Clinical Assistant Professor, Director, Cancer Genetics and Breast Health Clinic, Department of Obstetrics and Gynecology, University of Michigan, Ann Arbor, Michigan

LOBNA RAYA, MSEd
Tufts University, Medford, Massachusetts

WILLIAM F. RAYBURN, MD, MBA
Affiliate Professor, Department of Obstetrics and Gynecology and College of Graduate Studies, Medical University of South Carolina Charleston, South Carolina; Emeritus Distinguished Professor, Department of Obstetrics and Gynecology, University of New Mexico School of Medicine, Albuquerque, New Mexico

MONICA WOLL ROSEN, MD
Clinical Assistant Professor, Department of Obstetrics and Gynecology, Michigan Medicine, Ann Arbor, Michigan

KYRA W. SEIGER, BA
Yale School of Medicine, New Haven, Connecticut

SARRAH SHAHAWY, MD, MPH
Instructor in Obstetrics, Department of Obstetrics and Gynecology, Division of Global and Community Health, Harvard Medical School, Beth Israel Deaconess Medical Center, Boston, Massachusetts

COURTNEY D. TOWNSEL, MD, MSc
Assistant Professor, Department of Obstetrics, Gynecology and Reproductive Sciences, University of Maryland, Baltimore, Baltimore, Maryland

KEELY K. ULMER, MD (OGLALA SIOUX NATION OF SOUTH DAKOTA)
Gynecologic Oncology Fellow, University of Iowa Hospitals and Clinics, Iowa City, Iowa

VERSHA PLEASANT, MD, MPH
Clinical Assistant Professor, Director, Cancer Genetics and Breast Health Clinic, Department of Obstetrics and Gynecology, University of Michigan, Ann Arbor, Michigan

LORNA RAYA, MSEd
Tufts University, Medford, Massachusetts

WILLIAM F. RAYBURN, MD, MBA
Associate Professor, Department of Obstetrics and Gynecology, and College of Graduate Studies, Medical University of South Carolina, Charleston, South Carolina; Emeritus Distinguished Professor, Department of Obstetrics and Gynecology, University of New Mexico School of Medicine, Albuquerque, New Mexico

MONICA WOLL ROSEN, MD
Clinical Assistant Professor, Department of Obstetrics and Gynecology, Michigan Medicine, Ann Arbor, Michigan

IRYNA W. SEIGER, BA
Yale School of Medicine, New Haven, Connecticut

SARRAH SHAHAWY, MD, MPH
Instructor in Obstetrics, Department of Obstetrics and Gynecology, Division of Global and Community Health, Harvard Medical School, Beth Israel Deaconess Medical Center, Boston, Massachusetts

COURTNEY D. TOWNSEL, MD, MSc
Assistant Professor, Department of Obstetrics, Gynecology and Reproductive Sciences, University of Maryland, Baltimore, Baltimore, Maryland

KEELY K. ULMER, MD (OGLALA SIOUX NATION OF SOUTH DAKOTA)
Gynecologic Oncology Fellow, University of Iowa Hospitals and Clinics, Iowa City, Iowa

Contents

evidence-based policies and practices while empowering the next generation to chart the path forward to equity.

Pelvic floor disorders are a group of common conditions affecting women of all racial and ethnic groups. These disorders are undertreated in all women, but this is especially magnified in Black people who have been historically marginalized in the United States. This article seeks to highlight the prevalence of pelvic floor disorders in Black women, evaluate the clinical care they receive, examine barriers they face to equitable care, and present a strategic agenda to prioritize the care of Black women with pelvic floor disorders.

Institutional transformation and moving diversity from the periphery to the core of excellence have increased the representation of both female and racial and ethnic minoritized populations in academic obstetrics and gynecology (OB/GYN). Enabling the recruitment and retention of diverse residents and faculty, measuring their contributions to the department academic and social missions, and providing a supportive environment will be important in the coming years as the changing OB/GYN workforce progresses through their careers.

Stigma toward pregnant and postpartum people who use drugs is common and seeks to define addiction as a moral weakness rather than a chronic medical illness that requires resources and treatment. More concerning is the additive impact of substance use and racial discrimination, whose intersections present particularly challenging circumstances. In this article, the authors review the history of substance use in the United States and focus on 3 substances of abuse that illustrate the inequity faced by pregnant person of color who use drugs.

There is a long-standing history of reproductive oppression in the United States which impacts how patients, particularly those from marginalized communities, receive reproductive health services today. The reproductive justice (RJ) framework is a tool to support people to become pregnant, to not become pregnant, and to parent in safe communities. In this review, the authors provide essential background about this history and how those in reproductive health care can use the RJ framework through an intersectional lens to achieve inclusive reproductive goals and advocate for comprehensive access to family planning care, including contraceptive and abortion care.

OBSTETRICS AND GYNECOLOGY CLINICS

THE CLINICS ARE AVAILABLE ONLINE!
Access your subscription at:
www.theclinics.com

Foreword

Taking Health Care to the Next Level Through Practicing Diversity, Equity, and Inclusiveness

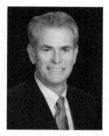

William F. Rayburn, MD, MBA
Consulting Editor

A generation and certainly two generations ago, the concept of diversity, equity, and inclusion (DEI) was not well recognized in medicine. It was not until recently that DEI in medicine became recognized as diversity, equity, and inclusiveness among health care providers and between providers, patients, and their families. The act or practice of including and accommodating people who have historically been excluded because of their race, ethnicity, gender, sexuality, and ability has become a *frontline* issue to encourage variety and freedom from bias or favoritism. This edition of Obstetrics and Gynecology Clinics of North America—capably edited by Versha Pleasant, MD, MPH from the University of Michigan—speaks to these pressing issues.

Since the recent Coronavirus disease 2019 (COVID-19) pandemic, more attention has been placed on people of all races and backgrounds and their health outcomes. People of color experienced higher rates of infection, hospitalization, and death attributed to COVID-19. Politically charged social issues brought more attention to everyone about racism and inequity in America. There is increased awareness of the human rights of people with different sexual orientations and gender expressions, fertility options, gender-affirming medications and surgeries, mental and physical disabilities, and reproductive justice within family planning.

This issue highlights several examples of practice in obstetrics and gynecology dating back to enslaved persons. Articles in this issue focus on pressing disparity issues, such as increased maternal mortality, breast cancer, pelvic floor disorders, and substance use in pregnancy among Black communities and cervical cancer among American Indian and Alaska Natives. Health disparities are also explored in other ethnic and cultural groups, such as Latinx and Muslim patients.

Obstet Gynecol Clin N Am 51 (2024) xi–xii
https://doi.org/10.1016/j.ogc.2023.12.001
0889-8545/24/© 2023 Published by Elsevier Inc.

One means for addressing health care delivery of our increasingly diverse population is to recruit more health care students with diverse backgrounds. Undergraduate and graduate medical programs are becoming more engaged in training about racial and ethnic diversity, as well as in culturally sensitive care. The field of OB/GYN has led recruiting students who are underrepresented in medicine. The resultant faculty, especially those who are junior, reflects this diversity of racial and ethnic groups, yet more is necessary to better reflect the patients we serve.

Preparing an article for this issue was educational to me. Terminology is important, and Dr Pleasant was instructive in the constantly evolving DEI language with significant social and medical consequences. Use of the words "race" and "ethnicity" and "female" and "woman" illustrates examples of common terms that do not fully encompass the breadth of our patients.

The manuscripts in this issue aim to highlight extreme disparities impacting vulnerable populations. The expert group of authors has been purposeful in offering actionable strategies in practicing inclusive, quality, and compassionate care. Simply reading about DEI or listening to lectures is insufficient. I concur with Dr Pleasant that practitioners must "live" diversity, equity, and inclusiveness in their clinics and hospital settings. Enhanced care for vulnerable and underserved populations must be better measured and reported but also may not produce immediate results. These efforts may require time and a long-term commitment to DEI to demonstrate improvements. I look forward to re-addressing this issue as we take health care to the next level by understanding and practicing DEI with our colleagues and patients.

William F. Rayburn, MD, MBA
Department of Obstetrics and Gynecology
University of New Mexico School of Medicine
Albuquerque, NM 87106, USA

Department of Obstetrics and Gynecology
Medical University of South Carolina
Charleston, SC 29425, USA

E-mail address:
wrayburnmd@gmail.com

Preface

The Time is Now: Diversity, Equity, and Inclusion in Obstetrics and Gynecology

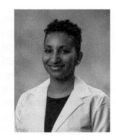

Versha Pleasant, MD, MPH
Editor

Diversity, equity, and inclusion (DEI)—the foundation of this issue of *Obstetrics and Gynecology Clinics of North America*—represents three enormous concepts that both individually and collectively hold incredible significance. The *Webster's Dictionary*[1] suggests the following definitions:

Diversity (noun) (də-'vər-sə-tē): The condition of having or being composed of differing elements: VARIETY, especially: the inclusion of people of different races, cultures, etc in a group or organization.

Equity (noun) (e-kwə-tē): Justice according to natural law or right specifically: freedom from bias or favoritism.

Inclusion (noun) (in-'klü-zhən): The act or practice of including and accommodating people who have historically been excluded (as because of their race, gender, sexuality, or ability).

While these words have existed for quite some time in isolation, recent events in our nation have propelled their unification. COVID-19 emerged as one of the most devastating pandemics the world has ever seen, claiming the lives of over 7 million across the globe.[2] While people of all races and backgrounds were affected by COVID-19, Black and Hispanic communities have experienced higher rates of infection, hospitalization, and COVID-19–related mortality compared with White communities.[3,4] In addition, educational attainment appeared to provide no protection, as the world witnessed

Dr Pleasant is the recipient of a MICHR K12 award (UM1TR004404; K12TR004374; and T32TR004371)

Obstet Gynecol Clin N Am 51 (2024) xiii–xvii
https://doi.org/10.1016/j.ogc.2023.11.004
0889-8545/24/© 2023 Published by Elsevier Inc.

obgyn.theclinics.com

Dr. Susan Moore video journaling her concerns of racist medical treatment and subsequently dying from COVID-19 complications following her hospital discharge.[5]

In parallel to the physical scourge, a concurrent epidemic has swept the country, with roots that far preceded 2019. The public was reminded of the longstanding, permeating institution of racism in the United States while actively witnessing the death of George Floyd on May 25, 2020 via cell phone video. While police brutality against Black people is not a new occurrence in the United States, the culmination of these two major events truly embodied the personifications of inequity and racism in America.[6] They painfully unearthed our nation's dark past of social injustice toward minority groups and medical mistreatment of people of color.

Obstetrics and gynecology (OB/GYN) is not exempt from these phenomena. Historically, the field of OB/GYN has wrestled with racism since the specialty's inception. With the banning of the transatlantic slave trade in 1808, there developed an increasing interest in the reproductive health of Black enslaved people in the United States as it pertained to the reliance on and perpetuation of the institution of slavery. Due to this heightened interest, physicians became more involved in births (where midwives were historically predominant). Furthermore, as discussed in several articles, the bodies of Black enslaved people were perpetually used for experimentative purposes, as was the case with Lucy, Betsy, and Anarcha, who underwent countless unanesthetized surgeries by J. Marion Sims—named the "father of modern gynecology."[7]

Unfortunately, these medical atrocities are not isolated or outdated. Racism in all of its forms continues to be perpetuated in our modern society and is interwoven in our nation's medical system. One of the most pressing issues of our time is Black maternal mortality, for which Black birthing people have a three-fold increased risk of death from pregnancy and its complications compared with White people.[8] "Black Pregnancy-related Mortality in the United States" confronts these disturbing statistics through addressing systemic racism and challenging how the medical system reports and records these disparities. Breast cancer represents another appalling disparity disproportionately impacting Black communities. While breast cancer affects people of all races and ethnic backgrounds, it carries a 40% increased mortality among Black people (the highest across all racial and ethnic groups).[9] The racial disparities in the diagnosis, care, and treatment of breast cancer among Black communities is illuminated in "A Public Health Emergency: Breast Cancer among Black Communities in the United States." These findings are not only disheartening but also unacceptable.

Other unique subspecialty areas that are largely underrepresented in medical literature are included in this issue. "Pelvic Floor Disorders in Black Women: Prevalence, Clinical Care, and a Strategic Agenda to Prioritize Care" highlights the racial disparities in the practice of pelvic floor medicine as well as the lack of research among Black communities, despite the prevalence of pelvic and genitourinary issues. In addition, "Substance Use in Pregnancy and its Impact on Communities of Color" outlines the history, legislation, and policing of substance use disorder in our nation and its complex intersection with pregnancy. Authors highlight these alarming disparities, in which Black birthing people are 10 times more likely to be reported to authorities after positive toxicology compared with their White counterparts despite similar rates of substance use.[10]

Health disparities among other racial, ethnic, and cultural groups are also explored in this collection. With Hispanic people representing the largest growing minority group in the nation, it is imperative that barriers to the provision of quality care (such as language and insurance coverage) are addressed. The article, "OB/GYN Care in Latinx Communities," outlines these disparities, highlights cultural considerations, and provides the way forward with strategic interventions. "Caring for Muslim Patients: A Primer for the OB/GYN" is another article that explores the intersection of culture and OB/GYN care—from fasting in pregnancy during Ramadan to considerations in the provision of family planning services to Muslim patients. Finally, "Cervical Cancer: Preventable Deaths Among American Indian/Alaska Native Communities" reveals sobering statistics regarding the high rates of cervical cancer and related mortality among the American Indian and Alaska Native group, a community that has been significantly marginalized and historically mistreated in our nation. Each of these articles provides a comprehensive lens into the cultural context of each community, with authors offering incredible perspective on these critical topics for which there is largely a dearth of literature. A common theme across each of these articles includes the importance of cultural sensitivity and awareness to build trust, foster compassion, and improve health outcomes.

DEI not only encompasses racial and ethnic diversity. This concept also includes diversity in regard to sexual orientation and gender expression. "Gynecologic Care for LGBTQ+ Patients" equips health care practitioners with the knowledge and tools to provide care to those who have been historically marginalized due to heteronormative structures in OB/GYN. Authors provide a comprehensive review of topics, including fertility options and gender-affirming medications and surgeries. In the same vein, DEI also includes those of diverse abilities, such as people with physical and mental disabilities. This is a community for which practitioners may feel ill-equipped to provide quality care, with authors from "Obstetric and Gynecologic Care for Individuals with Disabilities" offering key recommendations and strategies. Both of these articles provide frameworks for how to best deliver care in a way that is respectful and compassionate.

One of the common themes mentioned throughout this issue as an approach to addressing disparities involves expanding the medical workforce to include individuals from more diverse backgrounds, as data suggest that racial- and ethnic-concordant care could improve outcomes.[11–14] "Delivering Diversity and Inducing Inclusion: Evidence-based Perspectives on Charting a Future of Equity in Obstetrics and Gynecology Residency Programs" provides a bold perspective into diversity among OB/GYN residency programs, presents challenges in recruitment and retention, and provides examples of the positive impact of culturally sensitive training. "Diversity in Academic Obstetrics and Gynecology" similarly explores the changes in OB/GYN clinician demographics over time and how we can (and must) continue to improve representation of all racial-, ethnic-, and gender-diverse groups in this specialty. These articles truly speak to the role of diversity as a cornerstone for excellence in the field of OB/GYN.

Finally, it is nearly impossible to discuss OB/GYN as a specialty without concurrently addressing the human rights of all people. The two concepts are inextricably linked—with each serving as a proxy for the other and a collective gauge of the evolving human conscience. "Achieving Reproductive Justice Within Family Planning" presents an outstanding overview of the history of reproductive rights, legislation, and injustices in the United States. Authors demonstrate how people of color remain disproportionately impacted by barriers to care and how harmful legislation limits the realization of reproductive justice: the right to bodily autonomy, to have children, to not have children, and to raise children in healthy environments.[15]

Throughout the articles, we recognize that terminology is important. Language is constantly evolving as we evolve through a social, cultural, and ethical lens. The terms "race" and "ethnicity" are terms that are often at the root of dialogue surrounding DEI.

Race is indeed a social construct, but its implications still have significant social and medical consequences. While race cannot be ignored, racism is truly the cause of racial health disparities. In addition, we want to acknowledge that although the words "female" and "woman" have historically predominated in the field of OB/GYN and are utilized as needed throughout the articles, these words do not fully encompass the breadth of gender diversity of the patients we serve. We celebrate diversity in all of its forms and remain enthusiastic that our specialty will continue to move the needle in regard to DEI.

There is no better time for such an issue to be published. While these articles are not exhaustive of all of the medical inequities occurring in this nation, they aim to highlight some of the most extreme disparities impacting some of the most vulnerable groups in OB/GYN. Authors in this issue do not simply report on statistics. While knowledge is power, knowledge must also translate to action. The authors are intentional about equipping practitioners with tangible, actionable strategies regarding how to practice inclusive, quality, and compassionate care. Despite what our dictionary definitions tell us about the words diversity, equity, and inclusion—that these are all nouns—this issue of *Obstetrics and Gynecology Clinics of North America* challenges us all to see these concepts as verbs. It is no longer enough to discuss DEI. Rather, we must live it daily, act upon it, commit to it, and be persistently and unapologetically intentional about it. We can and must strive to want better for our patients and to be better as clinicians. The time is now.

DISCLOSURE

No disclosures to be made.

Versha Pleasant, MD, MPH
Cancer Genetics &
Breast Health Clinic
Department of Obstetrics and Gynecology
University of Michigan
1500 East Medical Center Drive
Ann Arbor, MI 48109, USA

E-mail address:
vershap@med.umich.edu

REFERENCES

1. Merriam-Webster. America's Most Trusted Dictionary. Merriam-Webster dictionary. Available at: https://www.merriam-webster.com. Accessed November 15, 2023.

2. Marks KM, Gulick RM. COVID-19. Ann Intern Med 2023;176(10):ITC145–60.

3. Mackey K, Ayers CK, Kondo KK, et al. Racial and ethnic disparities in COVID-19-related infections, hospitalizations, and deaths: a systematic review. Ann Intern Med 2021;174(3):362–73.

4. Vasquez Reyes M. The disproportional impact of COVID-19 on African Americans. Health Hum Rights 2020;22(2):299–307.

5. Stewart A. Black physician's COVID death underscores health disparities. American Academy of Family Physicians. January 15, 2021. Available at: https://www.aafp.org/news/blogs/leadervoices/entry/20210115lv-coviddisparities.html. Accessed November 16, 2023.

6. Merritt D. George Floyd's death and COVID-19: inflection points in the Anthropocene Era? J Anal Psychol 2021;66(3):750–62.
7. Owens DC. Medical bondage: race, gender, and the origins of American gynecology. Athens: University of Georgia Press; 2017.
8. Centers for Disease Control and Prevention. Working together to reduce Black maternal mortality. April 3, 2023. Available at: https://www.cdc.gov/healthequity/features/maternal-mortality/index.html. Accessed November 16, 2023.
9. American Cancer Society. Breast Cancer Facts and Figures 2022–2024. 2022. Available at: https://www.cancer.org/content/dam/cancer-org/research/cancer-facts-and-statistics/breast-cancer-facts-and-figures/2022-2024-breast-cancer-fact-figures-acs.pdf. Accessed September 7, 2023.
10. Chasnoff IJ, Landress HJ, Barrett ME. The prevalence of illicit-drug or alcohol use during pregnancy and discrepancies in mandatory reporting in Pinellas County, Florida. N Engl J Med 1990;322(17):1202–6.
11. Jetty A, Jabbarpour Y, Pollack J, et al. Patient-physician racial concordance associated with improved healthcare use and lower healthcare expenditures in minority populations. J Racial Ethn Health Disparities 2022;9(1):68–81.
12. Shen MJ, Peterson EB, Costas-Muñiz R, et al. The effects of race and racial concordance on patient-physician communication: a systematic review of the literature. J Racial Ethn Health Disparities 2018;5(1):117–40.
13. Greenwood BN, Hardeman RR, Huang L, et al. Physician-patient racial concordance and disparities in birthing mortality for newborns. Proc Natl Acad Sci USA 2020;117(35):21194–200.
14. Snyder JE, Upton RD, Hassett TC, et al. Black representation in the primary care physician workforce and its association with population life expectancy and mortality rates in the US. JAMA Netw Open 2023;6(4):e236687.
15. Ross LJ, Solinger R. Reproductive justice: an introduction. Oakland, CA: University of California Press; 2017.

Black Pregnancy-Related Mortality in the United States

Jasmine D. Johnson, MD

KEYWORDS

- Maternal mortality • Black maternal mortality • Racial disparities • Health equity
- Racism • Reproductive justice

KEY POINTS

- The maternal mortality rate for non-Hispanic Black birthing people is 69.9 deaths per 100,000 live births compared with 26.6 deaths per 100,000 live births for non-Hispanic White birthing people.
- Black pregnancy-related mortality has been underrepresented in research and the media; however, there is growing literature on the role of racism in health disparities.
- Those who provide care to Black patients should increase their understanding of racism's impact and take steps to center the experiences and needs of Black birthing people.

INTRODUCTION

The National Center for Health Statistics defines a maternal[a] death as "the death of a woman while pregnant or within 42 days of termination of pregnancy, irrespective of the duration and site of the pregnancy, from any cause related to or aggravated by the pregnancy or its management, but not from accidental or incidental causes."[1] The maternal mortality rate (MMR) is calculated as the number of deaths per 100,000 live births. In 2019, the MMR was 20.1 in 2019 and 23.8 in 2020. The most recent data for 2021 from the Centers for Disease Control and Prevention (CDC) reported an overall MMR in the United States of 32.9 deaths per 100,000 live births.[2]

Division of Maternal-Fetal Medicine, Indiana University School of Medicine, 550 North University Bloulevard, Suite 2440, Indianapolis, IN 46202, USA
E-mail address: Jadrans@iu.edu

[a] The author notes that there continues to be a need for more inclusive terminology to broaden the focus to include all individuals who may be affected by pregnancy-related and -associated mortality, not just those traditionally considered "maternal." This language acknowledges the diverse range of gender identities and experiences of people who may experience pregnancy-related issues. Throughout this review, the terms "pregnant person" or "birthing person" will be used whenever possible. When describing study populations used in research or initiatives, the author will use the gender terminology reported by the study investigators.

Obstet Gynecol Clin N Am 51 (2024) 1–16
https://doi.org/10.1016/j.ogc.2023.11.005
0889-8545/24/© 2023 Elsevier Inc. All rights reserved.

obgyn.theclinics.com

When the data are disaggregated by race and ethnicity, the MMR for non-Hispanic Black birthing people was 69.9 deaths per 100,000 live births, compared with 26.6 deaths per 100,000 live births for non-Hispanic White birthing people, representing an almost threefold increased risk.[3] Most importantly, behind every statistical is a family that has been devastated. Despite growing national discourse and ongoing initiatives aimed to decrease US maternal mortality,[4] including standardization of practices[5] and perinatal quality collaboratives,[6] Black birthing people continue to have worse outcomes.

The staggering rates of death experience during or within 1 year of pregnancy for Black birthing people in the United States is not a new problem. In a study examining maternal mortality in Chicago and Detroit from 1979 to 1984, the Black MMR was four times that of their White counterparts.[7] Similar to other racial and ethnic health disparities, the pregnancy mortality crisis for Black individuals has been historically underrepresented in research and the media. One study observing the media coverage trends for maternal mortality found that news reporting specifically on "Black maternal mortality" did not reach mainstream media prominence, and race-related coverage of the issue remained mostly stagnant until Serena Williams told her story to Vogue in 2018.[8] In her personal account, she repeatedly appealed to her health care team symptoms concerning for a pulmonary embolism—something she had previously experienced. Although her concerns were initially dismissed, she subsequently underwent imaging demonstrating that she did have a pulmonary embolism in additions to the complications from a delayed diagnosis. Her story spoke to the larger issue that Black birthing people—regardless of education, financial status, or influence—are not protected from racial health disparities. In addition, despite the historical underreporting and lack of recognition, Black birthing people have been acutely aware of the disproportionate burden they bear in the United States maternal mortality crisis. Not only is a collective awareness of these staggering and unacceptable statistics necessary, but also take active steps in clinical care, research, and advocacy to correct this unacceptable inequity. The following is an exploration on the current state of Black pregnancy-related and -associated mortality including data trends, updated research, and evidence-based care strategies that obstetrics and gynecology (OB/GYN) clinicians can consider when providing care to Black birthing people.

CAUSES

The top causes of maternal mortality in the United States include hemorrhage, hypertension, infection, venous thromboembolism, and cardiac conditions.[9] A review of racial and ethnic disparities in the United States using enhanced vital records from 2016 to 2017 found that the leading causes of death for non-Hispanic Black people were preeclampsia/eclampsia and postpartum cardiomyopathy, with rates noted to be five times that of non-Hispanic White people.[10]

Preeclampsia and Eclampsia

Hypertensive disorders of pregnancy can impact both morbidity and mortality among birthing people and represent a significant and alarming racial health disparity in obstetrics. Preeclampsia and eclampsia, the extremes of the hypertensive disorders spectrum, disproportionately impact Black birthing people. The prevalence of preeclampsia from 1980 to 2010 was estimated to be 2% to 8%,[11] and several studies have determined that this percentage is greatly increased among non-Hispanic Black people.[12,13] Data from the National Inpatient Sample demonstrated that 69.8 per 1000 deliveries by Black birthing people were complicated by preeclampsia (compared with

43.3 per 1000 for White people and 46.8 per 1000 for Hispanic people).[13] One retrospective cohort analysis using data from 2004 to 2012 showed that Black birthing people with preeclampsia or eclampsia carried an increased risk of inpatient mortality (OR = 3.70, 95% CI: 2.19–6.24), which persisted even after adjustment (OR = 2.85, 95% CI: 1.38–5.53).[14] A more recent literature search demonstrated that Black birthing people with preeclampsia demonstrated higher levels of severe hypertension, hemorrhage, and mortality, along with increased risk of preterm birth and intrauterine fetal demise.[15] The US Preventive Services Task Force, the American College of Obstetricians and Gynecologists (ACOG), and the Society for Maternal-Fetal Medicine (SMFM) recommend the use of aspirin to decrease the risk of recurrent preeclampsia. Alarmingly, a single-center study examining the impact of this recommendation on the incidence of preeclampsia demonstrated the relative proportion of Hispanic birthing people who experienced recurrent preeclampsia after the implementation of low-dose aspirin was lower in the post-aspirin group (76.4% vs 49.6%). However, there was no difference in recurrent preeclampsia in non-Hispanic Black birthing people (13.7 vs 18.1; $P = 252$).[16]

Within the postpartum period, one retrospective cohort study indicated that birthing people with new-onset postpartum preeclampsia were more likely to be of non-Hispanic Black race (31.4% vs 18.0%; $P < .01$).[17] A second single-center study found that although there were no statistically significant differences in the rates of postpartum readmission for hypertensive disorders of pregnancy, Black patients were more likely to be admitted for preeclampsia with severe features and more likely to have their initial evaluations in the emergency room compared with their White counterparts.[18]

Deaths from preeclampsia spectrum causes are some of the most preventable causes of maternal deaths as they are due to delays in diagnosis and timely treatment of severe range blood pressure. Several Black women's stories have been elevated who died during the perinatal period from complications of preeclampsia. In 2017, Dr Shalon Irving, an epidemiologist at the CDC, died after having a cardiac arrest caused by postpartum preeclampsia. Dr Irving's mother speaks of the days leading up to her daughter's death in which she had been pleading with her care team because she felt something was wrong; however, they ignored her concerns. She had been seen only 6 hours before her death.[19] In 2020, Amber Rose Isaac tweeted hours before her death from Hemolysis-Elevated Liver Enzymes-Low Platelets (HELLP) syndrome that her care team was not listening to her. Her story is shared in the documentary *Aftershock*.[20] To date, there are no genetic factors that have been identified to justify the persistent racial disparities in preeclampsia and preeclampsia-related morbidity. This serves as a call to action to expose and eliminate the downstream effects of systemic racism including biased treatment and barriers to care play a role.

Peripartum Cardiomyopathy

Peripartum cardiomyopathy (PPCM) is the development of heart failure during pregnancy or in the months following delivery in the absence of other causes. Data suggest that Black people have a higher incidence of PPCM compared with other racial and ethnic groups. This is multifactorial in etiology—including sequelae of preeclampsia—which may confer a higher risk of postpartum cardiomyopathy.[21,22] Multiple studies have found that Black patients are diagnosed with PPCM at younger ages, later in the postpartum period, and are more likely to have an ejection fraction less than 30% (being the most severe).[23,24] In addition, Black patients with PPCM are more likely to have implantable defibrillator placement and are less likely to have recovery of their ejection fraction compared with White patients.[25] Although management of PPCM by a cardiologist is associated with improved outcomes, one study found that Black patients admitted to the ICU for management of heart failure were less likely than White patients to receive their primary care by a cardiologist. Primary care by a cardiologist was associated with higher survival for both Black and White patients.[26] There is a significant need for more extensive examination of maternal deaths due to cardiovascular causes for Black patients.

Hemorrhage

A 2021 review found that non-Hispanic Black mortality rates from obstetric hemorrhage were 2.3 to 2.6 times that of non-Hispanic White populations.[10] One study using data from the National Inpatient Sample found that Black birthing people were at a higher risk of severe morbidity due to hemorrhage.[27] For non-Hispanic Black compared with non-Hispanic White, Hispanic, and Asian or Pacific Islander birthing people, risk was higher for disseminated intravascular coagulation (8.4% vs 7.1%, 6.8%, and 6.8%, respectively, $P < .01$) and transfusion (19.4% vs 13.9%, 16.1%, and 15.8%, respectively, $P < .01$). Black birthing people were also more likely than non-Hispanic White birthing people to undergo hysterectomy. Despite this greater risk for hemorrhage-related morbidity, a recent single-center study identified racial disparities in escalation of care for postpartum hemorrhages requiring blood transfusion. Black and Hispanic patients were less likely to have received higher levels of intervention compared with White patients. This difference persisted with increasing estimated blood loss up to ≥3000 mL, with Black and Hispanic patients being significantly less likely to receive higher levels of intervention compared with White patients.[28] Similar to preeclampsia, most of the pregnancy-related deaths due to hemorrhage are preventable. Alarmingly, one state-wide review suggested that almost all pregnancy-related deaths due to hemorrhage were potentially preventable.[29] Jarring racial and ethnic disparities in preventable pregnancy-related deaths further underscores this crisis is a human rights issue.

PREVENTABILITY

Unfortunately due to the limitations in data collection, statistics related to racial and ethnic disparities in perinatal outcomes is primarily ascertained through medical claims or birth certificates. This leaves significant gaps related to specific case-level contributors to each to adverse outcomes for Black birthing people. One crucial avenue for obtaining more specific information on pregnancy and postpartum-related deaths is through the efforts of maternal mortality review committees (MMRCs). During the in-depth reviews of individual cases, each is assessed for preventability. Preventability is defined as "having at least some chance of the death being prevented by one or more reasonable changes to patient, family, provider, facility, system, and/or community factors". In an examination of maternal mortality committee data across 36 states from 2017 to 2019, up to 84% of maternal deaths were determined to be preventable.[30] A single-state analysis in North Carolina found differences in preventability by cause of death—with 93% of hemorrhage and 60% of hypertension-related deaths found to be preventable.[29] Devastatingly, one study examining racial and ethnic differences in preventable maternal deaths found that for non-Hispanic Black birthing people who experienced pregnancy-related death, 59% of deaths were deemed potentially preventable, compared with 9% for non-Hispanic White birthing people.[31]

Given the limitations of review committee data, an assessment of the experience of prenatal, intrapartum, and postpartum care for Black birthing people can provide some opportunities for intervention. One study demonstrated that daily life experiences of microaggressions of Black pregnant people were associated with delay in seeking prenatal care, defined as initial entry of care at third trimester or no prenatal care at all.[32] Another study found that Black and Hispanic (vs White) pregnant people had higher odds of perceived discrimination due to their race or ethnicity during their delivery hospitalization. Interestingly, higher education was associated with more reported communication problems with their care team among Black pregnant people only.[33] With respect to peridelivery care, a review of multistate delivery records demonstrated that compared with White patients, Black patients were more likely to have a cesarean delivery, have a longer length of stay, and had higher odds of in-hospital mortality.[34] In the postpartum period, Black patients receiving Medicaid in California were less likely to attend a postpartum visit, less likely to receive any contraception, and less likely to receive highly effective methods of contraception compared with their White counterparts.[35]

In addition, it is important to highlight that there is a paucity of research focusing on identifying care team differences in clinical management during pregnancy and postpartum based on race or ethnicity, especially in conditions that can lead to pregnancy-related mortality, such as differences by race and ethnicity on the escalation of care for postpartum hemorrhage[28] or the treatment of postoperative pain after a cesarean delivery.[36] This knowledge gap is extremely problematic for raising awareness, and holding health care teams accountable in situations where unconscious bias and discrimination may play a role. Despite this barrier, through the growing influence of social media and the efforts of advocates, the experiences of Black birthing people who have tragically died during pregnancy or postpartum have been illuminated. Continuing research and transparent case reviews that are publicly available can shed light on differential treatment, including biases in medical practice and discrimination that patients may encounter. This heightened awareness serves as a crucial step in elimination of preventable death related to pregnancy.

"Minorities DIMINISHED RETURNS"

Prior critiques of pregnancy-related mortality disparity data have suggested that Black communities carry more risk factors during pregnancy and, therefore, are at a higher risk of poor outcomes. This argument highlights the importance of understanding how "racism and not race" impacts health outcomes when addressing Black pregnancy-related mortality. Multiple studies have demonstrated how the absence of traditionally held sociodemographic risk factors or the presence of traditional "protective factors" (such as having private insurance or higher educational attainment) do not confer the same protection for Black populations. For example, in a high socioeconomic status cohort, rates of preterm birth at each gestational age cutoff remained highest for those who identified as non-Hispanic Black, intermediate for those identifying as both non-Hispanic Black and White, and lowest for those identifying as non-Hispanic White.[37] In a California population, higher socioeconomic status was associated with a decreased rate of preterm birth for White people but the same decreases were not seen in Black people.[38] This same trend was observed with preeclampsia. Black people had a higher risk of developing preeclampsia independent of education or insurance status.[39] In addition, US maternal mortality data have shown that although White people demonstrate a decrease in MMR with increasing education, this trend is not observed in Black people. Instead, Black people with at least a college degree have a higher pregnancy-related mortality rate than White people who have not finished high school (**Fig. 1**).[40] This phenomenon, in which Black people do not receive

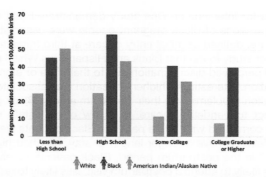

Fig. 1. Pregnancy related deaths and education. Previously published materials unchanged from the source: From Infographic: Racial/Ethnic Disparities in Pregnancy-Related Deaths — United States, 2007–2016. Centers for Disease Control and Prevention; with permission. Available at https://www.cdc.gov/reproductivehealth/maternal-mortality/disparities-pregnancy-related-deaths/infographic.html.

the same protective benefit from positive sociodemographic factors, is called "Minorities' Diminished Returns." This concept has been most devastatingly apparent in the stories of Dr Shalon Irving, Kira Johnson, and Dr Chaniece Wallace—who were all insured, educated, and resourced women who did not survive their pregnancies. Increasing ones awareness of this distinguishing facet of Black pregnancy-related mortality will shift improvement efforts from patient or "person blaming"[41] to addressing the root cause: racism and its downstream effects on structural and social determinants of health.

RACISM AND DISCRIMINATION

There is nothing inherent about Black birthing people that make them at risk for poor outcomes, including death in childbirth. Instead, it is the intersection between racism and health care that leads to health disparities. Dr Camara Jones allegory "The Gardner's Tale" describes three types of racism and how systems perpetuate inequities.[42] Institutionalized or structural racism is differential access to material conditions and access to power. Personally mediated racism is prejudice and discrimination, whereas prejudice means differential assumptions about the abilities, motives, and intentions of others according to their race, and discrimination means differential actions toward others according to their race. Internalized racism is defined as acceptance by members of the stigmatized races of negative messages about their own abilities or intrinsic worth.

Thompson and colleagues found that both structural and individual experiences of racism influenced the reproductive health care access, utilization, and experiences of Black people.[43] Among Black people of child-bearing age, participants reported experiencing all forms of racism over their life course, and childhood experiences were noted to have particularly enduring effects.[44] The experience of racism and discrimination during pregnancy has been associated with a number of adverse outcomes including increased depressive symptoms,[45] preterm birth,[46] and low birth weight infants.[47] In addition, "area racism" as determined by racial animus ascertained from Internet search query data demonstrated that each standard deviation increase in area racism was associated with relative increases of 5% in the prevalence of preterm birth and 5% in the prevalence of low birth weight among Black communities.[48]

Njoku and colleagues stress that racism is "a social construct, root cause, and determinant of maternal morbidity and mortality."[49] Most importantly, they also examine the connections of historical oppression to present-day social determinants of health that disproportionately effect Black birthing people and their families. Crear-Perry and colleagues suggest that expanding assessment of social determinants of health to include "structural determinants of health" and "root causes of inequities" will identify racism as a cause of inequities in maternal health outcomes, as many of the social and political structures and policies in the United States were born out of racism, classism, and gender oppression.[50] This is most clearly depicted in the Restoring Our Own Through Transformation Web of Causation theoretic framework developed by Roach.[51]

Despite race being a social construct, it has biologic consequences. Developed by Dr Arline Geronimus, the concept of weathering demonstrates how racism and discrimination increase physiologic inflammation and accelerate cellular aging. Data suggest that Black people experience higher allostatic load scores (a measure of stress through biometric and clinical measurements) compared with their White counterparts.[52] For instance, Krieger and colleagues demonstrated a higher mean arterial blood pressure in Black adults with self-reported experiences of racism and discrimination.[53] Interestingly, among Black professional adults, systolic blood pressure was 9 to 10 mm Hg lower among those reporting that they challenged unfair treatment or among those who had not experienced racial discrimination. Despite data reflecting the impact of racism on various areas of health (like blood pressure), it is important to highlight that there is a lack of data regarding allostatic load specifically in Black birthing people. This is a much needed area of further investigation.

RECOMMENDATIONS

There is an urgent need to eradicate racism in all of its forms to adequately address racial health disparities. Health care providers at all levels must make a commitment to providing equitable, anti-racist care to Black birthing patients to create safe and thriving environments for birthing people and their infants. This section addresses strategies to achieve this goal. **Table 1** summarizes these recommendations.

Elevating the Black Voice

Efforts to decrease Black maternal mortality and other health inequities will require engagement with Black birthing people and their support networks to address historical and present-day harms that have been committed by the medical institution. Although there is no scarcity of quantitative studies demonstrating health disparities in pregnancy for Black people, only a handful of qualitative studies have centered the voices of Black birthing people. One study found that during pregnancy regardless of socioeconomic status, marital status, or parity, Black people reported encountering assumptions that they had low incomes, were single, and had multiple children.[54] In addition, racialized pregnancy stigma influenced their access to and quality of services and contributed to overall stress. In exploring the lived experience of racism and how it effects the reproductive health experiences of Black people,[55] Treder and colleagues found that personal, vicarious, and historical experiences of racism within reproductive health care influenced study participants to reveal a number of self-protective actions they take when interacting with the health care system. This included behaviors such as seeking health care professionals of color, overpreparation for appointments to "show" a clinician that they are knowledgeable, and seeking care or intervention only when desperate.

Table 1 Key recommendations to eliminate black maternal mortality disparities	
Elevating the Black Voice	Engage Black birthing people and their support networks in the process of care delivery to address historical and present-day harms. Use the lived experiences of Black people to inform policy and practice changes that improve Black birthing outcomes. Understand that historical and present practices that marginalize vulnerable groups must be eliminated and replaced with more inclusive and equitable approaches.
No Quality without Equity	Train clinicians to recognize and address racism and impact on health outcomes. Require clearly defined equity-focused goals as quality metrics in reproductive health care services and discrete variables to capture root causes disparities research. Provide racial equity-focused training and encourage institutions to evaluate practices and policies at their institution or clinical settings that may be perpetuating racism.
Centering at the Margins	Implement community-informed models of care that reflect the racial, ethnic, and cultural diversity of the communities being served (such as pregnancy centering and multidisciplinary care teams including doulas). Promote cultural safety and inclusion in the health care environment.
Transparency and Accountability	Use validated tools like the PREM-OB Scale to capture instances of obstetric racism. Encourage accountability through data transparency and digital applications that allow patients to share their experiences. Develop a formal process for reporting and addressing medical racism and mistreatment.
Morbidity and Mortality Review Committees	Standardize the review process and data collection for maternal mortality review committees. Improve data collection on direct and indirect measures of racism. Apply a health equity framework and engage community members in the review process.
Clinicians as Advocates	Recognize the importance of policy and legislation in addressing the structural determinants of health and systemic change needed to improve pregnancy-related mortality disparities. Support legislation for formal bias and anti-racism training, Medicaid expansion, paid family leave, and funding for maternal mortality review committees. Participate in advocacy events and support initiatives like the Black Maternal Health Momnibus.

Abbreviations: PREM-OB (TM), the patient reported experience measure of obstetrc racism.

Canty and colleagues interviewed nine Black women who experienced severe maternal morbidity to better understand the psychological and emotional implications of suffering and surviving a life-threatening complication during childbirth and post-partum.[56] Up to one-third of participants described negative experiences with their health care team, and their race influenced how they presented themselves, the ways in which they responded to their health care providers, and how they perceived their health care providers responding to them. In conceptualizing a prenatal care model that *centers* the experience of the Black birthing person, a study at the Roots Community Birth Center in Minneapolis explored patient perceptions of what defines a good birthing experience.[57] Themes that arose in their focus groups included having agency or autonomy, having a historically and culturally safe experience, and experiencing relationship-centered care. These studies highlight an opportunity to listen to Black birthing people before they experience a sentinel event, giving insight to their needs and informing innovative solutions.

No Quality Without Equity

In a clinical opinion piece on lessons from mortality reviews,[58] a group of MMRC members emphasize that addressing US maternal mortality will require educating and training physicians to deal with the downstream consequences of upstream events. This involves increasing attention on educating themselves and their trainees about the effect of racism, social disadvantage, and poor coordination of care on health, as well as the role of the care team in resolving these issues. Trainings focused on racial equity are offered by organizations such as the Racial Equity Institute, National Birth Equity Collaborative, and March of Dimes.

Furthermore, a study in California demonstrated decreased hemorrhage associated maternal morbidity addressing through addressing knowledge deficits and implementation of standardized care practices.[6] When specifically examining the impact of similar changes on Black–White hemorrhage disparities and accounting for maternal risk factors, the Black–White relative risk for severe maternal morbidity excluding transfusion alone was reduced from a baseline of 1.33 (95% CI, 1.16–1.52) to 0.99 (0.76–1.29) in the post-intervention period.[5] In single health care system, the implementation of evidence-based practices driven solely to improve Black maternal morbidity rates was associated with significant reductions in maternal morbidity for Black people from pre-goal to post-goal development overall.[59] These studies support that institutions can and should develop clearly defined equity-focused goals when enacting changes that seek to improve disparate outcomes.

"Centering at the Margins"

Recommendations from Black Mamas Matter Alliance[60,61] and Julian and colleagues emphasize the importance of community-informed models of care.[62] "Centering at the margins" means that care provision is centric to the needs of communities who have been historically excluded or marginalized. This model of care should include team members that reflect the racial, ethnic, and cultural diversity of the communities they serve. As a result, this may foster a more inclusive and culturally safe pregnancy environment for Black birthing people. Teaching this type of care model and health care culture should start as early as medical and nursing school training.

Studies have highlighted that Black birthing people seek out Black care providers as a self-protective action against experiencing racism and adverse outcomes.[44,54,55,57] In addition, Black patients are more likely to seek preventative care from racial concordant providers,[63] and Black newborns had higher rates of survival when cared for by Black doctors.[64] The obvious recommendation is to continue to increase diversity in the medical workforce. The current reality, however, is that approximately 5% of practicing US physicians identify as Black,[65] and as a result, not every Black patient will be able to access a Black care team. Given this, non-Black providers should be better equipped to understand the experiences and address the needs of Black birthing people. In their paper, "This is Our Lane: Talking with Patients About Racism,"[66] Diop and colleagues suggest using trauma-informed care as a framework for talking to patients about their experiences of racism and discrimination. They highlight that acknowledging and gaining an understanding of structural racism's impact on health, providers can create safe spaces within the clinical encounter that build trust and engagement. Most importantly, team members should develop pathways to support patients who experience racism such as connecting patients to local advocacy programs and civil rights legal aid.

Transparency and Accountability

Calling out medical racism and mistreatment endured in the health care system should have a formal process, timely follow-up, and accountability. The PREM-OB Scale is a tool that captures instances of obstetric racism and harm endured by Black birthing people.[67] Using this validated tool, hospital systems can formally measure their patients' experiences of racism. In addition, leveraging technology with digital applications, such as IRTH[68] ("Taking the B for bias out of birth"), encourages Black birthing people to share their experiences in health care systems across the country with the goal of signaling to others which hospitals provide cultural supportive and safe care. Tools that give spotlight to the experiences of Black birthing people when receiving health care offer increased accountability for health systems as an impetus for change.

It is important for systems to take this one step further to clearly call out racism and health disparities related to each safety bundle (which represent collection of evidence-based literature and practices on a given topic). The Alliance for Innovation in Maternal Health has removed the Eliminating Racial and Ethnic Health Disparities Bundle, and in its place, added "Respectful, equitable, and supportive care" as a main tenant within all Obstetric care safety bundles. This change seeks to better integrate equity into every safety bundle. The SMFM summaries the anti-racism strategies to improve reproductive, maternal, and infant health.[69] Examples of this include creating a culture of safety, centralized reporting, and institutional response to identify and address instances of racism, thereby supporting community-based strategies as a complement to traditional medical care for specific populations.

Morbidity and Mortality Review Committees

The CDC provides oversight for maternal mortality data in the United States. They have defined three classifications of maternal death for determination by MMRCs.

1. Pregnancy-related death: a death during pregnancy or within 1 year of the end of pregnancy from a pregnancy complication, a chain of events initiated by pregnancy, or the aggravation of an unrelated condition by the physiologic effects of pregnancy.
2. Pregnancy-associated but not related death: a death during pregnancy or within 1 year of the end of pregnancy from a cause that is not related to pregnancy.
3. Pregnancy-associated but unable to determine pregnancy-relatedness death.

In 2018, the US Congress passed the "Preventing Maternal Deaths Act" which allowed the CDC to support state MMRCs.[70] This act was reaffirmed in 2023. Currently, 39 states and one US territory have been awarded funding support through the ERASE Maternal Mortality Program. On a state and local level, this analysis and discussion of maternal mortality cases occurs through MMRCs. However, with some states lacking an infrastructure for timely and thorough case review, there is no uniformity regarding who is selected for these committees or the committees' process for evaluating cases. Many times, hospitals or state organizations create their own review committees with little or no dedicated time or funding. The Maternal Mortality Review Information Application[71] (MMRIA) is a data system that helps to standardize review practices and data collection in regard to maternal mortality. It is available to all MMRCs to help organize available data and begin the critical steps necessary to comprehensively identify and assess maternal mortality cases. MMRIA also plays a critical role in data aggregation the dissemination of review committee findings for national improvement efforts.

Improving data collection on direct and indirect measures of racism should not only be a priority for state MMRCs, but for severe hospital morbidity review committees as well. In 2021, a work group appointed by the CDC defined types of racism and discrimination that should be considered as contributors to pregnancy-related mortality for inclusion on the MMRIA form.[72] The Black Mamas Matter Alliance published an executive summary of recommendations for better engaging community members in MMRC to promote equity.[60] Key recommendations from the report included (1) centering the experiences of community members, (2) diversifying MMRC membership, (3) increasing transparency of the MMRC process and data, and (4) strengthen the capacity of MMRCs to better examine and address racism and discrimination. Additional recommendations for MMRCs are to apply a health equity framework (**Fig. 2**) with social determinants of maternal health, socio-spatial measures of community context to potentially incorporate into individual maternal death review narratives, and illustrative policy and programmatic interventions that map community-based factors to possible MMRC recommendations for prevention.[73]

Clinicians as Advocates

In addition to speaking out against racism and all its forms in clinical settings, clinicians can be advocates by further addressing the structural determinants of health and root causes of inequities. There is an important role legislation and policy play in undoing the burden of racism on health. It is not enough to be educated on the ways in which society perpetuates inequities, but clinicians are also called to advocacy for vulnerable populations beyond the examination room. The ACOG and SMFM continue to support OB/GYN physicians and other reproductive health providers with resources for communicating with their local and national legislatures. By participating in events such as ACOG Congressional Leadership Conference,[74] as well as local and national advocacy days, clinicians can speak with policy makers to advocate for systemic change. This can be in the form of interventions such as required formal bias and anti-racism training, Medicaid expansion, paid family leave, and increased funding for MMRCs through the reauthorization of the Preventing Maternal Deaths Act.[75] One such large-scale policy initiative is the Black Maternal Health Momnibus which includes 13 individual bills created by members of the US House of Representatives Black Maternal Health Caucus. This initiative seeks to address Black pregnancy mortality through historic investments that comprehensively address every driver of

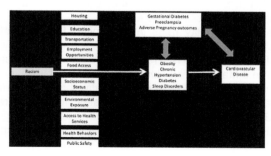

Fig. 2.

maternal mortality, morbidity, and disparities in the United States.[76] Increasing public awareness and non-partisan support for these initiatives will work toward improving health outcomes in Black birthing people.

SUMMARY

In order to successfully address the Black pregnancy-related mortality crisis in the United States, the direct and indirect role of racism on health outcomes must be acknowledged. Historical and present-day practices that continue to uphold systems that marginalize vulnerable groups must be addressed and eliminated. These practices should be replaced by radical change in governmental policy, innovation in care team education, directed research strategy and practice with respect to cultural humility, and elevating the lived experience Black people to improve Black birthing outcomes.

CLINICS CARE POINTS

- The US maternal mortality rate has increased since 2019, and significant racial and ethnic perinatal health disparities continue to exist.
- Preeclampsia and eclampsia, as well as postpartum cardiomyopathy, represent the large percentage of mortality burden among Black birthing people.
- Health disparities, including those during pregnancy, are the downstream result of historical and present-day racism.
- A better understanding of structural and social determinants of health due to racism can further elucidate the most impactful solutions to eradicate racial and ethnic disparities related to pregnancy.
- There are practical opportunities OB/GYN clinicians can use to combat racism and its resultant inequities in clinical spaces, particularly through statewide and local maternal mortality review committees, and health care advocacy.

DISCLOSURE

The author reports no conflicts of interest or financial disclosures. The author reports no funding sources.

REFERENCES

1. Organization WH. International statistical classification of diseases and related health problems, 10th revision. 2008 ed2009.
2. Hoyert D. Maternal mortality rates in the United States, 2019. NCHS Health E-Stats; 2022.
3. Simpson KR. Effect of the COVID-19 pandemic on maternal health in the United States. MCN Am J Matern Child Nurs 2023;48:61.
4. Ahn R, Gonzalez GP, Anderson B, et al. Initiatives to reduce maternal mortality and severe maternal morbidity in the united states : a narrative review. Ann Intern Med 2020;173:S3–s10.
5. Main EK, Chang SC, Dhurjati R, et al. Reduction in racial disparities in severe maternal morbidity from hemorrhage in a large-scale quality improvement collaborative. Am J Obstet Gynecol 2020;223:123, e1-.e14.

6. Main EK, Cape V, Abreo A, et al. Reduction of severe maternal morbidity from hemorrhage using a state perinatal quality collaborative. Am J Obstet Gynecol 2017;216:298, e1-.e11.
7. Siefert K, Martin LD. Preventing black maternal mortality: a challenge for the 90's. J Prim Prev 1988;9:57–65.
8. Walker D, Boling K. Black maternal mortality in the media: how journalists cover a deadly racial disparity. Journalism 2023;24:1536–53.
9. Davis NLSA, Goodman DA. Pregnancy-related deaths: data from 14 U.S. Maternal mortality review committees 2008-2017. Atlanta, GA: Centers for Disease Control and Prevention, U.S. Department of Health and Human Services; 2019.
10. MacDorman MF, Thoma M, Declcerq E, et al. Racial and ethnic disparities in maternal mortality in the united states using enhanced vital records, 2016–2017. Am J Publ Health 2021;111:1673–81.
11. Ananth CV, Keyes KM, Wapner RJ. Pre-eclampsia rates in the United States, 1980-2010: age-period-cohort analysis. BMJ 2013;347:f6564.
12. Gyamfi-Bannerman C, Pandita A, Miller EC, et al. Preeclampsia outcomes at delivery and race. J Matern Fetal Neonatal Med 2020;33(21):3619–26.
13. Fingar KR, Mabry-Hernandez I, Ngo-Metzger Q, et al. Delivery hospitalizations involving preeclampsia and eclampsia, 2005–2014. Rockville (MD): Agency for Healthcare Research and Quality (US); 2006.
14. Shahul S, Tung A, Minhaj M, et al. Racial disparities in comorbidities, complications, and maternal and fetal outcomes in women with preeclampsia/eclampsia. Hypertens Pregnancy 2015;34:506–15.
15. Zhang M, Wan P, Ng K, et al. Preeclampsia among african american pregnant women: an update on prevalence, complications, etiology, and biomarkers. Obstet Gynecol Surv 2020;75:111–20.
16. Tolcher MC, Chu DM, Hollier LM, et al. Impact of USPSTF recommendations for aspirin for prevention of recurrent preeclampsia. Am J Obstet Gynecol 2017; 217:365 e1–e8.
17. Redman EK, Hauspurg A, Hubel CA, et al. Clinical course, associated factors, and blood pressure profile of delayed-onset postpartum preeclampsia. Obstet Gynecol 2019;134:995–1001.
18. Oladipo V, Dada T, Suresh SC, et al. Racial differences in readmissions in hypertensive disorders of pregnancy. Reprod Sci 2022;29:2071–8.
19. Honoring Dr, Irving W, Irving S, et al. Shalon irving, a champion for health equity. Health Aff 2022;41:304–8.
20. Eiselt PE, Lewis Lee Tonya. Aftershock. 2022.
21. Bello N, Rendon ISH, Arany Z. The relationship between pre-eclampsia and peripartum cardiomyopathy: a systematic review and meta-analysis. J Am Coll Cardiol 2013;62:1715–23.
22. Levine LD, Lewey J, Koelper N, et al. Persistent cardiac dysfunction on echocardiography in African American women with severe preeclampsia. Pregnancy hypertension 2019;17:127–32.
23. Irizarry OC, Levine LD, Lewey J, et al. Comparison of clinical characteristics and outcomes of peripartum cardiomyopathy between African American and non-African American women. JAMA Cardiol 2017;2:1256–60.
24. Goland S, Modi K, Hatamizadeh P, et al. Differences in clinical profile of African-American women with peripartum cardiomyopathy in the United States. J Card Fail 2013;19:214–8.

25. Sinkey RG, Rajapreyar IN, Szychowski JM, et al. Racial disparities in peripartum cardiomyopathy: eighteen years of observations. J Matern Fetal Neonatal Med 2022;35:1891–8.

26. Breathett K, Liu WG, Allen LA, et al. African Americans are less likely to receive care by a cardiologist during an intensive care unit admission for heart failure. JACC (J Am Coll Cardiol): Heart Fail 2018;6:413–20.

27. Gyamfi-Bannerman C, Srinivas SK, Wright JD, et al. Postpartum hemorrhage outcomes and race. Am J Obstet Gynecol 2018;219:185.

28. Guan CS, Boyer TM, Darwin KC, et al. Racial disparities in care escalation for postpartum hemorrhage requiring transfusion. Am J Obstet Gynecol MFM 2023;5:100938.

29. Berg CJ, Harper MA, Atkinson SM, et al. Preventability of pregnancy-related deaths: results of a state-wide review. Obstet Gynecol 2005;106:1228–34.

30. Trost S, Beauregard J, Chandra G, et al. Pregnancy-related deaths: data from maternal mortality review committees in 36 US states, 2017–2019. Atlanta, GA: Centers for Disease Control and Prevention, US Department of Health and Human Services; 2022.

31. Mehta PK, Kieltyka L, Bachhuber MA, et al. Racial inequities in preventable pregnancy-related deaths in Louisiana, 2011–2016. Obstet Gynecol 2020;135:276–83.

32. Slaughter-Acey JC, Sneed D, Parker L, et al. Skin tone matters: racial microaggressions and delayed prenatal care. Am J Prev Med 2019;57:321–9.

33. Attanasio L, Kozhimannil KB. Patient-reported communication quality and perceived discrimination in maternity care. Med Care 2015;53:863–71.

34. Tangel V, White RS, Nachamie AS, et al. Racial and ethnic disparities in maternal outcomes and the disadvantage of peripartum black women: a multistate analysis, 2007-2014. Am J Perinatol 2019;36:835–48.

35. Thiel de Bocanegra H, Braughton M, Bradsberry M, et al. Racial and ethnic disparities in postpartum care and contraception in California's Medicaid program. Am J Obstet Gynecol 2017;217:47, e1-.e7.

36. Johnson JD, Asiodu IV, McKenzie CP, et al. Racial and ethnic inequities in postpartum pain evaluation and management. Obstet Gynecol 2019;134:1155–62.

37. Johnson JD, Green CA, Vladutiu CJ, et al. Racial disparities in prematurity persist among women of high socioeconomic status. Am J Obstet Gynecol MFM 2020;2:100104.

38. Braveman PA, Heck K, Egerter S, et al. The role of socioeconomic factors in Black-White disparities in preterm birth. Am J Publ Health 2015;105:694–702.

39. Ross KM, Dunkel Schetter C, McLemore MR, et al. Socioeconomic status, preeclampsia risk and gestational length in black and white women. J Racial Ethn Health Disparities 2019;6:1182–91.

40. Infographic: Racial/Ethnic Disparities in Pregnancy-Related Deaths — United States, 2007–2016. Centers for Disease Control and Prevention.

41. Scott KA, Britton L, McLemore MR. The ethics of perinatal care for black women: dismantling the structural racism in "mother blame" narratives. J Perinat Neonatal Nurs 2019;33:108–15.

42. Jones CP. Levels of racism: a theoretic framework and a gardener's tale. Am J Publ Health 2000;90:1212–5.

43. Thompson TM, Young YY, Bass TM, et al. Racism runs through it: examining the sexual and reproductive health experience of black women in the south. Health Aff 2022;41:195–202.

44. Nuru-Jeter A, Dominguez TP, Hammond WP, et al. "It's the skin you're in": African-American women talk about their experiences of racism. an exploratory study to develop measures of racism for birth outcome studies. Matern Child Health J 2009;13:29–39.

45. Ertel KA, James-Todd T, Kleinman K, et al. Racial discrimination, response to un-fair treatment, and depressive symptoms among pregnant black and African American women in the United States. Ann Epidemiol 2012;22:840–6.

46. Braveman P, Heck K, Egerter S, et al. Worry about racial discrimination: a missing piece of the puzzle of Black-White disparities in preterm birth? PLoS One 2017; 12:e0186151.

47. Mustillo S, Krieger N, Gunderson EP, et al. Self-reported experiences of racial discrimination and Black-White differences in preterm and low-birthweight deliv-eries: the CARDIA Study. Am J Publ Health 2004;94:2125–31.

48. Chae DH, Clouston S, Martz CD, et al. Area racism and birth outcomes among Blacks in the United States. Soc Sci Med 2018;199:49–55.

49. Njoku A, Evans M, Nimo-Sefah L, et al. Listen to the whispers before they become screams: addressing black maternal morbidity and mortality in the United States. Healthcare (Basel) 2023;11.

50. Crear-Perry J, Correa-de-Araujo R, Lewis Johnson T, et al. Social and structural determinants of health inequities in maternal health. J Wom Health 2021;30: 230–5.

51. ROOTT's theoretical framework of the Web of Causation between structural and social determinants of health and wellness. 2016, Available at: https://www.roottrj.org/web-causation. Accessed August 3, 2022.

52. Geronimus AT, Hicken M, Keene D, et al. "Weathering" and age patterns of allo-static load scores among blacks and whites in the United States. Am J Publ Health 2006;96:826–33.

53. Krieger N, Sidney S. Racial discrimination and blood pressure: the CARDIA Study of young black and white adults. Am J Publ Health 1996;86:1370–8.

54. Mehra R, Boyd LM, Magriples U, et al. Black pregnant women "get the most judg-ment": a qualitative study of the experiences of black women at the intersection of race, gender, and pregnancy. Wom Health Issues 2020;30:484–92.

55. Treder K, White KO, Woodhams E, et al. Racism and the reproductive health ex-periences of U.S.-Born Black Women. Obstet Gynecol 2022;139:407–16.

56. Canty L. The lived experience of severe maternal morbidity among Black women. Nurs Inq 2022;29:e12466.

57. Karbeah J, Hardeman R, Katz N, et al. From a place of love: the experiences of birthing in a black-owned culturally-centered community birth center. J Health Dispar Res Pract 2022;15:47–60.

58. Minkoff H, Chazotte C, Nathan LM. Lessons from Mortality Reviews: Nonbiologic Contributors to Maternal Deaths. Am J Perinatol 2023. https://doi.org/10.1055/s-0043-1769470.

59. Hamm RF, Howell E, James A, et al. Implementation and outcomes of a system-wide women's health 'team goal' to reduce maternal morbidity for black women: a prospective quality improvement study. BMJ Open Qual 2022;11(4):e002061.

60. Black Mamas Matter Alliance RaED. Maternal Mortality Review Committees: Sharing Power with Communities2021 November 2021. https://blackmamasmatter.org/wp-content/uploads/2022/04/BMMA_MMRCReport2021_Finalv2.pdf.

61. Alliance BMM. Setting the standard for holistic care of and for Black women. https://blackmamasmatter.org/wp-content/uploads/2018/04/BMMA_BlackPaper_April-2018.pdf.
62. Julian Z, Robles D, Whetstone S, et al. Community-informed models of perinatal and reproductive health services provision: a justice-centered paradigm toward equity among Black birthing communities. Semin Perinatol 2020;44:151267.
63. Ma A, Sanchez A, Ma M. The impact of patient-provider race/ethnicity concordance on provider visits: updated evidence from the medical expenditure panel survey. J Racial Ethn Health Disparities 2019;6:1011–20.
64. Greenwood BN, Hardeman RR, Huang L, et al. Physician-patient racial concordance and disparities in birthing mortality for newborns. Proc Natl Acad Sci U S A 2020;117:21194–200.
65. Physician Specialty Data Report. 2022. at https://www.aamc.org/data-reports/workforce/data/active-physicians-black-african-american-2021.
66. Diop MS, Taylor CN, Murillo SN, et al. This is our lane: talking with patients about racism. Womens Midlife Health 2021;7:7.
67. White VanGompel E, Lai JS, Davis DA, et al. Psychometric validation of a patient-reported experience measure of obstetric racism© (The PREM-OB Scale™ suite). Birth 2022;49:514–25.
68. IRTH App. at https://irthapp.com.
69. Green CL, Perez SL, Walker A, et al. The cycle to respectful care: a qualitative approach to the creation of an actionable framework to address maternal outcome disparities. Int J Environ Res Public Health 2021;18(9):4933.
70. Congress US. Preventing Maternal Deaths Act of 2018, H.R. 1318, 115th Cong, 132 Sess. 2018.
71. Maternal Mortality Review Information Application — MMRIA. at https://review-toaction.org/tools/mmria.
72. Hardeman RR, Kheyfets A, Mantha AB, et al. Developing tools to report racism in maternal health for the CDC maternal mortality review information application (MMRIA): FINDINGS from the MMRIA racism & discrimination working group. Matern Child Health J 2022;26:661–9.
73. Kramer MR, Strahan AE, Preslar J, et al. Changing the conversation: applying a health equity framework to maternal mortality reviews. Am J Obstet Gynecol 2019;221:609, e1-.e9.
74. Gynecologists ACoOa. Congressional Leadership Conference.
75. ACOG Action Center. (Accessed July 22, 2023, at https://acog.quorum.us/action-center/).
76. Caucus UHoRBMH. Black Maternal Health Momnibus.

Gynecologic Care for Sexual and Gender Minority Patients

Kyra W. Seiger, BA[a], Blair McNamara, MD[b],
Iman K. Berrahou, MD[c],*

KEYWORDS

- Sexual and gender minorities • LGBTQ • Gynecology • Gender-affirming care

KEY POINTS

- Sexual and gender minority (SGM) people, including lesbian, gay, bisexual, transgender, and queer people, have a wide spectrum of gynecologic needs, including cancer screening, family building, and gender-affirming care.
- SGM people face a disproportionate burden of health disparities, which are directly and indirectly related to pervasive discrimination.
- Gynecologists should use evidence-based care that incorporates an understanding of health disparities faced by SGM patients and addresses current gaps in knowledge.
- Gynecologists should actively work to dismantle institutionalized cisheteronormativity in their clinical practices, avoiding unnecessarily gendered language and clinical assumptions based on patients' sex, gender, gender identity, or sexual orientation identity.

INTRODUCTION

Sexual and gender minority (SGM) people, including lesbian, gay, bisexual, transgender, and queer (LGBTQ+) individuals, comprise at least 7% of adults in the United States.[1] This rate is increasing over time, particularly among US young adults aged 18 to 25 years, with 21% identifying as SGM.[1]

SGM people experience a disproportionate burden of health and health-care disparities, including higher rates of obesity, tobacco and substance use, underinsured or uninsured status, mental health morbidity, and lower utilization of preventative health services and cancer screening tests.[2–4] These disparities are directly and

[a] Yale University School of Medicine, 367 Cedar Street, New Haven, CT 06510, USA;
[b] Department of Obstetrics, Gynecology & Reproductive Sciences, Yale University School of Medicine, 333 Cedar Street, New Haven, CT 06520, USA; [c] Department of Obstetrics, Gynecology & Reproductive Sciences, Yale University School of Medicine, 333 Cedar Street, PO Box 208063, Suite 302 FMB, New Haven, CT 06520-806, USA
* Corresponding author.
E-mail address: iman.berrahou@yale.edu

Obstet Gynecol Clin N Am 51 (2024) 17–41
https://doi.org/10.1016/j.ogc.2023.10.001
0889-8545/24/© 2023 Elsevier Inc. All rights reserved.

obgyn.theclinics.com

indirectly related to pervasive discrimination faced by SGM populations, which include experiences of discrimination while seeking health care. Discrimination because of sexual orientation and gender identity begins at a young age; a recent survey showed that 75% of LGBTQ + youth experienced discrimination because of their sexual orientation or gender identity (SOGI) at least once in their lifetime.[5] Chronic exposure to stigma and discrimination, often referred to as minority stress, contributes to psychological stress and deteriorates coping skills with resultant adverse health effects and an inordinate burden of negative health outcomes among SGM people.[6-9] Additionally, there are few clinicians who feel educated and confident providing care to SGM people, leading this group to face a critical barrier to accessing health care. For example, in a recent survey of gynecology providers, only 42% reported prior training in LGBTQ health.[10] Finally, because most national health databases and registries do not routinely and comprehensively collect SOGI data, this population's health-care needs, including in the field of obstetrics and gynecology (OB/GYN), are often underdescribed and understudied.[11,12]

Health-care providers and systems must become safe, equitable, and proficient in addressing the clinical needs of this underserved and marginalized patient population. Health-care providers, including gynecologic providers and specialists, can play a critical role in creating inclusive care environments and supporting the development of resilience for SGM patients. In this article, we focus specifically on the provision of gynecologic care to SGM people. We review key topics in gynecology, including gynecologic cancers and cancer screening, sexually transmitted infection (STI) and intimate partner violence (IPV) screening, contraception and pregnancy prevention, family building and preconception counseling, and, finally, gender-affirming gynecologic care. We finally offer considerations toward improving gynecologic care environments and clinical spaces.

We use the following terminology and definitions throughout this review. We define sexual orientation as how a person identifies their physical, emotional, and romantic attachments to other people through the components of attraction, behavior, and identity.[13] Sexual minority is an umbrella term referring to anyone who is not heterosexual or straight; examples include those who identify as gay, lesbian, bisexual, queer, or pansexual, although there are many more.[13] Although we believe that sexual behavior categorizations (eg, men who have sex with men, women who have sex with women [WSW], women who have sex with men and women [WSMW]) should not be used to displace sexual orientation identity, we use these terms when discussing previously published studies that use these categorizations in their reporting.[14]

The "gender binary"—the concept that there are only 2 distinct genders, "man" and "woman," and that one's assigned sex at birth aligns with their gender identity—has long been the dominant discourse of gender in the United States.[15] However, this cultural belief does not accurately encapsulate the identities, expression, and experiences of many people. Transgender is an umbrella term for individuals whose gender identity differs from that typically associated with the sex they were assigned at birth.[13] Gender nonbinary is an umbrella term used to describe individuals whose gender falls outside of the gender binary.[13]

DISCUSSION
Cancers and Cancer Screening in Sexual and Gender Minority Patients

SGM people experience a disproportionate burden of health-care disparities, which translate to higher prevalence of cancer risk factors, such as higher rates of tobacco use, obesity, underinsured or uninsured status, and lower utilization of cancer screening tests.[2,16–19] Additionally, experiences and fear of discrimination adversely influence the care of SGM patients with cancer and patient-centered outcomes.[20–22] The impact of discrimination manifests not only during treatment but also during remission; higher rates of psychological distress are reported among LGBTQ cancer survivors compared with their heterosexual cisgender counterparts.[20] Based on American Cancer Society and National Cancer Institute estimates of a 40% lifetime risk of cancer for US adults, there are likely 9 million SGM adults with cancer in the United States.[23,24] However, the true incidence and prevalence of cancer in this population remain unknown because no national health surveys or cancer registries routinely and comprehensively collect SOGI data.[25,26] In this section, we will review the known evidence surrounding gynecologic and breast cancers and screening among SGM patients.

Cervical cancer

There has been widespread adoption of cervical cancer screening in the United States during the last several decades; however, despite advances in screening, it is estimated that there will still be 13,960 new cervical cancer diagnoses, and 4310 deaths from cervical cancer in 2023.[27] The incidence of cervical cancer among the SGM population is not known. Unfortunately, human papillomavirus (HPV)-associated risk factors are known to be higher in the SGM population, leading many to believe that patients may be of increased risk for dysplasia and cervical cancer.[28] Additionally, SGM people are known to be underscreened for cervical cancer and undervaccinated against HPV across several subpopulations.[29,30] Several barriers to SGM populations accessing cervical cancer screening have been identified in the literature, and barriers to presentation for gynecologic concerns in this population are discussed elsewhere in this review. Encouragement of HPV vaccination should occur for all members of the SGM community and cervical cancer screening recommended for all SGM people with a cervix.

Exogenous testosterone is known to cause atrophy of cervical tissues, leading to increased rates of insufficient Pap tests in SGM populations on testosterone therapy.[29] Because The American Cancer Society guidelines now recommend universal high-risk HPV screening for patients aged older than 30 years, insufficient Pap tests can now be more clinically meaningful for older patients. Some have proposed universal high-risk HPV screening for SGM patients on testosterone but this is not supported by evidence at this time.[28] Furthermore, given that presenting to a gynecologist and undergoing a speculum examination can contribute to gender dysphoria among transmasculine patients, many have proposed patients self-collect Pap smear results; the diagnostic accuracy of this strategy has been supported by several studies and meta-analyses.[31]

Endometrial cancer

Endometrial cancer is the most common gynecologic cancer in the United States with more than 66,000 new cases diagnosed annually.[24] In particular, higher rates of obesity and nulliparity, and lower rates of oral contraceptive use in the SGM population, are all risk factors for the development of endometrial hyperplasia (precancer) and cancer.[19,32] Tobacco use, which occurs at higher rates in the SGM population, has been associated with an increased risk of Type II (estrogen-independent) endometrial cancers.[32] For transgender or gender nonbinary patients with a uterus who use gender-affirming hormone therapy, there is a theoretic concern that the use of exogenous testosterone may create an environment of unopposed estrogen due to its aromatization to estrogen and the anovulatory state it induces, which may increase the risk of endometrial hyperplasia/cancer.[33] Based on very limited data, testosterone hormonal therapy alone without the use of estrogen and/or progesterone did not cause a difference in rates of proliferative versus atrophic endometrium in a retrospective review.[34] Furthermore, in that same review, longer duration of testosterone use was not associated with endometrial thickness or proliferation.[34] Although testosterone therapy seems to not modulate risk, providers should perform a thorough evaluation when patients present with abnormal uterine bleeding or postmenopausal bleeding, regardless of hormone therapy use.

Ovarian cancer

The American Cancer Society estimates that 19,710 new ovarian cancer cases and 13,270 ovarian cancer-related deaths will occur in the United States in 2023.[27] Of all gynecologic cancers in the United States, epithelial ovarian cancer is associated with the highest mortality.[35] Despite modest advancements in chemotherapy and surgical techniques for treating ovarian cancer, there is still no validated screening or early detection technology. Because of this, most patients present with advanced disease. There is a paucity of data on ovarian cancer incidence and prevalence among SGM populations.

Exogenous testosterone has been thought to possibly contribute to the development of ovarian cancer because it can be aromatized to estrogen. Several cases of ovarian cancer in transmasculine patients on testosterone have been described.[28] One nested case-control study of more than 1200 cases of ovarian cancer noted that higher serum levels of testosterone correlated with an increased risk of endometrioid and mucinous ovarian cancer subtypes[36]; however, a separate report from the same group noted that although endogenous testosterone levels were correlated with lower grade carcinomas, there was an inverse association with high-grade endometrial carcinomas.[37]

There is a critical need for research that investigates the prevalence, incidence, outcomes, and experiences of SGM people who develop cancer. Understanding differences in outcomes and experiences of SGM people with gynecologic cancer will influence care patterns and support health-care systems in moving toward visibility and equity in caring for this patient population.

Finally, gynecologists should be prepared to recommend cancer screenings appropriate to which organs a patient has, avoiding anatomic assumptions based on a patient's sex, gender expression, and/or gender identity. This is true, not just for transgender and gender nonbinary (TGNB) people but for all patients. Providers should maintain updated records of which organs are present and apply evidence-based cancer prevention and screening guidelines as applicable.

Breast cancer

Although there are no clearly established data that clearly estimate the prevalence of breast cancer among transgender individuals, some national and international studies have approximated risk. A Dutch retrospective study of transfeminine individuals demonstrated a lower incidence of breast cancer (4.1 per 100,000 person years) compared with cisgender women (155 per 100,000 person years), for which researchers compared the prevalence to male breast cancer among the transfeminine group.[38] A 2015 study of transgender veterans in the United States showed a breast cancer incidence rate of 20.0 per 100,000 person years (regardless of hormonal therapy use).[39]

Hormonal and surgical options among this patient population may influence breast cancer screening and diagnosis. To date, the impact of exogenous estrogen on breast cancer risk for transgender women individuals is unclear, although increased concentrations of prediagnostic endogenous estradiol have been found to be associated with breast cancer in those assigned male at birth.[40,41] However, it is hypothesized that transfeminine individuals have a lower lifetime exposure to estrogen that may decrease their risk.[38] Screening recommendations for those with enhanced breast tissue following exogenous hormone administration has not been established, although some organizations have proposed that transgender women undergo mammogram every 2 years starting at age 50 (having had 5–10 years of feminizing hormone therapy).[40] There should also be the consideration of lower mammographic sensitivity in those with breast implants, and data suggest that exogenous estrogen may increase breast density.[42]

For transgender men, the impact of testosterone on breast cancer risk is unclear. The aforementioned Dutch study also examined transgender men and found an incidence of 5.9 per 100,00 person years, which was lower than the incidence of breast cancer in the cisgender female group and comparable to the rates of breast cancer among people assigned male at birth (AMAB).[38] In regard to surgery, there should be consideration of possible discrepancies between gender-affirming chest surgery and risk-reducing mastectomy, for which the volume of tissue remaining in situ may differ and could have implications on the need for additional screening and residual increased lifetime risk of breast cancer (in those with germline mutations, strong family history, and so forth).[43]

Contraception and Unintended Pregnancy

Members of the SGM population have contraceptive needs that are both similar to and distinct from their cisgender, exclusively heterosexual counterparts. Because SGM assigned female at birth (AFAB) people engage in a variety of sexual behaviors across their life span, regardless of their sexual orientation identity or gender identity, this population can be at risk of becoming pregnant.

In this section, we discuss unintended pregnancies and the contraceptive needs of SGM AFAB patients, focusing first on sexual minority cisgender women, followed by transmasculine and gender nonbinary AFAB people. We discuss the critical skill of sexual history taking that is inclusive of SGM people as a tool to understand patients' contraceptive and noncontraceptive needs. Finally, we offer strategies for gynecology providers to create treatment plans that are aligned with patients' priorities and goals, particularly given the overlapping effects of treatment modalities.

Considerations for sexual minority women

Compared with their exclusively heterosexual peers, sexual minority women (SMW) are more likely to experience unintended pregnancy.[44–52] Several studies have documented an increased risk of teen pregnancy among sexual minority adolescent girls, particularly among bisexual adolescents who are 1.62 to 5.82 times more likely than heterosexual girls to experience teen pregnancy.[45,47] Although less research has focused on sexual minority adult women, studies have demonstrated higher rates of unwanted or mistimed pregnancies in this population. Using data from the 2006 to 2010 National Survey of Family Growth, Everett and colleagues[51] found that, compared with pregnancies in heterosexual women with exclusively male partners, heterosexual women who have sex with women and do not identify as bisexual or lesbian were more likely to have mistimed pregnancies and bisexual and lesbian women were more likely to have unwanted pregnancies. A small number of studies have investigated abortion rates among SMW with inconsistent results.[52] In a 2020 study, using data from the Nurses' Health and Growing Up Today Studies, Charlton and colleagues[46] demonstrated that SMW, except lesbians, were more likely than their heterosexual peers to have an abortion; bisexual women were 3 times as likely as heterosexuals to have had an abortion.

SMW have differences in patterns of contraceptive use, which may contribute to their increased risk of unintended pregnancy.[53] Ela and Budnick report that although SMW had more distinct partners and more intercourse with men in their study period, they had less frequent contraceptive use and more gaps in contraceptive coverage.[54] Additionally, SMW self-report use of less-effective contraceptive methods due to infrequent penile–vaginal intercourse.[55] Finally, SMW are inadequately counseled regarding contraceptive needs and options; Everett and colleagues[56] reported that although 87% of a sample of lesbians and bisexual women had a male partner in the prior 12 months, only 48% received contraceptive counseling at a routine gynecology visit.

Considerations for transmasculine and gender nonbinary assigned female at birth people

There are limited studies investigating rates of unintended pregnancy and contraceptive use among transmasculine and gender nonbinary AFAB people. In one survey of transgender men, 60% of participants used a form of contraception, most commonly condoms and pills.[57] Cipres and colleagues found that less than half of transgender study participants who were at risk of pregnancy and did not desire pregnancy used reliable contraception.[58] Another survey study comparing gender minority and cisgender college students found that gender minorities were less likely to use a method of contraception or consistently use barrier methods or emergency contraception.[59]

People using gender-affirming testosterone have had biologically confirmed ovulatory events and cases of unintended pregnancies, even when amenorrheic.[60,61] Testosterone is not a method of contraception. Consequently, all transgender and gender nonbinary patients who are engaged in sexual intercourse that places them at risk for pregnancy should be offered a contraceptive method if they desire to prevent pregnancy, even if they are amenorrheic on testosterone.

Improving contraceptive care for sexual and gender minority patients at risk of pregnancy

There are several likely contributors to underutilization of contraceptive methods and unintended pregnancy among SGM patients. First, there is a dearth of both patient-facing and provider-facing LGBTQ-inclusive sexual education programming and materials.[46,62–64] This can lead to misconceptions around pregnancy risk at both the patient and provider level. For example, Light and colleagues[57] reported that 16% of surveyed transgender men believed that testosterone was a form of contraception and 5.5% reported that their health-care providers advised testosterone as contraception.

It is critical for health-care providers to take inclusive sexual histories that ask about sexual behaviors, avoiding harmful heteronormative assumptions based on patients' sexual orientation and gender identities. **Table 1** offers examples of LGBTQ-inclusive clinical scripts. Several authors have offered frameworks for inclusive sexual histories; we agree with the recommendation to move away from the commonly taught "Do you have sex with men, women, or both?" in favor of open-ended questions that more specifically characterize patients' contraceptive needs.[63,65,66] Examples include "Do you have sex," "What are the genders and bodies of your sexual partners and which body parts do you use," "Do you use anything for pregnancy prevention," and "Do you desire pregnancy now or in the future?"[65] All patients who are at risk of pregnancy and do not desire pregnancy should receive contraceptive counseling.

Table 1
Recommendations for lesbian, gay, bisexual, transgender, and queer-inclusive clinical scripts

Recommendations/Best Practice	Examples
When addressing new patients, introduce yourself and your preferred pronouns Avoid using gendered terms such as "sir," "ma'am," "Mr ____," or "Ms ____" when referring to new patients	"Hello, my name is Dr Smith. I use she/they pronouns."
In a private setting, ask the patient their preferred name and pronouns	"How would you like to be addressed?" or "What name and pronouns would you like me to use?"
If relevant, ask about preferred names to refer to body parts. Avoid using gendered language. Use anatomy-based language and care	Instead of "breasts," patients may ask to use "chest." Instead of "vulva," patients may prefer "external pelvic area." Instead of "Pap smear" and "prostate examination," you can use "HPV screening" and "cancer screening," respectively
If a patient's name and gender identity do not match their medical record, you can respectfully ask further if necessary for a visit to proceed. Never ask about a "real" name or gender	"Could your chart/medical record/insurance policy be under any other name?"
If asking questions related to sexual history, sexuality, gender, or any potentially sensitive questions, let the patient know that you ask all patients these questions and why these questions are important	"I am now going to ask you a few questions about your sexual history and past partners. I ask all my patients these questions because sexual health and practices influence overall mental and physical health. Your answers are completely confidential."
Do not make assumptions about a patient's sexual or romantic partner(s). Ask politely	"Are you in a relationship? Are you currently sexually active?" "How would your partner(s) identify as in terms of gender?"
Always use a patient's correct name and pronouns, even when the patient is not present	
If you make any mistakes, apologize and demonstrate a willingness to learn and change	"I am so sorry for using the incorrect pronouns/name. I did not mean to be disrespectful. Please let me try again."

Providers should acknowledge the prevalence of marginalization, discrimination, and stigma experienced by SGM people in health-care contexts. In the context of contraceptive counseling, SGM patients may withhold their sexual orientation, gender identity, or details of their sexual behaviors for fear of discrimination or stigmatization. Trust building, longitudinal patient–provider relationships, and creating safe and inclusive clinical spaces are critical to overcoming these challenges.

Finally, all gynecologists are uniquely positioned to offer exceptional contraceptive counseling to SGM patients due to their extensive knowledge of the risks, benefits, and noncontraceptive effects of contraceptive methods. SGM patients may benefit from noncontraceptive aspects of a hormonal contraceptive method. This can include the use of hormonal treatment modalities for common gynecologic indications (eg, endometriosis, abnormal uterine bleeding, acne, and polycystic ovarian syndrome [PCOS]) or indications more specific to the needs of SGM people (eg, gender-affirming menstruation suppression for transmasculine patients). For SMW, many of whom may not conceive of themselves as needing contraception due to infrequent sexual interactions with cisgender men, qualitative studies have illustrated that contraception can align with queer identity by highlighting noncontraceptive benefits and being framed as sex positive.[55] For transgender and gender nonbinary patients, many individuals choose a contraceptive method of the basis of factors such as mitigation of gender dysphoria and rates of menstruation suppression.[65,67–69] Knowledge of these facilitators can aid gynecologic providers in providing SGM-inclusive contraceptive counseling.

Screening for Sexually Transmitted Infections

Table 2 indicates rates of STIs in SGM populations. Notably, prevalence rates of human immunodeficiency virus (HIV), chlamydia, and herpes simplex virus (HSV) were elevated

Table 2
Sexually transmitted infection rates among sexual and gender minority populations in the United States

HIV Rates	CDC, 2021 CDC, 2021
0.43% Prevalence in general population	Clark H et al., 2017; Becasen JS et al., 2019
17% Prevalence in cisgender MSM population	Becasen JS et al., 2019
17% Prevalence in transwomen	
2%–3% Prevalence in transmen	
Chlamydia trachomatis rates	CDC, 2021; Kreisel KM et al., 2021
1.22%–2.14% prevalence in general population	Gorgos LM and Marrazzo JM, 2011; Singh D et al., 2011
5.3% prevalence in heterosexual women	Gorgos LM and Marrazzo JM, 2011; Singh D et al., 2011
7.1% prevalence in WSW and WSMW	
Highest prevalence in WSMW	Singh D et al., 2011; Muzny CA et al., 2014
HSV rates	CDC, 2021
12.1% prevalence in general population	Tao G et al., 2008
8.7%–10% self-reported viral STI (HSV/HPV) in heterosexual women	Tao G et al., 2008
15%–17.2% self-reported in WSMW	Tao G et al., 2008
2.3%–6.7% self-reported in WSW	Muzny CA et al., 2014
HSV-2 seropositivity is higher in bisexual women than in lesbian women	
HPV rates	CDC, 2021
13.0% prevalence in general population	Marazzo JM et al., 2001
6.1% seropositivity in WSW	Marazzo JM et al., 2001
24.5% seropositivity in WSMW	
Gonorrhea rates	CDC, 2021; Kreisel KM et al., 2021
0.064% prevalence in general population	Weston EJ et al., 2019; Johnson Jones ML et al., 2019
4.5%–4.6% prevalence in MSM	Kirkaldy RD et al., 2019
26.5% self-reported gonococcal positivity rate in MSM	Pitasi MA et al., 2019
2.8%–9.8% positivity rate in transwomen	Pitasi MA et al., 2019
5.9%–14.7% positivity rate in transmen	
Hepatitis B rates	CDC, 2020
4.3% past or present prevalence in general population	
Limited prevalence data in SGM populations	
Hepatitis C rates	CDC, 2023
~1.0% prevalence in general population	
Limited prevalence data in SGM populations	

in various SGM patient subpopulations compared with the overall US population prevalence rates. Meanwhile, there is a paucity of research in prevalence rates of trichomoniasis and hepatitis B and C in SGM populations, particularly AFAB people. The prevalence of bacterial vaginosis, which is associated with an increased risk for STI acquisition, is also higher in WSW than in women who have never had sex with women.[70]

There are several contributors to increased rates of STIs in the SGM population. First, the SGM population experiences delays in STI screening and treatment related to limited access to affirming and respectful care, as well as underinsured status.[71-73] This is further perpetuated by anticipated discrimination and stigma related to sexual orientation, sexual behaviors, gender identity, and/or race.[74-77]

A lack of sexual and gender-expansive sexual health educational resources also contributes to underutilization of STI screening and participation in sexual behaviors that increase risk of STI acquisition, such as unprotected sex.[78] One recent study showed that lesbians believe that they are at relatively low risk for STIs because they are excluded from dominant sexual scripts.[79,80] Multiple studies have shown that transmen having sex with men experience lower perceived access to HIV prevention services and resources, lack of trans-specific knowledge among STI testing providers, and lack of transinclusive institutional policies.[81,82] Similar experiences and perceptions were also noted in SMW living with HIV.[83,84]

Redesigning heteronormative sexual health information to reflect gender and sexual orientation diversity is an important step to reducing STI transmission and increasing STI testing and treatment. Many gender nonconforming, trans, and lesbian/gay individuals report turning to other members of the LGBTQ community for sexual and reproductive health information.[76,85] Community involvement in the development of sexual health information for both providers and patients, STI prevention and testing resources, and safe provider directories designed by and for underrepresented SGM identities is thus a cornerstone of fostering more inclusive and effective OB/GYN resources and clinical settings.[86] Normalizing routine STI testing by incorporating HIV and other STI testing into gender-affirming and/or identity empowering settings—such as during hormone therapy monitoring—may further increase levels of effective STI identification and treatment.[85]

Screening for Intimate Partner Violence

Another vital service that OB/GYN clinics must provide is safe, respectful, and compassionate IPV screening. Research has shown that SGM individuals are more likely than their heterosexual counterparts to have experienced sexual violence and/or intimate partner violence in their lifetimes.[87,88] In cross-sectional survey studies, bisexual women were more likely than other SGM women and heterosexual women to experience sexual violence and verbal coercion but less likely to report it.[84,89] In a systematic review of existing literature, researchers found that transgender and gender-nonconforming individuals were also significantly more likely than cisgender individuals to experience any IPV, including physical IPV and sexual IPV.[90,91]

Additionally, IPV is underreported in the LGBTQ + population. Intracommunity concerns that speaking out about IPV in the LGBTQ community will strengthen systemic stigma and homophobia may lead to underreporting of IPV.[88] Internalized homophobia has been associated with higher rates of perpetrating and accepting IPV.[92,93] Socially constructed gender norms and gendered power narratives further serve to silence individuals in same-sex couples who may be experiencing IPV.[94,95] A literature review identified 3 barriers to seeking help for IPV: a lack of general understanding and research about LGBTQ IPV, fear of stigma from providers, and systemic inequities in the justice system and law enforcement.[96]

OB/GYN spaces have the potential to help address IPV endured by members of the LGBTQ community. Clinics should consider questioning their existing IPV screening and scripts that may isolate or exclude at-risk SGM groups. Stigma, heterosexism, and erasure from within the health-care system and expressed through existing IPV screening questions has been associated with underreporting of violence, leading to unaddressed harm and continued violence.[84,97] Screening for IPV regardless of SOGI and eradicating heteronormative assumptions and biases are essential to protecting and supporting SGM patients going through IPV.[98] When screening, providers should be aware of potential differences in IPV patterns due to the social contexts in which LGBTQ IPV occurs, including internalized and/or systemic homophobia. OB/GYN clinics must also be equipped to connect victims of IPV to competent and LGBTQ-welcoming legal counsel, shelters, and community-based support services.

Family Building and Preconception Counseling

One-third of SGM people are parents, and an estimated 63% of SGM people aged 18 to 35 years are considering expanding their families.[99,100] SGM people have many options for building their families, including conception from intercourse, use of assisted reproductive technology, gestational surrogacy, adoption, or foster care. With increasing numbers of SGM people expanding their families, family building providers, including OB/GYNs, must be prepared to address the specific needs of this population.

In this section, we review existing data on preconception health and obstetric outcomes of SGM people. Finally, we offer an evidence-based approach to preconception counseling for SGM patients grounded in a queer reproductive justice framework.

Sexual and gender minority preconception health, obstetric experiences, and perinatal outcomes

A lack of routine sexual orientation and gender identity data collection in perinatal and obstetric health databases has contributed to limited visibility of the perinatal outcomes and experiences of SGM people, and erasure of SGM people in national attention to obstetric health disparities.[11,12,101,102] This is despite the nonpregnant SGM population having documented health-care disparities that may adversely affect pregnancy.

A small number of studies have described the preconception health of SGM patients, predominantly focusing on SMW. In 2 studies examining sexual orientation disparities in preconception health, SMW were more likely to report adverse health conditions and behaviors before pregnancy compared with heterosexual women, including higher rates of depression, binge drinking and other substance use, having an STI diagnosis, and having unmet medical care needs owing to cost.[103,104] In contrast, using California birth certificate data, Berrahou and colleagues[105] found that parents giving birth in likely SGM parental structures were more likely to be 35 years or older, identify as White, and have higher educational attainment and commercial health insurance than those giving birth in mother–father parental structures. Likely SGM parents were more likely to conceive using assisted reproductive technologies, consistent with previous reports of increased assisted reproductive technology (ART) use for SMW in same-sex marriages, and had higher prepregnancy body mass index.[105–107] These findings indicate that the studied population of SGM people that became pregnant, delivered a live pregnancy, and disclosed an identifiable SGM parental structure on the birth certificate may benefit from an increased ability to access and navigate health-care systems. This is further evidenced by higher use of fertility treatments in this group. There are currently no published studies that specifically examine gender identity disparities in preconception health; therefore, providers must rely on health disparities data from nonpregnant transgender and gender nonbinary patients to inform preconception counseling.

A small but growing body of literature has sought to investigate perinatal experiences and outcomes in the SGM population. As compared with heterosexual women, SMW are more likely to report pregnancies affected by miscarriage, stillbirth, low birth weight, and preterm birth.[108,109] Two groups have used state birth certificate data to examine SGM perinatal health outcomes. Downing and colleagues[110] used Massachusetts birth certificate data to investigate perinatal outcomes of birthing people in same-sex marriages compared with different-sex marriages; they report increased risk of high birthweight infants among people birthing in same sex marriages. Using California birth certificate data, Leonard and colleagues[111] found that parents birthing in mother–mother parental structures were more likely than birthing parents in mother–father partnerships to have multifetal gestation, labor induction, postpartum hemorrhage, severe morbidity, and nontransfusion severe morbidity. These differences persisted after adjustment for sociodemographic factors, multifetal gestation, and comorbidities.

There is a critical need for research investigating the obstetric and birth outcomes of gender minority people. In their study, Leonard and colleagues found no statistically significant differences in outcomes between father birthing parents (thought to likely represent transmasculine individuals) and birthing parents in mother–father partnerships.[111] However, population-based research that directly collects sexual orientation and gender identities as distinct from reproductive anatomy is needed.[12,105,111] Several researchers have conducted qualitative studies to understand the pregnancy experiences of transgender men.[61,112,113] Their study has demonstrated that transgender men have children through planned and unplanned pregnancies but report a diverse range of challenges to positive pregnancy experiences, including the following: institutionalized cisnormativity embedded within medical norms and practices, stigmatization, loneliness, social isolation, lack of gender-affirming perinatal environments and experienced providers, distrust of medical systems, fear of childbirth, adverse mental health effects of pregnancy, and increased gender dysphoria for some patients.[61,112–114] These studies also revealed that some transgender men experienced strong therapeutic alliances with their providers that played a central role in promoting safety, empowerment, and improving their pregnancy experience; anticipatory guidance and preconception counseling (when applicable) were critical aspects of these positive clinical relationships.[113,115,116]

A model for preconception counseling

Fig. 1 outlines critical aspects of SGM-inclusive preconception counseling. When counseling SGM patients in the preconception period, we encourage providers to use an evidence-based approach that incorporates an understanding of the health disparities that SGM patients face before and during pregnancy, current gaps in knowledge, and the ways in which institutionalized cisheteronormativity adversely affects pregnancy experiences. We also advocate for use of a queer reproductive justice framework: enforcing patients' fundamental right to sexual and bodily autonomy, including the right to decide whether or when to become a parent, parent the children one has, and to do so with dignity and free from violence and discrimination—all while avoiding assumptions on the basis of sex, gender, sexual orientation, and gender identity.[117,118]

Transgender and gender nonbinary AFAB people on testosterone should be counseled around management of testosterone before, during and after pregnancy. Testosterone has unclear effects on fertility, fecundity, and fetal development.[115,119,120] Based on a limited number of case reports and theoretic concerns of teratogenicity, pregnancy

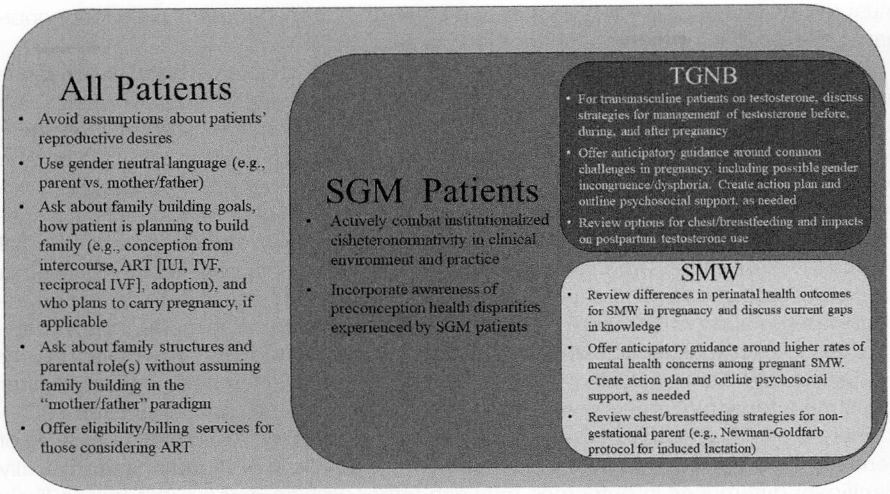

Fig. 1. A model for SGM inclusive preconception counseling. SGM, sexual and gender minorities; SMW, sexual minority women; TNGB, transgender and gender nonbinary.

is currently an absolute contraindication to testosterone use.[121–123] In the absence of evidence-based guidelines, providers should engage their patients in individualized discussions around preconception cessation of testosterone therapy. If a patient conceives a pregnancy while on testosterone and plans to continue the pregnancy, current guidelines recommend cessation of testosterone.[121]

We recommend preconception counseling around lactation and breastfeeding/chestfeeding for all SGM patients. For transgender birthing parents, infant feeding plans may affect the timing of reinitiation of gender-affirming testosterone in the postpartum period. Use of exogenous testosterone may decrease or delay milk production; therefore, patients wanting to breastfeed/chestfeed may opt to delay reinitiation of testosterone.[124,125] Birth parents who are not breastfeeding/chestfeeding are suggested to delay until 4 to 6 weeks postpartum, although there is limited evidence to support this.[61,115(P2)] We recommend an individualized discussion, incorporating infant feeding plans, to determine timing of postpartum testosterone reinitiation.[126]

Nongestational parents may be able to breastfeed/chestfeed if they desire. The Newman-Goldfarb protocol for lactation indication has been described for cisgender women using surrogacy or adoption and can easily be offered to nonbirthing cisgender women in same-sex partnerships who desire to breastfeed/chestfeed.[127] This protocol has been adapted by Reisman and Goldstein for use in transgender women and gender nonbinary AMAB people who want to induce lactation.[128]

Gender-Affirming Gynecologic Care for Transgender and Gender Nonbinary Patients

Gender affirmation is a multifaceted process by which a person is recognized and feels supported in their gender identity, expression, and role. This process may include but does not necessarily require social gender role transition, legal change in name or pronoun, and medical and/or surgical treatments.[129,130]

Gynecologists play an important role in the care of TGNB patients, both for their gender affirmation and routine gynecologic needs.[131–135] Gynecologists are uniquely skilled to perform certain gender-affirming surgeries, particularly for transmasculine patients, such as hysterectomy (typically including salpingectomy) with or without oophorectomy. When hysterectomy ± salpingo-oophorectomy is being performed for the indication of gender affirmation, the World Professional Association for Transgender Health (WPATH) outlines that patients must be consentable and have marked or sustained gender incongruence.[121] Patients should be informed of risks and benefits of surgical intervention, in particular effects of biological reproduction and offered reproductive/fertility preservation options preoperatively, if desired.[121] Finally, WPATH suggests that patients be stable on gender-affirming hormone therapy for at least 6 months before surgery unless hormone therapy is not desired by the patient or is medical contraindicated.[121] Data suggest that gender-affirming hysterectomy is a safe procedure with complication rates consistent with those performed for different diagnoses in cisgender women.[136]

Some TGNB patients may desire oophorectomy at the time of hysterectomy. The role of oophorectomy should be carefully considered, particularly given that many patients will seek gender-affirming gonadectomy at a young age. Oophorectomy has lifelong implications for patients' reproductive health, oncologic risk, endocrine management, cardiovascular health, bone density, and neurocognitive status. Testosterone therapy is thought to ameliorate these risks, although further research is needed to better understand long-term health outcomes of oophorectomy for TGNB patients on chronic testosterone therapy.[137] Oophorectomy should only be considered for patients who intend to remain on testosterone indefinitely; even so, patients may experience interruptions in their testosterone therapy for a variety of reasons, including changes in gender affirmation goals, undesired side effects, or loss of access to gender-affirming hormone therapy.[138] Additionally, patients should be aware that current evidence does not support regular reduction in testosterone dosing following oophorectomy.[137,139] Therefore, we recommend individualized discussion with patients regarding the risks and benefits of oophorectomy, including their long-term plans regarding use of gender-affirming testosterone.

Gynecologists are also often involved in the nonsurgical care of transgender patients. Transgender AMAB people may prefer to establish care with a gynecologist for routine health care, particularly after undergoing vaginoplasty because this helps them to affirm their gender. Gynecologists should be aware of common concerns after vaginoplasty, including granulation tissue, recurrent urinary tract infections, intravaginal hair growth, and pain with dilation or vaginal intercourse.[121,132,140,141] WPATH recommends routine speculum examinations to evaluate for neovaginal granulation tissue, hair growth, and lesions.[121]

Transgender AFAB people are also likely to be followed for routine gynecologic care. Providers should be aware of common gynecologic effects of testosterone therapy, in particular vaginal/frontal hole atrophy, which can lead to pain and dyspareunia. This can be effectively management with vaginal/frontal hole estrogens without affecting the gender-affirming effects of testosterone; however, some transmasculine patients may find estrogen-based therapies to be incongruent with gender identity, regardless of lack of impact on testosterone efficacy/dosing. Additionally, transmasculine patients may present for contraceptive counseling, menstruation suppression, breakthrough bleeding on testosterone, or any routine gynecologic complaint or concern. Gynecologists should offer inclusive, sensitive care that demonstrates knowledge of the intersections of gynecology and transgender health.

Considerations and Improvements in Gynecologic Clinical Spaces

Stigma and discrimination in health care, cisheteronormative medical systems and institutions, and limited accessibility to health services are major barriers to the provision of equitable gynecologic care for SGM individuals.[74,142,143] In this section, we review strategies and interventions at the individual clinical practice, institutional, and structural levels that can be implemented to improve the obstetric and gynecologic care of SGM patients.

Creating a safe and welcoming environment for SGM patients begins before patients physically enter a clinical space. Because OB/GYN has been historically positioned to serve "women," particularly cisgender, heterosexual women, it can be challenging for SGM patients to navigate these clinical settings. First, a clinic's name can be signal of inclusivity or exclusivity to SGM patients. We encourage gender-inclusive clinic names, avoiding unnecessarily gendered language such as "Women's Health Clinic" when possible.[144] OB/GYN clinics should also express their commitment to serving SGM patients in public-facing mission statements, websites, publications, and LGBTQ-friendly provider and clinic directories.[145–149]

It is important to also consider the multiple ways that patients interface with clinical environments before interacting with their provider; each of these is opportunity to demonstrate inclusivity to SGM patients. Clinics should use gender-neutral language throughout the physical space, including in restrooms, pamphlets, signage, and other provided resources.[144,150] Careful rooming processes to provide privacy can also foster safety, such as offering a separate waiting area for those who may not feel comfortable in an OB/GYN waiting room. Intake forms must provide adequate options and open-ended questions to allow patients to indicate their name, pronouns, and, if applicable, sexual orientation and gender identity. Intake questions can be reframed to indicate inclusivity of relationship status, gender identity, and sexual orientation, for example, by asking for names of spouse/partner or parent/guardian rather than wife/husband or mother/father, respectively. The electronic medical records should be updated to reflect these responses.[145,147,151,152] Finally, all clinic support staff, including registration/front desk staff, medical assistants, billing, and security, should receive training on LGBTQ +-affirming communication and care.[153]

On the institutional level, changes within hospital and health-care delivery organizations, structures, and operations must also be considered, including instituting new policies and resources to address health disparities. The United States Department of Health and Human Services, the federal Affordable Care Act, the Joint Commission, the Human Rights Campaign, and the American College of Physicians all reinforce the rights to confidentiality, visitation rights, and quality health care for sexual and gender minority patients.[154–156] Given both their legal and ethical responsibilities, hospitals should institute explicit nondiscrimination policies to provide institutional protection to patients' confidentiality and equal rights to visitation.[157] Additionally, institutions and health-care systems can partner with LGBTQ + community organizations and work to hire and retain staff and providers who are LGBTQ + identified and/or are committed to proficiency in SGM health care. Another effective institutional strategy is the establishment of a low-cost or no-cost legal team specifically equipped to address the unique legal situations that members of the LGBTQ community face, such as pursuing legal gender and name changes, filing discrimination litigation, and negotiating for insurance coverage of life-saving gender-affirming procedures.[158]

Ultimately, achieving health equity for SGM patients requires eradicating structural level inequities and institutionalized discrimination. Despite federal protection against discrimination based on sexual orientation and gender, there has been a surge in anti-LGBTQ bills introduced to and passed in state legislatures, including but not limited to laws HB648 in Louisiana, HB254 in Florida, and SB14 in Texas, which have been signed to ban gender-affirming care of transgender youth.[159] Laws in an additional 16 states have restricted or banned gender-affirming care.160 Furthermore, insurance policies provide SGM individuals with varying and inconsistent access to reproductive health care and life-saving gender-affirming care.[161–163] Given the data we highlight throughout this article describing sexuality-associated and gender-associated health disparities, there is a critical need for federal and state-level legislation that aims to protect and improve access to health care for SGM patients. Individuals and institutions that act as patient advocates as well as lawmakers have the responsibility to advocate for laws that increase access to gender-affirming high-quality care, while striking down legislation that would restrict it. To combat national inaccessibility of quality health-care for SGM people, effective structural strategies must center around dismantling cisheteronormativity and bias across legal, political, social, economic, and health-care systems.

One critical aspect to structural change is the role of medical education and how it can be used to advance health equity. Across survey studies of first year medical students, OB/GYN residents, and gynecologists, participants expressed biases against SGM individuals, low levels of comfort in providing care to SGM people, and insufficient curricular exposure to LGBTQ health issues and considerations.[10,164–166] Several educators have introduced effective SGM health learning tools in medical school and OB/GYN residency curricula. These include practicing sensitivity and accountability in clinical interviews and history taking using interactive standardized patient cases at the medical school and residency level, using and normalizing LGBTQ-inclusive clinical scripts, and repeated curricular exposure to clinical cases involving gender and sexually diverse patients.[63,167–170]

Collectively, these multilevel interventions seek to create inclusivity and safety for SGM patients in OB/GYN clinical spaces and health-care systems more generally with the goal of higher utilization and quality of care for this marginalized patient population.

SUMMARY

Sexual and gender minority people, including LGBTQ+ individuals, are a diverse population with a wide spectrum of gynecologic needs. Institutionalized cisheteronormativity, stigmatization, lack of provider training, and fear of discrimination contribute to health disparities in this patient population. Gynecologists play a critical role in providing SGM people with equitable and inclusive full spectrum reproductive health care.

CLINICS CARE POINTS

- SGM people, including LGBTQ + people, have a wide spectrum of gynecologic needs, including cancer screening, family building, and gender-affirming care.
- SGM people face a disproportionate burden of health disparities, which are directly and indirectly related to pervasive discrimination.
- Gynecologists should use evidence-based care that incorporates an understanding of health disparities faced by SGM patients and addresses current gaps in knowledge.
- Gynecologists should actively work to dismantle institutionalized cisheteronormativity in their clinical practices, avoiding unnecessarily gendered language and clinical assumptions based on patients' sex, gender, gender identity, or sexual orientation identity.

DISCLOSURES

The authors do not report any conflicts of interest.

REFERENCES

1. Jones J. U.S. LGBT Identification Steady at 7.2%. Gallup.com. 2023. Available at:. https://news.gallup.com/poll/470708/lgbt-identification-steady.aspx. Accessed July 12, 2023.
2. Johnson SE, Holder-Hayes E, Tessman GK, et al. Tobacco Product Use Among Sexual Minority Adults: Findings From the 2012-2013 National Adult Tobacco Survey. Am J Prev Med 2016;50(4):e91–100.
3. Eliason MJ. Chronic Physical Health Problems in Sexual Minority Women: Review of the Literature. LGBT Health 2014;1(4):259–68.
4. Grant JM, Motter LA, Tanis J. Injustice at Every Turn: A Report of the National Transgender Discrimination Survey. 2011. Available at:. https://dataspace.princeton.edu/handle/88435/dsp014j03d232p. Accessed December 3, 2020.
5. The Trevor Project National Survey. Available at:. https://www.TheTrevorProject.org/survey-2021/. Accessed November 12, 2021.
6. Hendricks ML, Testa RJ. A conceptual framework for clinical work with transgender and gender nonconforming clients: An adaptation of the Minority Stress Model. Prof Psychol Res Pract 2012;43(5):460–7.
7. Lefevor GT, Boyd-Rogers CC, Sprague BM, et al. Health disparities between genderqueer, transgender, and cisgender individuals: An extension of minority stress theory. J Counsel Psychol 2019;66(4):385–95.
8. Bockting WO, Miner MH, Swinburne Romine RE, et al. Stigma, mental health, and resilience in an online sample of the US transgender population. Am J Public Health 2013;103(5):943–51.
9. Kelleher C. Minority stress and health: Implications for lesbian, gay, bisexual, transgender, and questioning (LGBTQ) young people. Counsell Psychol Q 2009;22(4):373–9.
10. Mehta PK, Easter SR, Potter J, et al. Lesbian, Gay, Bisexual, and Transgender Health: Obstetrician-Gynecologists' Training, Attitudes, Knowledge, and Practice. J Womens Health 2018;27(12):1459–65.
11. Cahill S, Makadon H. Sexual Orientation and Gender Identity Data Collection in Clinical Settings and in Electronic Health Records: A Key to Ending LGBT Health Disparities. LGBT Health 2014;1(1):34–41.
12. Zhang A, Berrahou I, Leonard SA, et al. Birth registration policies in the United States and their relevance to sexual and/or gender minority families: Identifying existing strengths and areas of improvement. Soc Sci Med 2022;293:114633.
13. Foundational Concepts and Affirming Terminology Related to Sexual Orientation, Gender Identity, and Sex Development. Available at: https://lgbt.hms.harvard.edu/terminology. Accessed July 12, 2023.
14. Young RM, Meyer IH. The Trouble With "MSM" and "WSW": Erasure of the Sexual-Minority Person in Public Health Discourse. Am J Publ Health 2005;95(7):1144–9.
15. Vaid-Menon A. Beyond the gender binary. Penguin Workshop; 2020. Available at:. https://www.penguinrandomhouse.com/books/611537/beyond-the-gender-binary-by-alok-vaid-menon-illustrated-by-ashley-lukashevsky/. Accessed November 19, 2021.
16. Tang H, Greenwood GL, Cowling DW, et al. Cigarette smoking among lesbians, gays, and bisexuals: how serious a problem? (United States). Cancer Causes Control CCC 2004;15(8):797–803.

17. Lunn MR, Cui W, Zack MM, et al. Sociodemographic Characteristics and Health Outcomes Among Lesbian, Gay, and Bisexual U.S. Adults Using Healthy People 2020 Leading Health Indicators. LGBT Health 2017;4(4):283–94.
18. Fredriksen-Goldsen KI, Kim HJ, Barkan SE, et al. Health Disparities Among Lesbian, Gay, and Bisexual Older Adults: Results From a Population-Based Study. Am J Publ Health 2013;103(10):1802–9.
19. Zaritsky E, Dibble SL. Risk factors for reproductive and breast cancers among older lesbians. J Womens Health 2010;19(1):125–31.
20. Kamen CS, Smith-Stoner M, Heckler CE, et al. Social Support, Self-Rated Health, and Lesbian, Gay, Bisexual, and Transgender Identity Disclosure to Cancer Care Providers. Oncol Nurs Forum 2015;42(1):44–51.
21. Margolies, L & Scout, NFN. National LGBT cancer network LGBT patient-centered outcomes. 2013. Available at: https://cancer-network.org/resources/lgbt-patient-centered-outcomes/. Accessed October 6, 2020.
22. Alexander, K and Banerjee, S. Older Sexual and Gender Minorities With Cancer: A Population Hidden in the Open - Google Search. 2019. Available at:. https://ascopost.com/issues/october-10-2019/older-sexual-and-gender-minorities-with-cancer/. Accessed October 6, 2020.
23. Cancer Statistics - NCI. 2015. Available at:. https://www.cancer.gov/about-cancer/understanding/statistics. Accessed February 8, 2023.
24. Cancer Facts & Figures 2023| American Cancer Society. Available at:. https://www.cancer.org/research/cancer-facts-statistics/all-cancer-facts-figures/2023-cancer-facts-figures.html. Accessed February 8, 2023.
25. Obedin-Maliver J. Time to change: supporting sexual and gender minority people – an underserved understudied cancer risk population. J Natl Compr Cancer Netw JNCCN 2017;15(11):1305–8.
26. Berrahou IK, Snow A, Swanson M, et al. Representation of Sexual and Gender Minority People in Patient Nondiscrimination Policies of Cancer Centers in the United States. J Natl Compr Cancer Netw JNCCN 2022;20(3):253–9.
27. Siegel RL, Miller KD, Wagle NS, et al. Cancer statistics, 2023. CA Cancer J Clin 2023;73(1):17–48.
28. Stenzel AE, Moysich KB, Ferrando CA, et al. Clinical needs for transgender men in the gynecologic oncology setting. Gynecol Oncol 2020;159(3):899–905.
29. Peitzmeier SM, Reisner SL, Harigopal P, et al. Female-to-Male Patients Have High Prevalence of Unsatisfactory Paps Compared to Non-Transgender Females: Implications for Cervical Cancer Screening. J Gen Intern Med 2014;29(5):778–84.
30. Agénor M, Muzny CA, Schick V, et al. Sexual orientation and sexual health services utilization among women in the United States. Prev Med 2017;95:74–81.
31. Arbyn M, Verdoodt F, Snijders PJF, et al. Accuracy of human papillomavirus testing on self-collected versus clinician-collected samples: a meta-analysis. Lancet Oncol 2014;15(2):172–83.
32. Practice Bulletin No. 149. Endometrial cancer. Obstet Gynecol 2015;125(4):1006–26.
33. Ovarian and endometrial cancer considerations in transgender men | Gender Affirming Health Program. Available at:. https://transcare.ucsf.edu/guidelines/ovarian-cancer. Accessed February 7, 2023.
34. Grimstad FW, Fowler KG, New EP, et al. Uterine pathology in transmasculine persons on testosterone: a retrospective multicenter case series. Am J Obstet Gynecol 2019;220(3):257.e1–7.
35. Cannistra SA. Cancer of the ovary. N Engl J Med 1993;329(21):1550–9.

36. Ose J, Poole EM, Schock H, et al. Androgens Are Differentially Associated with Ovarian Cancer Subtypes in the Ovarian Cancer Cohort Consortium. Cancer Res 2017;77(14):3951–60.
37. Ose J, Fortner RT, Rinaldi S, et al. Endogenous androgens and risk of epithelial invasive ovarian cancer by tumor characteristics in the European Prospective Investigation into Cancer and Nutrition. Int J Cancer 2015;136(2):399–410.
38. Gooren LJ, van Trotsenburg MAA, Giltay EJ, et al. Breast Cancer Development in Transsexual Subjects Receiving Cross-Sex Hormone Treatment. J Sex Med 2013;10(12):3129–34.
39. Brown GR, Jones KT. Incidence of breast cancer in a cohort of 5,135 transgender veterans. Breast Cancer Res Treat 2015;149(1):191–8.
40. Bedrick BS, Fruhauf TF, Martin SJ, et al. Creating Breast and Gynecologic Cancer Guidelines for Transgender Patients With BRCA Mutations. Obstet Gynecol 2021;138(6):911.
41. Brinton LA, Key TJ, Kolonel LN, et al. Prediagnostic Sex Steroid Hormones in Relation to Male Breast Cancer Risk. J Clin Oncol 2015;33(18):2041–50.
42. Weyers S, Villeirs G, Vanherreweghe E, et al. Mammography and breast sonography in transsexual women. Eur J Radiol 2010;74(3):508–13.
43. Jaber C, Ralph O, Hamidian Jahromi A. BRCA Mutations and the Implications in Transgender Individuals Undergoing Top Surgery: An Operative Dilemma. Plast Reconstr Surg Glob Open 2022;10(1):e4012.
44. Stoffel C, Carpenter E, Everett B, et al. Family Planning for Sexual Minority Women. Semin Reprod Med 2017;35(5):460–8.
45. Charlton BM, Corliss HL, Missmer SA, et al. Sexual orientation differences in teen pregnancy and hormonal contraceptive use: an examination across 2 generations. Am J Obstet Gynecol 2013;209(3):204.e1–8.
46. Charlton BM, Everett BG, Light A, et al. Sexual Orientation Differences in Pregnancy and Abortion Across the Lifecourse. Womens Health Issues Off Publ Jacobs Inst Womens Health 2020;30(2):65–72.
47. Goldberg SK, Reese BM, Halpern CT. Teen Pregnancy Among Sexual Minority Women: Results From the National Longitudinal Study of Adolescent to Adult Health. J Adolesc Health Off Publ Soc Adolesc Med 2016;59(4):429–37.
48. Lindley LL, Walsemann KM. Sexual Orientation and Risk of Pregnancy Among New York City High-School Students. Am J Publ Health 2015;105(7):1379–86.
49. Tornello SL, Riskind RG, Patterson CJ. Sexual orientation and sexual and reproductive health among adolescent young women in the United States. J Adolesc Health Off Publ Soc Adolesc Med 2014;54(2):160–8.
50. Saewyc EM, Bearinger LH, Blum RW, et al. Sexual intercourse, abuse and pregnancy among adolescent women: does sexual orientation make a difference? Fam Plann Perspect 1999;31(3):127–31.
51. Everett BG, McCabe KF, Hughes TL. Sexual Orientation Disparities in Mistimed and Unwanted Pregnancy Among Adult Women. Perspect Sex Reprod Health 2017;49(3):157–65.
52. Hodson K, Meads C, Bewley S. Lesbian and bisexual women's likelihood of becoming pregnant: a systematic review and meta-analysis. BJOG An Int J Obstet Gynaecol 2017;124(3):393–402.
53. Everett BG, Turner B, Hughes TL, et al. Sexual Orientation Disparities in Pregnancy Risk Behaviors and Pregnancy Among Sexually Active Teenage Girls: Updates from the Youth Risk Behavior Survey. LGBT Health 2019;6(7):342–9.
54. Ela EJ, Budnick J. Non-Heterosexuality, Relationships, and Young Women's Contraceptive Behavior. Demography 2017;54(3):887–909.

55. Higgins JA, Carpenter E, Everett BG, et al. Sexual Minority Women and Contraceptive Use: Complex Pathways Between Sexual Orientation and Health Outcomes. Am J Publ Health 2019;109(12):1680–6.
56. Everett BG, Higgins JA, Haider S, et al. Do Sexual Minorities Receive Appropriate Sexual and Reproductive Health Care and Counseling? J Womens Health 2019;28(1):53–62.
57. Light A, Wang LF, Zeymo A, et al. Family planning and contraception use in transgender men. Contraception 2018;98(4):266–9.
58. Cipres D, Seidman D, Cloniger C, et al. Contraceptive use and pregnancy intentions among transgender men presenting to a clinic for sex workers and their families in San Francisco. Contraception 2017;95(2):186–9.
59. Reynolds CA, Charlton BM. Sexual Behavior and Contraceptive Use Among Cisgender and Gender Minority College Students Who Were Assigned Female at Birth. J Pediatr Adolesc Gynecol 2021;34(4):477–83.
60. Taub RL, Ellis SA, Neal-Perry G, et al. The effect of testosterone on ovulatory function in transmasculine individuals. Am J Obstet Gynecol 2020;223(2):229.e1–8.
61. Light AD, Obedin-Maliver J, Sevelius JM, et al. Transgender men who experienced pregnancy after female-to-male gender transitioning. Obstet Gynecol 2014;124(6):1120–7.
62. Gowen LK, Winges-Yanez N. Lesbian, gay, bisexual, transgender, queer, and questioning youths' perspectives of inclusive school-based sexuality education. J Sex Res 2014;51(7):788–800.
63. Mayfield JJ, Ball EM, Tillery KA, et al. Beyond Men, Women, or Both: A Comprehensive, LGBTQ-Inclusive, Implicit-Bias-Aware, Standardized-Patient-Based Sexual History Taking Curriculum. MedEdPORTAL J Teach Learn Resour 2017; 13:10634.
64. Baker AM, Jahn JL, Tan ASL, et al. Sexual Health Information Sources, Needs, and Preferences of Young Adult Sexual Minority Cisgender Women and Non-Binary Individuals Assigned Female at Birth. Sex Res Soc Policy J NSRC SR SP 2021;18(3):775–87.
65. Krempasky C, Harris M, Abern L, et al. Contraception across the transmasculine spectrum. Am J Obstet Gynecol 2020;222(2):134–43.
66. Bates CK, Carroll N, Potter J. The challenging pelvic examination. J Gen Intern Med 2011;26(6):651–7.
67. Berrahou IK, Grimes A, Autry AM, et al. Management of Menstruation in Transgender and Gender Nonbinary Adolescents. Clin Obstet Gynecol 2022;65(4): 753–67.
68. Bonnington A, Dianat S, Kerns J, et al. Society of Family Planning clinical recommendations: Contraceptive counseling for transgender and gender diverse people who were female sex assigned at birth. Contraception 2020;102(2): 70–82.
69. Agénor M, Cottrill AA, Kay E, et al. Contraceptive Beliefs, Decision Making and Care Experiences Among Transmasculine Young Adults: A Qualitative Analysis. Perspect Sex Reprod Health 2020;52(1):7–14.
70. Koumans EH, Sternberg M, Bruce C, et al. The Prevalence of Bacterial Vaginosis in the United States, 2001–2004; Associations With Symptoms, Sexual Behaviors, and Reproductive Health. Sex Transm Dis 2007;34(11):864.
71. Clark KD, Luong S, Lunn MR, et al. Healthcare Mistreatment, State-Level Policy Protections, and Healthcare Avoidance Among Gender Minority People. Sex Res Soc Pol 2022;19(4):1717–30.

72. White Hughto JM, Reisner SL, Pachankis JE. Transgender stigma and health: A critical review of stigma determinants, mechanisms, and interventions. Soc Sci Med 2015;147:222–31.

73. Kcomt L, Gorey KM, Barrett BJ, et al. Healthcare avoidance due to anticipated discrimination among transgender people: A call to create trans-affirmative environments. SSM Popul Health 2020;11:100608.

74. Gonzales G, Henning-Smith C. Barriers to Care Among Transgender and Gender Nonconforming Adults. Milbank Q 2017;95(4):726–48.

75. Logie CH, Navia D, Loutfy MR. Correlates of a lifetime history of sexually transmitted infections among women who have sex with women in Toronto, Canada: results from a cross-sectional internet-based survey. Sex Transm Infect 2015; 91(4):278–83.

76. Agénor M, Zubizarreta D, Geffen S, et al. "Making a Way Out of No Way:" Understanding the Sexual and Reproductive Health Care Experiences of Transmasculine Young Adults of Color in the United States. Qual Health Res 2022; 32(1):121–34.

77. Magee JC, Bigelow L, DeHaan S, et al. Sexual Health Information Seeking Online: A Mixed-Methods Study Among Lesbian, Gay, Bisexual, and Transgender Young People. Health Educ Behav 2012;39(3):276–89.

78. Reisner SL, White JM, Mayer KH, et al. Sexual risk behaviors and psychosocial health concerns of female-to-male transgender men screening for STDs at an urban community health center. AIDS Care 2014;26(7):857–64.

79. Power J, McNair R, Carr S. Absent sexual scripts: lesbian and bisexual women's knowledge, attitudes and action regarding safer sex and sexual health information. Cult Health Sex 2009;11(1):67–81.

80. Rubinsky V, Cooke-Jackson A. "It Would Be Nice to Know I'm Allowed to Exist:" Designing Ideal Familial Adolescent Messages for LGBTQ Women's Sexual Health. Am J Sex Educ 2021;16(2):221–37.

81. Scheim AI, Travers R. Barriers and facilitators to HIV and sexually transmitted infections testing for gay, bisexual, and other transgender men who have sex with men. AIDS Care 2017;29(8):990–5.

82. Scheim AI, Santos GM, Arreola S, et al. Inequities in access to HIV prevention services for transgender men: results of a global survey of men who have sex with men. J Int AIDS Soc 2016;19(3S2):20779.

83. Teti M, Bowleg L. Shattering the Myth of Invulnerability: Exploring the Prevention Needs of Sexual Minority Women Living with HIV/AIDS. J Gay Lesb Soc Serv 2011;23(1):69–88.

84. Flanders CE, Anderson RE, Tarasoff LA, et al. Bisexual Stigma, Sexual Violence, and Sexual Health Among Bisexual and Other Plurisexual Women: A Cross-Sectional Survey Study. J Sex Res 2019;56(9):1115–27.

85. Seelman KL, Poteat T. Strategies used by transmasculine and non-binary adults assigned female at birth to resist transgender stigma in healthcare. Int J Transgender Health 2020;21(3):350–65.

86. Reisner SL, Perkovich B, Mimiaga MJ. A Mixed Methods Study of the Sexual Health Needs of New England Transmen Who Have Sex with Nontransgender Men. AIDS Patient Care STDS 2010;24(8):501–13.

87. Messinger AM. Invisible victims: same-sex IPV in the National Violence Against Women Survey. J Interpers Violence 2011;26(11):2228–43.

88. Rollè L, Giardina G, Caldarera AM, et al. When Intimate Partner Violence Meets Same Sex Couples: A Review of Same Sex Intimate Partner Violence. Front Psychol 2018;9:1506.

89. McCauley HL, Silverman JG, Decker MR, et al. Sexual and Reproductive Health Indicators and Intimate Partner Violence Victimization Among Female Family Planning Clinic Patients Who Have Sex with Women and Men. J Womens Health 2015;24(8):621–8.

90. Peitzmeier SM, Malik M, Kattari SK, et al. Intimate Partner Violence in Transgender Populations: Systematic Review and Meta-analysis of Prevalence and Correlates. Am J Publ Health 2020;110(9):e1–14.

91. Disparities in Exposure to Intimate Partner Violence Among Transgender/Gender Nonconforming and Sexual Minority Primary Care Patients - PubMed. Available at:. https://pubmed-ncbi-nlm-nih-gov.yale.idm.oclc.org/28719246/. Accessed July 11, 2023.

92. Badenes-Ribera L, Sánchez-Meca J, Longobardi C. The Relationship Between Internalized Homophobia and Intimate Partner Violence in Same-Sex Relationships: A Meta-Analysis. Trauma Violence Abuse 2019;20(3):331–43.

93. Eric S Reyes M, Camille M Alday A, Jay J Aurellano A, et al. Minority Stressors and Attitudes Toward Intimate Partner Violence Among Lesbian and Gay Individuals. Sex Cult 2023;27(3):930–50.

94. Eaton L, Kaufman M, Fuhrel A, et al. Examining Factors Co-Existing with Interpersonal Violence in Lesbian Relationships. J Fam Violence 2008;23(8):697–705.

95. Cannon C. Illusion of Inclusion: The Failure of the Gender Paradigm to Account for Intimate Partner Violence in LGBT Relationships. Partn Abuse 2015;6(1):65–77.

96. Calton JM, Cattaneo LB, Gebhard KT. Barriers to Help Seeking for Lesbian, Gay, Bisexual, Transgender, and Queer Survivors of Intimate Partner Violence. Trauma Violence Abuse 2016;17(5):585–600.

97. Helfrich CA, Simpson EK. Improving Services for Lesbian Clients: What Do Domestic Violence Agencies Need to Do? Health Care Women Int 2006;27(4):344–61.

98. Bermea AM, Slakoff DC, Goldberg AE. Intimate Partner Violence in the LGBTQ+ Community: Experiences, Outcomes, and Implications for Primary Care. Prim Care 2021;48(2):329–37.

99. Family Equality | LGBTQ Family Building Survey. Family Equality. Available at: https://www.familyequality.org/resources/lgbtq-family-building-survey/. Accessed July 12, 2023.

100. Gates G. LGBT parenting in the United States. Williams Institute. Available at:. https://williamsinstitute.law.ucla.edu/publications/lgbt-parenting-us/. Accessed December 3, 2020.

101. Cahill S, Singal R, Grasso C, et al. Do ask, do tell: high levels of acceptability by patients of routine collection of sexual orientation and gender identity data in four diverse American community health centers. PLoS One 2014;9(9):e107104.

102. Grasso C, McDowell MJ, Goldhammer H, et al. Planning and implementing sexual orientation and gender identity data collection in electronic health records. J Am Med Inform Assoc JAMIA 2019;26(1):66–70.

103. Gonzales G, Quinones N, Attanasio L. Health and Access to Care among Reproductive-Age Women by Sexual Orientation and Pregnancy Status. Womens Health Issues Off Publ Jacobs Inst Womens Health 2019;29(1):8–16.

104. Limburg A, Everett BG, Mollborn S, et al. Sexual Orientation Disparities in Preconception Health. J Womens Health 2020;29(6):755–62.

105. Berrahou IK, Leonard SA, Zhang A, et al. Sexual and/or gender minority parental structures among California births from 2016 to 2020. Am J Obstet Gynecol MFM 2022;4(4):100653.

106. Downing J. Pathways to Pregnancy for Sexual Minority Women in Same-sex Marriages. Am J Obstet Gynecol 2019;221(3):281–2.
107. Thoma ME, Boulet S, Martin JA, et al. Births resulting from assisted reproductive technology: comparing birth certificate and National ART Surveillance System Data, 2011. Natl Vital Stat Rep Cent Dis Control Prev Natl Cent Health Stat Natl Vital Stat Syst 2014;63(8):1–11.
108. Barcelona V, Jenkins V, Britton LE, et al. Adverse pregnancy and birth outcomes in sexual minority women from the National Survey of Family Growth. BMC Pregnancy Childbirth 2022;22(1):923.
109. Everett BG, Kominiarek MA, Mollborn S, et al. Sexual orientation disparities in pregnancy and infant outcomes. Matern Child Health J 2019;23(1):72–81.
110. Downing J, Everett B, Snowden JM. Differences in Perinatal Outcomes of Birthing People in Same-Sex and Different-Sex Marriages. Am J Epidemiol 2021;190(11):2350–9.
111. Leonard SA, Berrahou I, Zhang A, et al. Sexual and/or gender minority disparities in obstetric and birth outcomes. Am J Obstet Gynecol 2022;226(6):846.e1–14.
112. Besse M, Lampe NM, Mann ES. Experiences with Achieving Pregnancy and Giving Birth Among Transgender Men: A Narrative Literature Review. Yale J Biol Med 2020;93(4):517–28.
113. Hoffkling A, Obedin-Maliver J, Sevelius J. From erasure to opportunity: a qualitative study of the experiences of transgender men around pregnancy and recommendations for providers. BMC Pregnancy Childbirth 2017;17(Suppl 2):332.
114. MacLean LRD. Preconception, Pregnancy, Birthing, and Lactation Needs of Transgender Men. Nurs Womens Health 2021;25(2):129–38.
115. McCracken M, DeHaan G, Obedin-Maliver J. Perinatal considerations for care of transgender and nonbinary people: a narrative review. Curr Opin Obstet Gynecol 2022;34(2):62–8.
116. Obedin-Maliver J, Makadon HJ. Transgender men and pregnancy. Obstet Med 2016;9(1):4–8.
117. Reproductive Justice. Sister Song. Available at: https://www.sistersong.net/reproductive-justice. Accessed July 30, 2023.
118. Queering Reproductive Justice. National LGBTQ Task Force. Available at:. https://www.thetaskforce.org/programs/queering-equity/queering-reproductive-justice/. Accessed July 30, 2023.
119. Leung A, Sakkas D, Pang S, et al. Assisted reproductive technology outcomes in female-to-male transgender patients compared with cisgender patients: a new frontier in reproductive medicine. Fertil Steril 2019;112(5):858–65.
120. Adeleye AJ, Cedars MI, Smith J, et al. Ovarian stimulation for fertility preservation or family building in a cohort of transgender men. J Assist Reprod Genet 2019;36(10):2155–61.
121. Coleman E, Radix AE, Bouman WP, et al. Standards of Care for the Health of Transgender and Gender Diverse People, Version 8. Int J Transgender Health 2022;23(sup1):S1–259.
122. Wolf CJ, Hotchkiss A, Ostby JS, et al. Effects of prenatal testosterone propionate on the sexual development of male and female rats: a dose-response study. Toxicol Sci Off J Soc Toxicol 2002;65(1):71–86.
123. Patel A, Rivkees SA. Prenatal virilization associated with paternal testosterone gel therapy. Int J Pediatr Endocrinol 2010;2010:867471.
124. Glaser RL, Newman M, Parsons M, et al. Safety of maternal testosterone therapy during breast feeding. Int J Pharm Compd 2009;13(4):314–7.

125. Betzold CM, Hoover KL, Snyder CL. Delayed lactogenesis II: a comparison of four cases. J Midwifery Wom Health 2004;49(2):132–7.

126. Brandt JS, Patel AJ, Marshall I, et al. Transgender men, pregnancy, and the "new" advanced paternal age: A review of the literature. Maturitas 2019;128:17–21.

127. The Newman Goldfarb Protocols for Induced Lactation. Available at:. https://www.asklenore.info/breastfeeding/induced_lactation/protocols4print.shtml. Accessed July 31, 2023.

128. Reisman T, Goldstein Z. Case Report: Induced Lactation in a Transgender Woman. Transgender Health 2018;3(1):24–6.

129. Reisner SL, Radix A, Deutsch MB. Integrated and Gender-Affirming Transgender Clinical Care and Research. J Acquir Immune Defic Syndr 2016;72(Suppl 3):S235–42.

130. Sevelius JM. Gender Affirmation: A Framework for Conceptualizing Risk Behavior among Transgender Women of Color. Sex Roles 2013;68(11–12):675–89.

131. Schmidt M, Ditrio L, Shute B, et al. Surgical management and gynecologic care of the transgender patient. Curr Opin Obstet Gynecol 2019;31(4):228–34.

132. Unger CA. Care of the transgender patient: the role of the gynecologist. Am J Obstet Gynecol 2014;210(1):16–26.

133. Crissman H, Randolph JF. Role for OBGYNs in Gender-Affirming Surgical Care of Transgender and Gender Nonconforming Individuals. Clin Obstet Gynecol 2018;61(4):722–30.

134. Dendrinos ML, Budrys NM, Sangha R. Addressing the Needs of Transgender Patients: How Gynecologists Can Partner in Their Care. Obstet Gynecol Surv 2019;74(1):33–9.

135. Grimstad F, Boskey ER, Taghinia A, et al. Gender-Affirming Surgeries in Transgender and Gender Diverse Adolescent and Young Adults: A Pediatric and Adolescent Gynecology Primer. J Pediatr Adolesc Gynecol 2021;34(4):442–8.

136. Bretschneider CE, Sheyn D, Pollard R, et al. Complication Rates and Outcomes After Hysterectomy in Transgender Men. Obstet Gynecol 2018;132(5):1265–73.

137. Kumar S, Mukherjee S, O'Dwyer C, et al. Health Outcomes Associated With Having an Oophorectomy Versus Retaining One's Ovaries for Transmasculine and Gender Diverse Individuals Treated With Testosterone Therapy: A Systematic Review. Sex Med Rev 2022;10(4):636–47.

138. Barrera EP, Grimstad FW, Boskey ER. Young Adult Patients with Testosterone Management Concerns after Gender-Affirming Hysterectomy and Bilateral Oophorectomy: A Case Series. J Pediatr Adolesc Gynecol 2023;36(1):89–91.

139. Grimstad FW, Fraiman E, Garborcauskas G, et al. Retrospective review of changes in testosterone dosing and physiologic parameters in transgender and gender-diverse individuals following hysterectomy with and without oophorectomy. J Sex Med 2023;20(5):690–8.

140. Gaither TW, Awad MA, Osterberg EC, et al. Postoperative Complications following Primary Penile Inversion Vaginoplasty among 330 Male-to-Female Transgender Patients. J Urol 2018;199(3):760–5.

141. Massie JP, Morrison SD, Van Maasdam J, et al. Predictors of Patient Satisfaction and Postoperative Complications in Penile Inversion Vaginoplasty. Plast Reconstr Surg 2018;141(6):911e–21e.

142. Harb CYW, Pass LE, De Soriano IC, et al. Motivators and Barriers to Accessing Sexual Health Care Services for Transgender/Genderqueer Individuals Assigned Female Sex at Birth. Transgender Health 2019;4(1):58–67.

143. Hoffmann J, Bergin A. Contraception, Abortion and More: Understanding Health Disparities for LBGTQ Patients in their Own Words [10G]. Obstet Gynecol 2019; 133:76S.

144. Jung C, Hunter A, Saleh M, et al. Breaking the Binary: How Clinicians Can Ensure Everyone Receives High Quality Reproductive Health Services. Open Access J Contracept 2023;14:23–39.

145. DeMeester RH, Lopez FY, Moore JE, et al. A Model of Organizational Context and Shared Decision Making: Application to LGBT Racial and Ethnic Minority Patients. J Gen Intern Med 2016;31(6):651–62.

146. Wilkerson JM, Rybicki S, Barber CA, et al. Creating a Culturally Competent Clinical Environment for LGBT Patients. J Gay Lesb Soc Serv 2011;23(3):376–94.

147. Sheedy CA. Clinic and Intake Forms. In: Eckstrand K, Ehrenfeld JM, editors. Lesbian, gay, bisexual, and transgender healthcare: a clinical guide to preventive, primary, and specialist care. Springer International Publishing; 2016. p. 51–63.

148. Adakama M, Love A, Kyeong Y, et al. Bridging the gap: online availability of gynecological care for lesbian, gay, bisexual, transgender, and questioning communities. Am J Obstet Gynecol 2022;226(3):S1309–10.

149. Nowaskie DZ. Development, Implementation, and Effectiveness of a Self-sustaining, Web-Based LGBTQ+ National Platform: A Framework for Centralizing Local Health Care Resources and Culturally Competent Providers. JMIR Form Res 2021;5(9):e17913.

150. Moseson H, Zazanis N, Goldberg E, et al. The Imperative for Transgender and Gender Nonbinary Inclusion: Beyond Women's Health. Obstet Gynecol 2020; 135(5):1059.

151. Deutsch MB, Buchholz D. Electronic Health Records and Transgender Patients—Practical Recommendations for the Collection of Gender Identity Data. J Gen Intern Med 2015;30(6):843–7.

152. Brooks H, Llewellyn CD, Nadarzynski T, et al. Sexual orientation disclosure in health care: a systematic review. Br J Gen Pract 2018;68(668):e187–96.

153. May 2021 PP on 4. Ten Strategies for Creating Inclusive Health Care Environments for LGBTQIA+ People (2021) » LGBTQIA+ health education center. LGBTQIA+ Health Education Center. Available at:. https://www.lgbtqiahealtheducation.org/publication/ten-strategies-for-creating-inclusive-health-care-environments-for-lgbtqia-people-2021/. Accessed July 12, 2023.

154. Attacks on Gender-Affirming and Transgender Health Care | ACP Online. 2023. Available at:. https://www.acponline.org/advocacy/state-health-policy/attacks-on-gender-affirming-and-transgender-health-care. Accessed July 6, 2023.

155. New antidiscrimination rule aims to advance health equity and ensure protections for transgender people. https://doi.org/10.26099/3gec-5m40.

156. HEI 2022. HRC digital reports. Available at: https://reports.hrc.org/hei-2022?_ga=2.88333915.1773524868.1688672792-2012374607.1686588348. Accessed July 6, 2023.

157. Dean MA, Victor E, Guidry-Grimes L. Inhospitable Healthcare Spaces: Why Diversity Training on LGBTQIA Issues Is Not Enough. J Bioethical Inq 2016;13(4): 557–70.

158. Nisly NL, Imborek KL, Miller ML, et al. Developing an Inclusive and Welcoming LGBTQ Clinic. Clin Obstet Gynecol 2018;61(4):646.

159. Roundup of Anti-LGBTQ+ Legislation Advancing In States Across the Country. Human Rights Campaign. 2023. Available at:. https://www.hrc.org/press-releases/roundup-of-anti-lgbtq-legislation-advancing-in-states-across-the-country. Accessed July 27, 2023.

160. 19 states have laws restricting gender-affirming care, some with the possibility of a felony charge | CNN Politics. Available at: https://www.cnn.com/2023/06/06/politics/states-banned-medical-transitioning-for-transgender-youth-dg/index.html. Accessed October 15, 2023.

161. Lo W, Campo-Engelstein L. Expanding the Clinical Definition of Infertility to Include Socially Infertile Individuals and Couples. In: Campo-Engelstein L, Burcher P, editors. Reproductive ethics II. Springer International Publishing; 2018. p. 71–83.

162. Neyra O. Reproductive Ethics and Family: An Argument to Cover Access to ART for the LGBTQ Community. Voices Bioeth 2021;7. https://doi.org/10.52214/vib.v7i.8559.

163. Chin MG, LaGuardia JS, Morgan KBJ, et al. United States Health Policies on Gender-Affirming Care in 2022. Plast Reconstr Surg 2023. https://doi.org/10.1097/PRS.0000000000010594.

164. Qin LA, Estevez SL, Radcliffe E, et al. Are Obstetrics and Gynecology Residents Equipped to Care for Transgender and Gender Nonconforming Patients? A National Survey Study. Transgender Health 2021;6(4):194–200.

165. Unger CA. Care of the Transgender Patient: A Survey of Gynecologists' Current Knowledge and Practice. J Womens Health 2015;24(2):114–8.

166. Guerrero-Hall KD, Muscanell R, Garg N, et al. Obstetrics and Gynecology Resident Physician Experiences with Lesbian, Gay, Bisexual, Transgender and Queer Healthcare Training. Med Sci Educ 2021;31(2):599–606.

167. Lackritz K, Braverman A, Leubner E, et al. Teaching Lesbian, Gay, Bisexual, Transgendered, and Queer Family Building in a Third Year OBGYN Clerkship. Obstet Gynecol 2018;132:43S.

168. Minturn MS, Martinez EI, Le T, et al. Early Intervention for LGBTQ Health: A 10-Hour Curriculum for Preclinical Health Professions Students. MedEdPORTAL J Teach Learn Resour 2021;17:11072.

169. Strategies to Improve the Cervical Cancer Screening Experience of LGBTQ Patients: a Film-Based Curriculum. Available at:. https://dash.harvard.edu/handle/1/37006476. Accessed July 6, 2023.

170. March 2020 PP on 9. Affirmative Services for Transgender and Gender Diverse People - Best Practices for Frontline Health Care Staff » LGBTQIA+ Health Education Center. LGBTQIA+ Health Education Center. Available at:. https://www.lgbtqiahealtheducation.org/publication/affirmative-services-for-transgender-and-gender-diverse-people-best-practices-for-frontline-health-care-staff/. Accessed October 16, 2023.

Obstetric and Gynecologic Care for Individuals with Disabilities

Kathleen E. O'Brien, MD*, Monica Woll Rosen, MD,
Susan Dwyer Ernst, MD

KEYWORDS

- Intellectual disability • Physical disability • Reproductive health • Sexuality
- Education • Family planning • Disparity

KEY POINTS

- Individuals with disabilities are less likely to receive appropriate breast and cervical cancer screening, sexual health education, and comprehensive contraceptive counseling.
- Barriers to appropriate care include provider biases and lack of training, difficulties with transportation, and inaccessible health care facilities and equipment.
- People with disabilities engage in consensual sexual activity and desire future pregnancy at rates similar to peers without disabilities.
- Individuals with disabilities enter pregnancy with unique health risks and have higher rates of severe obstetric morbidity and mortality.
- More formalized medical education and training are needed to provide patients with disabilities with optimal obstetric and gynecologic care.

INTRODUCTION

According to the Centers for Disease Control and Prevention (CDC), more than 61 million individuals and 27% of adults in the United States are living with a disability.[1] The CDC defines a disability as any condition of the body or mind (impairment) that makes it more difficult for the person with the condition to do certain activities (activity limitation) and interact with the world around them (participation restrictions).[1] Disabilities can be physical, intellectual, or sensory, and individuals often have impairment in two or more of these categories.

When caring for individuals with disabilities, special considerations for support and guidance should be given to their unique needs, abilities, and barriers. The American College of Obstetricians and Gynecologists (ACOG) states, "excellent gynecologic

---

Michigan Medicine, 1500 East Medical Center Drive, Ann Arbor, MI 48104, USA
* Corresponding author.
E-mail address: katobr@med.umich.edu

Obstet Gynecol Clin N Am 51 (2024) 43–56
https://doi.org/10.1016/j.ogc.2023.10.002
0889-8545/24/© 2023 Elsevier Inc. All rights reserved.

healthcare for women and adolescents with disabilities is comprehensive; maintains confidentiality; is an act of dignity and respect toward the patient; maximizes the patient's autonomy; avoids harm; and assesses and addresses the patient's knowledge of puberty, menstruation, sexuality, safety, and consent."[2] Despite these recommendations, people with disabilities experience several inequalities when receiving reproductive health care.

HISTORY

Forced sterilization of people with intellectual disabilities (IDs) was common and became a legally protected procedure in many cultures throughout Western society in the twentieth century. This includes the United States, which has a long history of forced sterilization and legal oppression of the reproductive rights of individuals with disabilities. This practice is deeply rooted in the eugenics movement and the fear that individuals with cognitive disabilities were reproducing at a greater pace and outnumbering individuals of "normal" intelligence. One of the many goals of the eugenics movement was to promote the procreation of "fit" members of society and breeding out less desired traits. This led to the targeted sterilization of people with disabilities, immigrants, people of color, indigenous people, and people living in poverty.[3]

A common argument used to justify sterilization was that people with ID were not fit to parent children and that sterilization would protect them from the dangers of pregnancy.[3] Several laws and programs promoting segregation and sterilization were set into place in the late 1800s in the United States. Thirty-two states developed eugenics laws that legally allowed for sterilization operations to be performed on individuals with ID, with most of these procedures occurring in the 1930s to 1950s.[3] More than 64,000 forced sterilizations occurred in the United States under these eugenics laws, disproportionately impacting individuals with disabilities and people of color.[4]

In the last several decades, human rights activism has largely curbed the practice of nonconsensual sterilization. However, several states still have laws in place that can allow sterilization of individuals with disabilities if it is deemed to be in their best interest. Applications for sterilization typically require review through local courts and medical ethics committees, thereby serving as a safeguard from nonconsensual sterilization.[5]

In the United States, people assigned female at birth (AFAB) with both intellectual and physical disabilities continue to undergo sterilization at higher rates than people without disabilities. Individuals with cognitive disabilities have significantly higher odds of female sterilization and hysterectomy, and they undergo sterilization at significantly younger ages than people with other types of disabilities and people without disabilities.[6]

BACKGROUND

Despite advances in the reproductive rights of people with disabilities, individuals with disabilities continue to experience significant stigma and barriers to reproductive health care in the United States. Numerous barriers to appropriate health care exist, including but not limited to implicit biases and discomfort among health care providers,[7] a lack of training in caring for individuals with disabilities,[8] structural barriers such as inaccessibility of medical offices and diagnostic equipment,[9] and difficulty with transportation to medical appointments. These barriers lead to several inequities in patient care and poor patient experiences. People with disabilities are more likely to perceive a lack of being heard, comprehensive explanation of their treatment, respect, adequate time, and shared decision-making with their physician.[10]

Inadequate Medical Training

Both in medical school and in residency, medical trainees consistently report a lack of adequate dedicated training in caring for individuals with disabilities. In regard to caring for those with disabilities, 81% of graduating medical students[11] reported that they had no experience or training in this area. There is significant variation in US medical school education regarding care for patients with disabilities, and demonstration of competency in caring for individuals with disabilities is not required for medical school accreditation. It was not until 2014 that the Association of American Medical Colleges directly addressed the need for competency in disability care.[12]

Providers in obstetrics and gynecology (OB/GYN) often do not feel trained or equipped to meet the needs of patients with physical disability and ID.[8] In a 2022 survey of obstetric care providers, only 12% of respondents reported having received an hour or more of training in caring for patients with ID.[13] A similar survey of gynecologic care providers in 2020 found that none of the respondents had ever received formal education or training on caring for individuals with disabilities who require a gynecologic examination. Those surveyed endorsed departing from screening guidelines and frustration regarding uncertainty of how to proceed with examination frequency.[14]

Inaccessible Medical Facilities

In addition to a lack of adequate training, the dearth of accessible facilities and equipment make provision of care to communities with disabilities more challenging. A 2020 survey of gynecologic care providers identified several perceived barriers to providing care for individuals with disabilities. They cited difficulty with completion of the gynecologic examination both with modifications required to the examination and transfers on and off the gynecologic examination table. They reported inadequate facilities and physical space for gynecologic examinations as a barrier to equitable care. This included narrow hallways, manual doors, small rooms, and a lack of adjustable examination tables.[14]

Unique Gynecologic Needs

Gynecologic care for people with disabilities should incorporate their unique medical, physical, and emotional needs while providing the same standard of care provided for all patients. Individuals with disabilities are at an increased risk of disability-related gynecologic conditions including catamenial seizures, medication-related hyperprolactinemia, and other endocrinopathies including insulin resistance and thyroid abnormalities. Adolescents and adults with disabilities may have difficulty at the time of menarche and subsequent tolerance of menses, leading to behavioral disruptions and distress. Nonverbal individuals with disabilities may be unable to communicate their experience of dysmenorrhea, which can lead to behavioral changes secondary to pain.

Catamenial Seizures

Patients with disabilities are more likely to have seizure disorders. Individuals with seizure disorders may experience cyclic seizure clusters. When the seizure exacerbations align with the menstrual cycle, this is referred to as catamenial epilepsy. Few studies have been published regarding treatment options for catamenial epilepsy, with some benefit demonstrated with continuous or cyclic progestin use, gonadotropin-releasing hormone agonists, acetazolamide, clobazam, lamotrigine, and clomiphene citrate.[15] If menstrual suppression is desired for treatment of catamenial epilepsy or other indications, care should be taken to choose the method of menstrual suppression as several antiepileptic medications have interactions with estrogen-containing contraceptive agents.

Inequities in Standard Screening

Individuals with disabilities are less likely to receive routine gynecologic examinations including pelvic examinations (**Box 1**) at regular intervals, screening for sexually transmitted infections (STIs), and screening for breast and cervical cancer.

Cervical cancer screening

Cervical cancer screening should be completed according to standard consensus guidelines. Pap testing is completed at significantly lower rates for patients with disabilities.[16] Individuals with physical disabilities report a lack of knowledge of cervical cancer screening and information regarding access, difficulties in accessing cancer screening providers and undergoing screening procedures, and discomfort during the screening examinations. Patients were more likely to use cervical cancer screening if there were available attendant services, wheelchair-accessible facilities, and longer appointment times.[17] Among people with ID, rates of cervical cancer screening are higher in those who live in residential facilities and in rural communities. Furthermore, higher rates of cervical cancer screening were also observed in those who had an OB/GYN compared with other individuals with ID.[18]

Breast cancer screening

People with disabilities should be screened for breast cancer at the same recommended intervals as those for AFAB people. Routine breast cancer screening is less likely to be completed at the recommended intervals for individuals with ID compared with the general population and individuals with physical disabilities.[19] Barriers to routine screening include lower perceived risk for breast cancer from health care providers and difficulty with positioning for mammography.[20] For patients who are unable to use standard mammography equipment due to issues with physical mobility, ultrasound has been proposed as an alternative screening method.[21] Ultrasound is not a comparable screening examination to mammography in terms of sensitivity or specificity, but this is the best alternative available at this time. Clinical breast examinations are important and recommended for patients with disabilities who are unable to perform regular self-breast examinations or participate in breast awareness.[22]

Box 1
Tips for the pelvic examination

- Not needed for sole purpose of initiating contraception or menstrual suppression
- Consider urine STI screening rather than vaginal swabs
- Perform only when necessary, such as for Pap screening
- Consider transabdominal ultrasound for evaluation of abnormal uterine bleeding
- Use other positions as necessary including side lying or frog leg
- Be mindful of contractures, impaired balance, weakness, and spasticity
- Choose the speculum carefully and start with more narrow width
- For difficult examinations, consider blind Pap over one finger with a cytobrush
- For patients with intellectual disabilities, pelvic examinations may require sedation

Although the incidence of breast cancer is similar in people with ID compared with people without disabilities, breast cancer among this community tends to be diagnosed at later stages.[23] A 2006 study found that individuals with Social Security Disability Insurance (SSDI) and Medicare coverage had higher rates of all-cause mortality and breast cancer-specific mortality following breast cancer diagnosis. Patients with SSDI and Medicare coverage had lower rates of breast conserving surgery and were less likely to receive radiotherapy and axillary lymph node dissection.[24]

Screening for sexually transmitted infections

Research has shown that the rates of STIs among AFAB people with disabilities are higher than in their nondisabled peers.[25] Increased rates of sexual assault and sexual violence among people with disabilities place individuals at an increased risk of contracting STIs. Finally, individuals with ID are less likely to receive sexual education regarding prevention and testing for STIs.[26] According to CDC guidelines, screening for STIs is important in patients with disabilities.

Contraceptive Needs

Clinicians should inquire regarding the patient's needs for contraception as well as desires for future fertility. Individuals with disabilities of reproductive age engage in sexual activity at similar or higher rates compared with those without disabilities.[27] However, individuals with disabilities are commonly viewed as asexual or not as sexual beings,[28] which may lead to biases in provision of contraceptive and preconception care. Patients should receive unbiased comprehensive education regarding all available methods of contraception, including long-acting reversible contraception (LARC). In a 2013 questionnaire, AFAB people with disabilities reported a similar rate of contraceptive use at last intercourse compared with respondents without disabilities, but they were statistically more likely to use permanent sterilization as their form of contraception.[29] Patients with intellectual and developmental disabilities are less likely to be provided LARC and moderately effective methods of contraception. Data also suggest that they are prescribed depot medroxyprogesterone injections at higher rates than people without disabilities.[30]

Family Planning

People with disabilities frequently endorse being discouraged from becoming pregnant and having children, possibly due to concerns for the individual's health and/or beliefs that people with disabilities should not become parents.[31] Individuals with disabilities who are of reproductive age endorse a similar rate of desire to conceive in the future as those without disabilities, at 61% and 60%, respectively.[32] Therefore, it is critical to assess and address the reproductive health plan for patients with disabilities.

Sexual and Physical Abuse

People with disabilities experience higher rates of physical abuse and sexual violence, both during childhood and as adults. One meta-analysis of 17 studies including children with disabilities found a pooled prevalence of violence of 27% and 14% pooled prevalence of sexual violence. Children with disabilities in this meta-analysis were found to be three to four times more likely to be victims of violence than their peers without disabilities.[33] Children with disabilities are at the highest risk of sexual abuse by their caregivers and have primarily male perpetrators. Of those AFAB people with developmental disabilities, 39% to 68% will experience sexual abuse before they reach adulthood. Approximately 65% of sexual abuse cases involve masturbation and or touching, and 31% involve actual or attempted penetration.[34]

People with ID experience the highest rates of sexual violence. According to the US Department of Justice Crime Statistics from 2009 to 2019, individuals with IDs have the highest rates of total violent crime, serious violent crime, and simple assault among the types of disability measured.[35] Individuals with ID were found to be at least seven times more likely to be sexually assaulted than individuals without disabilities. In addition to victimization through rape and sexual assault, those with ID were also more likely than their peers without disabilities to experience sexual coercion or manipulation.[35]

Sexual Health Education

Sexual education and monitoring for signs of physical or sexual abuse are within the purview of gynecologic care and should occur at routine gynecologic visits for patients with disabilities. Providers should initiate a discussion by evaluating the patient's understanding of sex and sexuality. For individuals with ID, providers should assess the patient's capacity to provide consent to sexual activity. If developmentally appropriate, a confidential interview should be completed with the patient, and the limits of confidentiality should be discussed. Sexual education should include simple but accurate terms for anatomy, sex and sexual development, sexuality, gender identity, consent, healthy expectations in romantic relationships, and sexual abuse.[36] For patients who are unable to provide consent to intimate contact and are at risk of sexual assault, patients and/or their families should be provided with strategies such as "NO-GO-TELL." Patients are taught to say "no" at attempted sexual contact, "go" and remove themselves from the situation, and "tell" a trusted adult.[37]

Menstrual Suppression

Individuals with disabilities often seek care from a gynecologist due to a desire to initiate menstrual suppression. This may be initiated by the patient or by parents or caregivers. When initiated by the patient, they should be treated like any other adolescent or adult who comes to the clinic requesting menstrual suppression. Providers should inquire about how menstrual periods affect the patient's life, including independence with toileting, menstrual hygiene, and impact on daily activities (**Table 1**). The patient should be questioned in private regarding the need for contraception. If the patient is currently sexually active, the provider should assess whether the relationship is consensual. Patients should be screened for high-risk behaviors at this time and offered appropriate STI screening if indicated.

When initiated by the patient's parent or caregiver, the provider should evaluate their motivation for requesting menstrual suppression. They should discuss whether menstrual periods are problematic for the patient or caregiver, and if behavioral changes and distress occur at the time of menses. The provider should question whether the parent or caregiver has a concern for underlying sexual abuse or risk of unwanted pregnancy. The patient's safety in their home and school environments should be assessed.

For adolescents with developmental disabilities, parents may seek out the initiation of menstrual suppression before the onset of menarche. Medication for menstrual suppression should not be initiated before menarche. This could expose the patient to several years of hormonal medication that are not required as menses have not yet begun. The patient should be allowed to undergo typical pubertal development without the use of exogenous hormones. Once menarche occurs, the provider should assess whether hormonal menstrual suppression is indicated at that time.

Table 1
Comparing methods of menstrual suppression

Method	Pros	Cons
Combined oral contraceptive pills	Higher rates of amenorrhea compared with progesterone only pills May use extended cycling or continuously	Increased risk of VTE Interacts with some antiepileptic medications Requires daily administration
Contraceptive patch	Weekly administration	May cause sensory issues Increased risk of VTE Interacts with some antiepileptic medications Continuous use is off-label
Contraceptive ring	Monthly administration	Interacts with some antiepileptic medications Increased risk of VTE
Progesterone-only pills	Less impact on VTE risk Fewer interactions with antiepileptic medications	Higher rates of breakthrough bleeding Bone mineral density loss with prolonged use Requires daily administration
Depot medroxyprogesterone	Administration every 12 wk	Weight gain Bone mineral density loss with prolonged use Longer duration of side effects
Etonogestrel implant	Administration every 3–5 y Superior contraceptive efficacy Less impact on VTE risk	May require sedation for placement Higher rates of breakthrough bleeding
Levonorgestrel IUD	Administration every 3–8 y Superior contraceptive efficacy Less impact on VTE risk	May require sedation for placement Several months of breakthrough bleeding following insertion
Endometrial Ablation	Variable amenorrhea rate	Legal and ethical implications Lower efficacy in menstrual suppression in younger adults
Hysterectomy	Complete amenorrhea	Legal and ethical implications

Combined hormonal contraceptives

Combined hormonal contraceptive pills, transdermal patches, and vaginal rings may be offered for menstrual suppression in the absence of medical contraindications. This may be used in a continuous fashion or with extended cycling to limit the number of periods experienced per year. With the use of a continuous method of combined hormonal contraceptives, complete amenorrhea is achieved in 66% to 88% of patients with 1 year of use.[38] Combined hormonal contraceptive methods may be used to treat dysmenorrhea or cyclic symptoms such as mood changes, worsening seizure activity, or migraines. Transdermal patches may be offered in a continuous fashion as well, though this is an off-label use and may be associated with increased odds of developing venous thromboembolism (VTE). The contraceptive ring may be offered if appropriate, though application of an intravaginal ring is often not possible or practical due to mobility limitations and the need for involvement of caregivers for administration. The most common side effect of combined hormonal contraceptives is breakthrough bleeding, particularly if being used continuously or in extended cycling. This may be treated with a 4-day hormone-free interval if breakthrough bleeding is heavy or persists longer than 48 hours.

Combined hormonal contraceptives do confer an increased risk of VTE, which may be increased at baseline for individuals who use wheelchairs or otherwise have limited mobility. The risk of VTE should be taken into consideration in the setting of additional risk factors including obesity and family history of VTE. Compared with patients who do not have multiple sclerosis (MS), patients with MS have an approximately threefold increased risk of deep vein thrombosis or VTE.[39]

PROGESTERONE-ONLY PILLS

Progesterone-only options of menstrual suppression may be considered, particularly in the presence of contraindications to estrogen use. Of contraceptives approved by the US Food and Drug Administration (FDA), progesterone-only pills may include norethindrone and drospirenone, as well as progestins used primarily for menstrual suppression. The norethindrone package insert suggests the possibility of complete amenorrhea in approximately 20% of patients. However, a more recent assessment of our patient data suggests a rate of amenorrhea in adolescent patients closer to 40%. Patients frequently report bothersome breakthrough bleeding with the use of low-dose norethindrone.[40] Other progestins used for menstrual suppression may include norethindrone acetate or oral medroxyprogesterone. Patients should be counseled regarding possible mood side effects.

DEPOT MEDROXYPROGESTERONE ACETATE INJECTIONS

Depot medroxyprogesterone acetate is an intramuscular injection that is typically given every 12 weeks but may be given in closer intervals for menstrual suppression and treatment of abnormal uterine bleeding. It is associated with a 60% to 70% rate of amenorrhea with regular use.[41] Prolonged use may cause lower bone mineral density, which may be cause for concern in patients with limited weight-bearing and mobility concerns. It may also result in mood side effects. If this is a major concern, oral medroxyprogesterone may be used first on a trial basis before administration of depot medroxyprogesterone acetate injection due to its long-acting nature.

ETONOGESTREL IMPLANTS

The etonogestrel implant is a superior option particularly in patients who also require reliable contraception. The implant is FDA-approved for 3 years of use, but may provide contraceptive benefit for up to 5 years in selected populations.[42] It is associated with amenorrhea rates of 11% to 22%, but can be associated with significant unscheduled and breakthrough bleeding. As the etonogestrel implant requires a minor procedure for placement, sedation may be required for placement in some patients with ID.

Intrauterine Devices

Levonorgestrel-containing intrauterine devices (IUDs) are another excellent option for patients desiring both amenorrhea and reliable contraception. As the 52-mg levonorgestrel-containing IUD is associated with the highest rates of amenorrhea, this is typically recommended as first line if the patient is considering an IUD for menstrual suppression. It is now FDA-approved for 8 years of use. Placement under intravenous (IV) sedation or general anesthesia may be considered for patients who would not tolerate placement in office.

Surgical Management

Patients with disabilities should be offered endometrial ablation for the same clinical indications as their peers without disabilities. Endometrial ablation is not recommended by ACOG for adolescents with disabilities for purposes of menstrual suppression or hygiene.[2] An endometrial ablation consists of a minor surgical procedure that causes destruction of the endometrial lining with the purpose of eliminating or lightning menses. This results in achievement of amenorrhea and approximately 25% to 40% of patients. This should only be considered for patients who have no desire for future fertility, as future pregnancy is contraindicated following an endometrial ablation due to the increased risk of abnormal placentation.

Hysterectomy is frequently requested by both individuals with disabilities and their parents and caregivers. Caregivers may question the utility of keeping the patient's uterus in situ if they would not be able to parent children and may experience difficulties secondary to menses. Hysterectomy should be completed only for medical indications and should not be performed solely for the purpose of sterilization or menstrual suppression.[2] A hysterectomy is a sterilization procedure, and the legal consent process must follow sterilization laws which vary between states. This typically involves court approval and possible involvement of an ethics committee if the patient is unable to provide their own consent due to ID. Although a hysterectomy would achieve complete amenorrhea and pregnancy prevention, it represents a major surgery that has a 4% to 10% rate of major complications depending on the route of hysterectomy.[43] In addition, a hysterectomy would not include a bilateral oophorectomy unless medically indicated, and thus, cyclical mood disturbances and behavioral changes would likely persist as the patient would continue to experience fluctuations in estrogen and progesterone.

Obstetric Care

Preconception counseling

People with disabilities are more likely to report fair or poor health compared with their peers. They have higher rates of diabetes, obesity, mental distress, asthma, and lack of emotional support compared with their nondisabled counterparts. They are less likely to receive routine dental care or health maintenance examinations.[44] Individuals with disabilities who desire pregnancy, therefore, should be provided with preconception counseling before conceiving as they may have risk factors that are associated with adverse pregnancy outcomes.

Unique factors must be considered when providing preconception counseling to people with disabilities. Medical comorbidities should be optimized before conception. Patients should be counseled regarding the natural history of medical comorbidities in pregnancy, including medical conditions that could improve or worsen while pregnant. Care should be taken to discuss possible difficulty in differentiating between pregnancy-related symptoms and problems arising from the patient's specific disability. Medication lists should be reviewed carefully to minimize teratogenic medication exposures to the fetus. Some disabilities are associated with established or increased risk of heritable genetic conditions, and thus genetic counseling referrals should be placed when indicated.[45]

Preconception care is associated with improved pregnancy outcomes. A team approach is recommended when caring for a pregnant patient with a disability, including the patient's primary physician, an obstetrician, anesthesiologist, neurologist, physiatrist, and other outside health professionals including occupational and physical therapists (**Box 2**).[46] Evidence suggests that many pregnant people with disabilities encountered negative attitudes toward their pregnancies and report difficulty receiving comprehensive prenatal care.[47] Before conception, patients should be provided with information regarding health care providers and health services to facilitate appropriate prenatal and intrapartum care. Providers should assist patients with identifying potential needs and challenges during the antepartum, intrapartum, and postpartum periods.

Unique Peripartum Needs

A qualitative study including interviews of 25 individuals with physical disabilities identified several unmet needs during and around the time of pregnancy. The three main themes identified from the interviews included a lack of clinician knowledge and poor clinician attitudes, need for physical accessibility of health care facilities and equipment, and the need for information related to pregnancy and postpartum support. Their recommendations to other individuals with physical disabilities considering becoming pregnant included finding a clinician one trusts, seeking peer support, self-advocating, and preparing for the baby.[48]

Pregnancy Outcomes

A 2021 study from the National Institutes of Health found that individuals with disabilities are at higher risk of severe maternal morbidity and mortality. This includes higher rates of gestational diabetes, premature rupture of membranes, preterm premature rupture of membranes, placenta previa, postpartum fever, severe preeclampsia and eclampsia, and postpartum hemorrhage. Individuals with disabilities were at a sixfold increased risk of thromboembolic events and fourfold increased risk of cardiovascular events. People with disabilities also experienced more interventions at the time of birth including oxytocin augmentation, operative vaginal delivery, and cesarean birth. Cesarean deliveries were less likely to be performed for true medical indications. These adverse outcomes and increased risk of intervention were present in all categories of disability including physical, intellectual, and sensory.[49]

In a 2015 study of people with disabilities in Rhode Island who had recently given birth, several disparities were identified in pregnancy complications and birth outcomes. They were more likely to report stressful life events and medical complications during their most recent pregnancy, less likely to receive prenatal care in the first trimester, and more likely to have preterm births and low birth weight babies.[50]

Box 2
Approach to care for individuals with disabilities

- Speak directly to your patient with a normal adult tone
- Ask how your patient communicates best
- Assume and assess patient competence
- Treat assistive devices as personal space and ask before assisting
- Assess patient's physical abilities, cognitive level, and independence with activities of daily living
- Minimize sensory stimulation within the clinic

Strategies to Improve Outcomes

Several strategies may be considered to improve obstetric outcomes and patient experiences during pregnancy and birth. Dedicated education to the care of individuals with disabilities should be implemented in all medical school curricula, including dedicated courses or modules and the use of standardized patients with intellectual and physical disabilities. Quality improvement efforts should directly include the input of individuals with disabilities to address their perceived needs and feedback regarding their obstetric care. Obstetric providers should collaborate and communicate with the pregnant patient's other medical providers to safely tailor care during pregnancy. Trainings on implicit bias may help practitioners to recognize and correct negative attitudes toward individuals with disabilities. When developing or remodeling clinical spaces in offices and in birth centers, rooms should be tailored to promote accessibility for individuals with physical disabilities. Although these strategies will not eliminate systemic inequities faced by individuals with disabilities, they may serve to close the gap in quality of care experienced during pregnancy and childbirth.

SUMMARY

In summary, people with disabilities deserve respectful and equitable OB/GYN care that lives up to the standard of care recommended for all patients. Barriers to appropriate reproductive health care include provider biases and discomfort, lack of medical education in caring for patients with disabilities, difficulties with transportation, and inaccessible health care facilities and equipment. Individuals with disabilities engage in consensual sexual activity and desire future pregnancy at rates similar to people without disabilities. They experience physical violence and sexual abuse at higher rates. They enter pregnancy with unique health risks and have higher rates of severe maternal morbidity and mortality. More formalized medical education and training are needed to provide patients with disabilities with optimal care that incorporates their unique health risks, desires for family planning, and obstetric needs.

CLINICS CARE POINTS

- Patients with disabilities should be screened for cervical cancer, breast cancer, and sexually transmitted infections at the same recommended intervals as those for all people.

- Comprehensive contraceptive counseling should be provided to all people with disabilities, as they engage in consensual sexual activity at rates similar to or higher than their nondisabled peers. Individuals with disabilities continue to undergo sterilization procedures at higher rates, and hysterectomies should only be offered for the typical medical indications.

- People with intellectual disabilities are at particularly increased risk of physical abuse and sexual violence, and obstetrician and gynecologists should assess for safety concerns at routine visits.

- When choosing a method of menstrual suppression, consideration should be paid to the individual's personal risks, including increased risk of venous thromboembolism with immobilization and interactions with antiepileptic medications.

- Owing to the increased risks of maternal mortality and all severe maternal morbidities during pregnancy and postpartum, individuals with disabilities should receive tailored preconception counseling and comprehensive obstetric care.

DISCLOSURES

The authors have no financial disclosures.

REFERENCES

1. CDC. Disability and health overview. Centers for Disease Control and Prevention. Published September 16, 2020. Accessed June 14, 2023. https://www.cdc.gov/ncbddd/disabilityandhealth/disability.html.
2. American College of Obstetricians and Gynecologists' Committee on Adolescent Health Care. Committee opinion no. 668: Menstrual manipulation for adolescents with physical and developmental disabilities. Obstet Gynecol 2016;128(2):e20–5.
3. Grekul J, Krahn A, Odynak D. Sterilizing the "feeble-minded": Eugenics in Alberta, Canada, 1929-1972. J Hist Sociol 2004;17(4):358–84.
4. Lombardo P. Eugenic sterilization laws. Published online May 10, 2007. Accessed July 30, 2023. https://repository.library.georgetown.edu/handle/10822/524974.
5. Rowlands S, Amy JJ. Sterilization of those with intellectual disability: Evolution from non-consensual interventions to strict safeguards. J Intellect Disabil 2019;23(2):233–49.
6. Li H, Mitra M, Wu JP, et al. Female Sterilization and Cognitive Disability in the United States, 2011–2015. Obstet Gynecol 2018;132(3):559.
7. Smeltzer SC, Mitra M, Long-Bellil L, et al. Obstetric clinicians' experiences and educational preparation for caring for pregnant women with physical disabilities: A qualitative study. Disabil Health J 2018;11(1):8–13.
8. Taouk LH, Fialkow MF, Schulkin JA. Provision of Reproductive Healthcare to Women with Disabilities: A Survey of Obstetrician–Gynecologists' Training, Practices, and Perceived Barriers. Health Equity 2018;2(1):207–15.
9. Nosek MA, Young ME, Rintala DH, et al. Barriers to Reproductive Health Maintenance Among Women with Physical Disabilities. J Womens Health 1995;4(5):505–18.
10. Smith DL. Disparities in patient-physician communication for persons with a disability from the 2006 Medical Expenditure Panel Survey (MEPS). Disabil Health J 2009;2(4):206–15.
11. Holder M, Waldman HB, Hood H. Preparing health professionals to provide care to individuals with disabilities. Int J Oral Sci 2009;1(2):66–71.
12. Santoro JD, Yedla M, Lazzareschi DV, et al. Disability in US medical education: Disparities, programmes and future directions. Health Educ J 2017;76(6):753–9.
13. Amir N, Smith LD, Valentine AM, et al. Clinician perspectives on the need for training on caring for pregnant women with intellectual and developmental disabilities. Disabil Health J 2022;15(2):101262.
14. Sonalkar S, Chavez V, McClusky J, et al. Gynecologic Care for Women With Physical Disabilities: A Qualitative Study of Patients and Providers. Wom Health Issues 2020;30(2):136–41.
15. Herzog AG. Catamenial epilepsy: definition, prevalence pathophysiology and treatment. Seizure 2008;17(2):151–9.
16. Iezzoni LI, Kurtz SG, Rao SR. Trends in Pap Testing Over Time for Women With and Without Chronic Disability. Am J Prev Med 2016;50(2):210–9.
17. Chan DNS, Law BMH, So WKW, et al. Factors associated with cervical cancer screening utilisation by people with physical disabilities: A systematic review. Health Pol 2022;126(10):1039–50.

18. Parish SL, Swaine JG, Son E, et al. Determinants of cervical cancer screening among women with intellectual disabilities: evidence from medical records. Publ Health Rep 2013;128(6):519–26.

19. Iezzoni LI, Kurtz SG, Rao SR. Trends in mammography over time for women with and without chronic disability. J Womens Health 2015;24(7):593–601.

20. Shin DW, Yu J, Cho J, et al. Breast cancer screening disparities between women with and without disabilities: A national database study in South Korea. Cancer 2020;126(7):1522–9.

21. Breastcancer.org. Detection rates similar to mammograms, ultrasound may be option if mammography isn't available. Breastcancer.org. Published January 9, 2016. Accessed July 30, 2023. https://www.breastcancer.org/research-news/ultrasound-may-be-alternative-to-mammo.

22. Wisdom JP, McGee MG, Horner-Johnson W, et al. Health Disparities Between Women With and Without Disabilities: A Review of the Research. Soc Work Publ Health 2010;25(3–4):368–86.

23. Batchelor NC. Breast cancer incidence and stage at diagnosis in ontarians with and without intellectual disabilities. University of Ontario Institute of Technology; 2017. https://api.core.ac.uk/oai/oai:ir.library.dc-uoit.ca:10155/799.

24. McCarthy EP, Ngo LH, Roetzheim RG, et al. Disparities in breast cancer treatment and survival for women with disabilities. Ann Intern Med 2006;145(9):637–45.

25. Brennand EA, Santinele Martino A. Disability is associated with sexually transmitted infection: Severity and female sex are important risk factors. Can J Hum Sex 2022;31(1):91–102.

26. Tilley E, Walmsley J, Earle S, et al. "The silence is roaring": sterilization, reproductive rights and women with intellectual disabilities. Disabil Soc 2012;27(3):413–26.

27. 2015 Oregon Healthy Teen Data.; 2016.

28. Esmail S, Darry K, Walter A, et al. Attitudes and perceptions towards disability and sexuality. Disabil Rehabil 2010;32(14):1148–55.

29. Haynes RM, Boulet SL, Fox MH, et al. Contraceptive use at last intercourse among reproductive-aged women with disabilities: an analysis of population-based data from seven states. Contraception 2018;97(6):538–45.

30. Wu J, Zhang J, Mitra M, et al. Provision of Moderately and Highly Effective Reversible Contraception to Insured Women With Intellectual and Developmental Disabilities. Obstet Gynecol 2018;132(3):565–74.

31. Personal experiences of pregnancy and fertility in individuals with spinal cord injury. Sex Disabil 2014;32(1):65–74.

32. Bloom TL, Mosher W, Alhusen J, et al. Fertility Desires and Intentions Among U.S. Women by Disability Status: Findings from the 2011–2013 National Survey of Family Growth. Matern Child Health J 2017;21(8):1606–15.

33. Jones L, Bellis MA, Wood S, et al. Prevalence and risk of violence against children with disabilities: a systematic review and meta-analysis of observational studies. Lancet 2012;380(9845):899–907.

34. Bowman RA, Scotti JR, Morris TL. Sexual abuse prevention: a training program for developmental disabilities service providers. J Child Sex Abuse 2010;19(2):119–27.

35. Harrell E. Crime against persons with disabilities, 2009–2019 – statistical tables. Published online 2021. Accessed June 30, 2023. https://calio.dspacedirect.org/handle/11212/5269.

36. Breuner CC, Mattson G. Committee on adolescence, committee on psychosocial aspects of child and family health. sexuality education for children and adolescents. Pediatrics 2016;138(2). https://doi.org/10.1542/peds.2016-1348.
37. Holland-Hall C, Quint EH. Sexuality and Disability in Adolescents. Pediatr Clin North Am 2017;64(2):435–49.
38. Wright KP, Johnson JV. Evaluation of extended and continuous use oral contraceptives. Therapeut Clin Risk Manag 2008;4(5):905–11.
39. Houtchens MK, Zapata LB, Curtis KM, et al. Contraception for women with multiple sclerosis: Guidance for healthcare providers. Mult Scler 2017;23(6):757–64.
40. Fei YF, Ernst SD, Dendrinos ML, et al. Preparing for Puberty in Girls With Special Needs: A Cohort Study of Caregiver Concerns and Patient Outcomes. J Pediatr Adolesc Gynecol 2021;34(4):471–6.
41. Dural Ö, Taş İS, Akhan SE. Management of Menstrual and Gynecologic Concerns in Girls with Special Needs. J Clin Res Pediatr Endocrinol 2020;12(Suppl 1):41–5.
42. Ali M, Akin A, Bahamondes L, et al. Extended use up to 5 years of the etonogestrel-releasing subdermal contraceptive implant: comparison to levonorgestrel-releasing subdermal implant. Hum Reprod 2016;31(11):2491–8.
43. Settnes A, Moeller C, Topsoee MF, et al. Complications after benign hysterectomy, according to procedure: a population-based prospective cohort study from the Danish hysterectomy database, 2004-2015. BJOG 2020;127(10):1269–79.
44. Mitra M, Clements KM, Zhang J, et al. Disparities in Adverse Preconception Risk Factors Between Women with and Without Disabilities. Matern Child Health J 2016;20(3):507–15.
45. Ruhl C, Moran B. The clinical content of preconception care: preconception care for special populations. Am J Obstet Gynecol 2008;199(6 Suppl 2):S384–8.
46. Thierry JM. The importance of preconception care for women with disabilities. Matern Child Health J 2006;10(5 Suppl):S175–6.
47. Rogers J. *ReadHowYouWant.com, Demos Health*. 2010.
48. Mitra M, Long-Bellil LM, Iezzoni LI, et al. Pregnancy among women with physical disabilities: Unmet needs and recommendations on navigating pregnancy. Disabil Health J 2016;9(3):457–63.
49. Gleason JL, Grewal J, Chen Z, et al. Risk of Adverse Maternal Outcomes in Pregnant Women With Disabilities. JAMA Netw Open 2021;4(12):e2138414.
50. Mitra M, Clements KM, Zhang J, et al. Maternal Characteristics, Pregnancy Complications, and Adverse Birth Outcomes Among Women With Disabilities. Med Care 2015;53(12):1027–32.

Caring for Muslim Patients
A Primer for the Obstetrician Gynecologist

Sarrah Shahawy, MD, MPH[a],*, Lobna Raya, MSEd[b],
Leen Al Kassab, MD[c]

KEYWORDS

- Muslim patients • Muslim health • Cross-cultural care • Modesty • Discrimination
- Contraception • Abortion • Sexual and reproductive health

KEY POINTS

- Studies show that Muslims face discrimination and challenges when accessing health care in the United States.
- Physicians are often uncomfortable or ill-equipped to provide cross-cultural sexual and reproductive health care to Muslim patients.
- Obstetrician-gynecologists need to be aware of Muslim norms around sexual and reproductive health topics while keeping in mind the great cultural, generational, and religious diversity of Muslim patients to provide informed, individualized, and holistic care.

INTRODUCTION

A small number of studies exploring Muslim patients' health needs in the United States suggest a failure of health care providers to understand and accommodate their beliefs and customs.[1,2] This article highlights the important role religion plays in delivering health care to Muslim patients, as well as the needs of a continuously growing and diverse Muslim patient population in the United States. This is particularly important since Muslims in the United States face social and political disadvantages as well as discrimination that extend to the healthcare setting.

A better understanding of Islamic cultural and religious beliefs can help prevent health care provider misconceptions and stereotypes. However, there are two major barriers to improved understanding. The first is the vast diversity of Muslims, who are not a monolithic group with a homogenous set of beliefs and practices. The second is the distinction between the scholarly religious viewpoint on a certain topic and

[a] Division of Global and Community Health, Department of Obstetrics and Gynecology, Harvard Medical School, Beth Israel Deaconess Medical Center, 330 Brookline Avenue, Boston, MA 02115, USA; [b] Tufts University, 419 Boston Avenue, Medford, MA 02155, USA; [c] Department of Obstetrics & Gynecology, Harvard Medical School, Brigham and Women's Hospital, 75 Francis Street, Boston, MA 02115, USA
* Corresponding author. 330 Brookline Avenue, Boston, MA 02215.
E-mail address: sshahawy@bidmc.harvard.edu

Obstet Gynecol Clin N Am 51 (2024) 57–67
https://doi.org/10.1016/j.ogc.2023.10.003
0889-8545/24/© 2023 Elsevier Inc. All rights reserved.

obgyn.theclinics.com

individual patient practice and belief. Islam has no clergy or a singular set of laws. The history of Islamic law is built on a tradition of different concurrent schools of religious thought that provide frameworks for Muslims to make their own day-to-day decisions. In this article, we discuss starting principles shared by many Muslims as well as opinions endorsed by various Islamic bioethical bodies and religious schools of thought with the understanding that this may not necessarily represent individual patient beliefs or practices.

Our goal in this article is to offer obstetrician-gynecologists (OB/GYNs) the necessary knowledge and tools to provide cross-cultural care to Muslim patients while keeping in mind their great cultural, generational, and religious diversity. We propose that the best way to do this is by enhancing awareness and education of each patient's background and context without overgeneralizing or stereotyping. Throughout this article, the authors strive to use gender-inclusive language, and in certain cases, the authors use the term "Muslim women" to specify individuals who identify as both Muslim and female.

BACKGROUND
Muslims in the United States

According to the Pew Research Center, there are approximately 3.45 million Muslims living in the United States as of 2017.[3] By 2040, the Muslim population is expected to become the second-largest religious group in the United States. By 2050, the Muslim population in the United States is estimated to reach 8.1 million, approximately 2.1% of the US total population.[3] The Muslim population is the most ethnically diverse faith community in the United States, with 28% identifying as Black or African American, 23% identifying as Asian/Chinese/Japanese, 19% identifying as White, 14% identifying as Arab, 8% identifying as Hispanic, 2% identifying as Native American/American Indian/Alaska Native, and 5% as Other.[4] Of note, immigrants from the Middle East/North Africa (MENA) and Iran are underrepresented in the census because they are currently identified as White. Although nearly 75% of American Muslims are immigrants or born to immigrants, 50% are born in the United States and 36% are naturalized citizens.[3] As such, many Muslims consider themselves very much a part of the American fabric and society and not as outsiders, as they are often portrayed in the media.

Religious Discrimination and Racism

Discrimination in the post-9/11 and Trump presidency eras has negatively impacted Muslim patients seeking health care in the United States. Muslims may be easily identifiable and subject to bias due to religious wear such as the *hijab*, or headscarf. Given that a quarter of Muslims in the United States identify as Black, the compounded impact of racism and religious discrimination on these patients' sexual and reproductive health (SRH) outcomes as well as health care experiences must be considered. Unfortunately, studies confirm that Muslim patients tend to be uncomfortable with physicians in the United States due to the religious, racial, and gender discrimination they experience.[4] As a result, Muslim patients may receive poor treatment or fail to seek the appropriate health care they need.[1]

Arab-American and Muslim patients face various barriers that prevent them from seeking necessary medical attention. For example, a 2016 Canadian study highlighted the fact that Muslims are more likely to be at risk of cervical cancer due to barriers such as not having access to gender-concurrent physicians and preventative health care measures.[5] Similarly, a 2021 US study found that "preventable female cancers were more prevalent among Muslim women than non-Muslim women and were also diagnosed at more advanced stages."[6] A 2016 US study surveying 254 Muslim women of various ethnic backgrounds (Black, Arab, and South Asian) found that 53% of respondents shared that they have delayed seeking health care when not given the option to see a gender-concordant physician.[7] In addition, they found that Muslims who had a stronger tendency toward modesty practices and who had lived in the United States for a shorter duration also had a higher rate of postponing their health care needs. A 2020 systematic review that included 59 studies from 22 countries identified 11 major themes in factors that affect Muslim women's SRH, which included:

> ...Insufficient knowledge and misconceptions about contraception and reproductive health services, sources of information on contraception, barriers to SRH education and information needs, socio-demographic factors influencing contraceptive use, attitudes toward family planning, women's lack of control over reproductive choices, religious and cultural barriers to family planning, marital status, access to reproductive health services, the role of healthcare providers, and privacy/confidentiality in health services.[8]

Health and Health Care in Islam

Medicine, science, and the importance of health are viewed in a positive light in Islam. Core Islamic mandates include caring for one's body and avoiding harm, as well as discovering the surrounding world. The human body is considered a precious gift, so Muslims experiencing physical or mental illness are encouraged to seek the necessary medical help to ensure their health and well-being.[9] Medical discovery flourished during the Islamic Golden Age (eight to thirteenth century CE) with various notable achievements, such as the prevention, diagnosis, and treatment of smallpox and measles, as well as the combination of the fields of medicine and surgery.[10,11] The medical and scientific achievements taking place during the Islamic Golden Age, and Islam's emphasis on the importance of science and health care is a point of pride for many Muslims.

Communitarian ethics, which "considers the consequence of any medical decision on the family and community resources," plays an important role in Islamic biomedical ethics.[12] As a result, it is not uncommon for Muslim patients to include their family members in their decision-making process when it comes to their health care needs; this should be acknowledged and respected by the health care team.

Providers' Cultural Awareness

Evidence shows that physicians' attitudes and confidence levels toward treating Muslim patients in non-Muslim majority countries is generally low. A 2020 US study surveyed medical students and residents at Michigan Medicine and found that only 41% of the respondents felt comfortable documenting history from Arab patients, whereas 55% of respondents felt comfortable caring for patients who chose to fast for the Islamic month of Ramadan.[13] Only 24% of respondents felt comfortable answering questions from patients about fasting, whereas 64% shared they had not been professionally trained to care for Arab patients and 81% shared they had not received any training regarding patients who are fasting. One study found that American physicians might be hesitant to discuss religion, especially Islam, in their provision of health care.[14]

In an effort to address this lack of culturally aware care in treating Arab-American and Muslim patients, a 2014 study created an online, interactive simulation that allowed second-year Michigan State University College of Osteopathic Medicine students to complete a questionnaire about their cross-cultural care skills.[15] The results of the study showed that enrolling medical students in cross-cultural care courses that involved similar online simulations could improve students' skills when caring for Arab American and Muslim patients. A 2020 UK study surveying health care professionals' experiences with pregnant Muslim patients identified that physicians believed they would benefit from in-depth learning of cross-cultural care through group discussion and learning directly from one another's experience.[16]

In this discussion, we hope to offer OB/GYNs a background on Islamic perspectives on SRH norms that informs recommendations for providing informed, individualized, and wholistic care to Muslim patients.

DISCUSSION
Modesty and Privacy

Muslim women's clothing is highly politicized and judged in various cultural and professional contexts, including health care. Addressing the assumptions made by health care professionals about Muslim patients is essential to provide them nonjudgmental care. Modesty is of particular cultural emphasis in regard to Muslim women's clothing; however, dressing modestly in Islam actually applies to all Muslims regardless of gender identity, who are expected to cover in public spaces and around people of all genders to varying degrees, excluding spouses. Approximately one-third of Muslim women in the United States wear the *hijab*, which is an article of clothing that covers their hair.[17] Some Muslims may also wear the *abaya*, a dress-like article of clothing that covers the body, or a *niqab,* which covers the hair, body, and face, excluding the eyes. There are various reasons why Muslims choose to wear the hijab, including religious piety, cultural reasons, protection, or to outwardly identify as Muslim. Many Muslims find dressing modestly to be a sign of independence, showing that their bodies belong to themselves and are not to be objectified. In reality, modesty is not only practiced through the *hijab*, *abaya*, or *niqab*, but also by other kinds of clothing or behavior that protect interpersonal boundaries.

Although respecting patients' personal beliefs is essential when delivering health care, it can be difficult to complete a physical examination while a patient is dressed modestly. Muslims in the United States are usually comfortable undressing for gender-concordant physicians, but some may otherwise feel less comfortable.[18] To accommodate a Muslim patient's needs in this scenario, physicians could offer gender-concordant staff to be present during the physical examination, complete the physical examination without asking the patient to undress if medically appropriate, or ask if the patient would like their family to be in the room. A health care worker, such as a gender-concordant nurse or medical assistant, could take note of the patient's preferences before the visit with the physician, which would allow time for the patient to share personal preferences for the medical encounter. If patients are comfortable with a medical examination performed by a gender non-concordant physician, it is still possible that the patient would want to limit any medically unnecessary physical touch. For instance, the physician should take no offense to the patient's preference should the patient choose not to shake hands. In order to properly identify Muslim patients, it may be beneficial to include relevant questions on intake or social history forms to ensure their needs are being met, as opposed to simply relying on appearance and name.

It is important to note that Muslim patients' preferences for gender-concordant physicians are not unique to this population alone. A 2016 US sub-analysis of studies from 1999 onward found that 8.4% of the population sample of 9861 women preferred a male physician, whereas 53.2% preferred a female physician and 38.5% had no preference.[19] Many Muslim patients might be comfortable with gender non-concordant physicians because many Islamic scholars believe that modesty guidelines do not apply as strictly in the health care setting. Again, it is essential to approach Muslim patients with their religious and cultural frameworks in mind, whereas also understanding that not every Muslim will have the same preferences. Therefore, asking questions and talking to patients about their preferences will help minimize discomfort and encourage Muslims to seek appropriate medical care.

Gynecology

Sexual health

Islam celebrates sex as an act of love, pleasure, giving, and spirituality independent of just its childbearing purposes. However, culturally, some Muslims may be hesitant to discuss sexual health and activity. Because premarital or extramarital sex is religiously forbidden, some patients may feel the need to hide their sexual activity. However, in the health care setting, it is essential to continue to ask the routine questions. It may be beneficial to approach the question sensitively and reassure the patient that these questions are standard for all patients and confidential. Some Muslims may be hesitant to undergo pelvic examinations, pap smears, or transvaginal ultrasounds due to an assumption that they are not required until they are sexually active or that these procedures may disrupt the integrity of the hymen. This is a topic that health care providers should approach sensitively by sharing standard of care recommendations, preparing patients for what these procedures involve, and reassuring patients that these are not "discoverable" later. When ordering an ultrasound, providers should specify if it will be transvaginal to set expectations and norms before the visit. If a patient refuses a transvaginal approach after appropriate counseling, an abdominal approach should be offered with the caveat that it may not be as accurate. It is not uncommon for some patients undergoing pap smears to ask for a chaperone's presence in the room, whereas other patients may prefer the presence of only essential personnel to ensure privacy.

Last, although sex is traditionally celebrated in Islam within the context of heterosexual marriages, it is essential to address the specific sexual health needs of lesbian, gay, bisexual, transgender, queer (LGBTQ) Muslims while continuing to take into consideration their religious and cultural needs within a health care setting, without making harmful assumptions about sexual practices.[20]

Contraception

Reversible forms of contraception are widely accepted by Muslims with 79.5% of American Muslim women using contraception.[21] Islamic religious scholars believe that contraception is lawful and allows for population control and the advancement of one's standards of living, especially in poverty-stricken societies.[12] Reversible contraceptives such as intrauterine devices, oral contraceptives, diaphragms, spermicide, and condoms are generally preferred over irreversible forms like tubal ligation and vasectomy (outside the context of medical necessity). A 2015 survey-based study conducted at the University of Alabama at Birmingham with a sample size of 224 sexually active Muslim women living in the United States found that American Muslims' contraception use was similar to both Americans' use in general and disadvantaged minority groups.[21] Identifying as generally "Muslim" coincided with a greater chance of using contraception than identifying as "Sunni" (the majority Islamic sect).

Identifying as "Shia" (a minority Islamic sect) coincided with a greater chance of using oral contraceptive pills than identifying as "Sunni." South Asians had higher odds of using oral contraceptive pills compared with MENA groups. This illustrates that differences in practice may exist within the diversity of sects in Islam, as well as within cultural and ethnic groups. It is important to remember not to make any assumptions that cast blanket guidelines, but rather providers should aim to deliver personalized health care to each patient.

Abortion

Muslims and Islamic scholars have had a wide range of legal and ethical views on abortion. Both maternal and fetal welfare are considered in the context of core Islamic bioethical principles: "no harm, no harassment" (the Islamic equivalent of beneficence and nonmaleficence), as well as "public good" (maslaha). Through this lens, some religious scholars have argued that abortion is permitted only when the life of the mother is in danger,[22] whereas others consider abortion justifiable in cases of rape, severe fetal anomalies, or unwanted pregnancies, especially when the family situation or social context could harm the mother or child's well-being and fulfillment.[12] After a certain period of time, a fetus is considered to have a soul; abortions after this date tend to be discouraged except for compelling reasons. Muslim scholars have differed on the timing of "ensoulment": at conception, 40 days postconception (approximately 8 weeks of gestation), or, most commonly, at 120 days postconception (approximately 19 weeks of gestation).

Religion often plays a central role in how Muslims navigate abortion in non-Muslim majority countries. A 2011 Canadian study surveyed 53 Muslims from diverse backgrounds presenting to abortion clinics and found that patients could see religion either as a source of comfort or guilt; patients who believed abortion was against Islamic principles had higher anxiety and guilt scores, while others were comforted by their sense that abortion was Islamically justifiable.[16] In a 2022 national survey by the Institute for Social Policy and Understanding, 56% of Muslim Americans believed that abortion should be legal in most or all cases.[23] Usually, Muslims in non-Muslim majority countries experience personal, rather than legal, barriers when seeking an abortion. However, in light of the 2022 US Supreme Court decision to overturn Roe v Wade, some Muslims actually believe that abortion bans restrict their religious freedom.[24]

It is important for health care providers to be aware of how religion might influence a Muslim patient's views but not to make assumptions, offering all termination options and fully discussing risks and benefits.

Obstetrics

Infertility

Pregnancy and childbearing are highly revered in Islam, which can make infertility particularly devastating on a spiritual level for Muslim patients. Muslim scholars have encouraged the research and use of infertility treatments and consider most currently available assisted reproductive technologies permissible in the context of marriage.[25] For instance, the Sunni tradition allows for artificial insemination and in vitro fertilization, so long as the treatment does not include a third party, such as donor sperm, egg, or surrogacy, given the importance placed on known parental lineage.[12] Although many Shia scholars would support this view, some have permitted third-party involvement, specifically in Lebanon and Iran. As a result, Muslim patients from these countries may be more open to third-party involvement in infertility treatments than Muslim patients from Sunni-majority countries.

Pregnancy and delivery

As with all our patients, caring for Muslim patients during pregnancy and delivery requires open communication and respect. During prenatal care, the patient's preferences for their delivery plan, clothing, and gender of providers should be adequately and respectfully identified in the medical chart and during sign out on labor and delivery. All medical teams, including OB/GYN, nursing, anesthesia, and neonatal intensive care unit (NICU) should have an open line of communication to understand the patient's needs. Muslims who choose to dress modestly may want to continue dressing modestly as much as possible on labor and delivery, which should be accommodated to the extent that it is possible and medically safe. Patients who indicate a gender preference should be informed ahead of time that every effort will be made to accommodate this, but that in certain cases, it may not be possible or medically safe depending on the available health care team members.

A common birth practice is the recitation of the *adhan,* or the call to prayer, in the newborn's ear, often performed by the father.[26] Although male circumcision is religiously proscribed, female circumcision or female genital cutting is considered Islamically forbidden.[26]

Fasting Ramadan

Fasting during the lunar month of Ramadan is an essential Islamic religious practice and requires those who are able to abstain from food, drink (including water), and sexual activity from sunrise to sunset. Pregnant Muslims may be religiously exempt from fasting, especially if there is concern for undue hardship or harm to maternal or fetal health.[22,27] Nevertheless, studies show that most pregnant Muslims choose to fast, with rates of 70% to 85% reported.[28–30] Some Muslims avoid discussing fasting with their providers, who often lack familiarity with the evidence regarding fasting in pregnancy and do not feel comfortable counseling pregnant Muslim patients in Ramadan.[31,32] A study of pregnant Muslims in Germany found that only 49% of individuals who did fast and 38% of individuals who did not fast shared this information with their physicians.[33] Less than 2% of patients reported being proactively approached about this by their doctor.

Based on meta-analysis and systematic review data, fasting during Ramadan in pregnancy likely does not have a significant effect on neonatal birth weight, preterm birth, or mode of delivery.[34,35] However, fasting Muslims may experience increased fatigue and dehydration, and antenatal fetal testing may show lower frequency of large accelerations, lower amniotic fluid indices, and lower biophysical profile scores. A few studies have shown the possibility of decreased long-term health and economic outcomes in individuals whose mothers chose to fast while pregnant.[36] Interpretation of current evidence is limited by several factors including the misclassification of actual fasting during Ramadan versus simply having a pregnancy that overlaps with Ramadan, the misclassification of Muslim patients versus using other demographic surrogates such as language and ethnicity as proxies for religion, and lastly, small and limited study sizes and designs.

In order to aid perinatal care providers, we developed a five-point framework to effectively counsel and support pregnant Muslim patients during Ramadan (**Fig. 1**).[37]

1. Demonstrate cultural and religious awareness: Providers should know when Ramadan falls each year and ask patients about their plans to fast. This conversation should involve an open-ended, respectful approach to ensure the patient feels safe sharing their plans, which will allow physicians to better support or counsel their patients. Fasting has specific parameters that cannot be modified, so providers should not recommend altering the fasting ritual by drinking water or fasting for fewer hours. Physicians should also be aware of the chaplain services available to them and connect their patients to them.

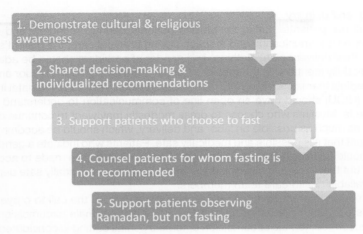

Fig. 1. Fasting Ramadan and pregnancy: counseling framework for providers.

2. Shared decision-making and individualized recommendations: Although it is certainly reasonable for providers to recommend against prolonged fasting while pregnant—both to avoid potentially adverse outcomes and undue hardship—strong blanket prohibitions against fasting are discouraged given the lack of strong evidence to support this. Patients with specific risk factors should be counseled to fully understand their risks.
3. Support patients who choose to fast: Providers should recommend practices that might decrease maternal and fetal harm, such as engaging in healthy eating, exercise and sleeping habits, discontinuing addictive substances, avoiding strenuous activity, staying cool, and consuming nutritious bedtime snacks and pre-sunrise meals. Providers should ensure they discuss warning signs with their patients for breaking their fast and seeking medical attention, such as preterm contractions, decreased fetal movement, vaginal bleeding, leakage of fluid, severe headache, or dizziness.
4. Counsel pregnant patients for whom fasting may not be medically recommended.
5. Support pregnant patients observing Ramadan, but not fasting.

SUMMARY

Studies show that Muslims face discrimination and challenges when accessing health care in the United States. Physicians are often uncomfortable or ill equipped to provide cross-cultural sexual and reproductive health care to Muslims. OB/GYNs need to be aware of Muslim norms around SRH topics while keeping in mind the great cultural, generational, and religious diversity of Muslim patients to provide informed, individualized, and holistic care. Providers must continuously educate themselves on the frameworks and experiences that may affect the Muslim patient in the OB/GYN setting to deliver high-quality, culturally appropriate care.

CLINICS CARE POINTS

- Due to discrimination and limited cultural awareness of health care providers, Muslim patients are at risk of receiving poor treatment or failing to seek appropriate health care.

- Although US physicians are hesitant to discuss religion, especially Islam, in relation to health care, religion is often vital to how Muslim patients perceive their health and health care.
- Islamic perspectives on modesty and privacy may affect the Muslim patient's experience with the US health care system. Obstetrician-gynecologists (OB/GYNs) should provide a safe space for respectful accommodation of Muslim patients' needs.
- Reversible contraceptives and infertility treatments are widely accepted among Muslims.
- Islamic views on abortion are varied and more expansive than might be expected.
- OB/GYNs should be prepared to counsel and support pregnant Muslim patients during Ramadan, both those who choose to fast and those who do not.

DISCLOSURES

The authors report no conflicts of interest.

REFERENCES

1. Padela AI, Gunter K, Killawi A, et al. Religious values and healthcare accommodations: voices from the American Muslim community. Gen Intern Med 2012;27:708–15.
2. Hasnain M, Connell KJ, Menon U, et al. Patient- centered care for Muslim women: provider and patient perspectives. J Womens Health (Larchmt) 2011;20:73–83.
3. Mohamed B. Muslims are a growing presence in U.S., but still face negative views from the public. Pew Research Center. Available at: https://www.pewresearch.org/short-reads/2021/09/01/muslims-are-a-growing-presence-in-u-s-but-still-face-negative-views-from-the-public/. Accessed November 12, 2023.
4. Center PR. 1. Demographic portrait of Muslim Americans. Pew Research Center's Religion & Public Life Project. Published July 26, 2017. Available at: https://www.pewresearch.org/religion/2017/07/26/demographic-portrait-of-muslim-americans/. Accessed November 12, 2023.
5. Vahabi M, Lofters A. Muslim immigrant women's views on cervical cancer screening and HPV self-sampling in Ontario, Canada. BMC Publ Health 2016;16(1):868.
6. Namoos A, Abosamak NE, Abdelkarim M, et al. Muslim Women and Disparities in Cancer Diagnosis: A Retrospective Study. J Muslim Minority Aff 2021;41(3):541–7.
7. Vu M, Azmat A, Radejko T, et al. Predictors of Delayed Healthcare Seeking Among American Muslim Women. J Wom Health 2016;586–93.
8. Alomair N, Alageel S, Davies N, et al. Factors influencing sexual and reproductive health of Muslim women: a systematic review. Reprod Health 2020;17:33.
9. Inhorn MC, Serour GI. Islam, medicine, and Arab-Muslim refugee health in America after 9/11. Lancet 2011;378(9794):935–43. ISSN 0140-6736.
10. Ashimi TA. The Contribution of Muslim Scholars To The Field of Medicine (With Particular Reference To Ibn Sina And Al-Razi During The Islamic Golden Age). J Educ Soc 2018;9(3):73–7.
11. Yale School of Medicine. From the Middle East, in the Middle Ages. Yale Medicine Magazine. 2005 - Autumn. Available at: https://medicine.yale.edu/news/yale-medicine-magazine/article/from-the-middle-east-in-the-middle-ages/#:~:text=Perhaps%20the%20most%20concrete%20legacy,of%20sex%2C%20religion%20or%20ethnicity. Accessed Nov 12, 2023.
12. Sachedina A. Islamic biomedical ethics: principles and applications. New York: Oxford University Press; 2009.

13. Sarsour NY, Ballouz D, Mokbel M, et al. Medical Trainees Comfort and Confidence in Providing Care to Arab and Muslim Patients at a Large Academic Medical Center. Teach Learn Med 2022;34(3):246–54.

14. Amin MEK, Abdelmageed A. Clinicians' Perspectives on Caring for Muslim Patients Considering Fasting During Ramadan. J Relig Health 2020;59:1370–87.

15. Smith BD, Silk K. Cultural Competence Clinic: An Online, Interactive, Simulation for Working Effectively With Arab American Muslim Patients. Acad Psychiatr 2011;35:312–6.

16. Hassan SM, Leavey C, Rooney JS, et al. A qualitative study of healthcare professionals' experiences of providing maternity care for Muslim women in the UK. BMC Pregnancy Childbirth 2020;20:400.

17. Center PR. U.S. Muslims Concerned About Their Place in Society, but Continue to Believe in the American Dream. Pew Research Center's Religion & Public Life Project. Published July 26, 2017. Available at: https://www.pewresearch.org/religion/2017/07/26/findings-from-pew-research-centers-2017-survey-of-us-muslims/. Accessed November 12, 2023.

18. Shahawy S, Deshpande NA, Nour NM. Cross-Cultural Obstetric and Gynecologic Care of Muslim Patients. Obstet Gynecol 2015;126(5):969–73.

19. Tobler KJ, Wu J, Khafagy AM, et al. Gender preference of the obstetrician gynecologist provider: a systematic review and meta-analysis [1E]. Obstet Gynecol 2016;127:43S.

20. Khan M, Mulé NJ. Voices of Resistance and Agency: LBTQ Muslim Women Living Out Intersectional Lives in North America. J Homosex 2021;68(7):1144–68.

21. Budhwani H, Anderson J, Hearld KR. Muslim Women's use of contraception in the United States. Reprod Health 2018;15(1):1.

22. Hathout H. Islamic perspectives in obstetrics and gynecology. Cairo (Egypt): Alam al-Kutub; 1988.

23. Wiebe E, Najafi R, Soheil N, et al. Muslim women having abortions in Canada: attitudes, beliefs, and experiences. Canadian family physician Medecin de famille canadien 2011;57(4):e134–8.

24. Quraishi-Landes A. Abortion bans trample on the religious freedom of Muslims, too. San Francisco Chronicle 2022. Available at: https://www.sfchronicle.com/opinion/openforum/article/abortion-bans-religion-17259119.php.

25. Inhorn MC, Gurtin ZB. Infertility and assisted reproduction in the Middle East: social, religious, and resource considerations. Facts Views Vision Obstet Gynecol 2012;24–9.

26. GATRAD AR, SHEIKH A. Muslim birth customs. Arch Dis Child Fetal Neonatal Ed 2001;84:F6–8.

27. Nasr SH, Dagli CK, Dakake MM, et al. The study quran: a new translation and commentary. New York: Harper Collins; 2015. p. 79–85.

28. Safari K, Piro TJ, Ahmad HM. Perspectives and pregnancy outcomes of maternal Ramadan fasting in the second trimester of pregnancy. BMC Pregnancy Childbirth 2019;19:128.

29. Seiermann AU, Al-Mufti H, Waid JL, et al. Women's fasting habits and dietary diversity during Ramadan in rural Bangladesh. Matern Child Nutr 2021;17:e13135.

30. van Bilsen LA, Savitri AI, Amelia D, et al. Predictors of Ramadan fasting during preg- nancy. J Epidemiol Glob Health 2016;6:267–75.

31. Robinson T, Raisler J. "Each one is a doctor for herself": Ramadan fasting among pregnant Muslim women in the United States. Ethn Dis 2005;15:S1–99.

32. Lou A, Hammoud M. Muslim patients' ex- pectations and attitudes about Ramadan fasting during pregnancy. Int J Gynaecol Obstet 2016;132:321–4.

33. Leimer B, Pradella F, Fruth A, et al. Ramadan Observance during Pregnancy in Germany: a Challenge for Prenatal Care. Geburtshilfe Frauenheilkd 2018;78(7):684–9.
34. Glazier JD, Hayes DJL, Hussain S, et al. The effect of Ramadan fasting during pregnancy on perinatal outcomes: a systematic review and meta-analysis. BMC Pregnancy Childbirth 2018;18:421.
35. Oosterwijk VNL, Molenaar JM, van Bilsen LA, et al. Ramadan fasting during pregnancy and health outcomes in offspring: a systematic review. Nutrients 2021;13: 3450.
36. Mahanani MR, Abderbwih E, Wendt AS, et al. Long-Term Outcomes of in Utero Ramadan Exposure: A Systematic Literature Review. Nutrients 2021;13(12):4511.
37. Shahawy S, Al Kassab L, Rattani A. Ramadan Fasting and Pregnancy: An Evidence-Based Guide for the Obstetrician. Am J Obstet Gynecol 2023;228(6): 689–95.

A Public Health Emergency
Breast Cancer Among Black Communities in the United States

Versha Pleasant, MD, MPH

KEYWORDS

- Black • Breast cancer • Mortality • Racial disparities • Genetics

KEY POINTS

- Black people have a 40% higher breast cancer–related mortality compared to White people.
- Black patients are more likely to have delays in breast cancer care and barriers to treatment.
- While Black people are more likely to be diagnosed with biologically aggressive breast cancers, systemic racism and social determinants of health also play a significant role in breast cancer-related racial health disparities.
- While genetic testing represents a critical tool in precision medicine, challenges among the Black community include low uptake of genetic testing and higher likelihood of equivocal, nonactionable results.
- Breast cancer–related racial disparities are unacceptable and require urgent national attention.

INTRODUCTION

Breast cancer represents the most commonly diagnosed cancer among people assigned female at birth (AFAB) and one of the leading causes of cancer deaths among people in the United States.[1] With an incidence of 12%, 1 in 8 will be impacted by breast cancer in their lifetime. Despite its high prevalence, most breast cancers are diagnosed at stage I and carry a good prognosis.[2] This is likely multifactorial, due to increased breast cancer awareness among the public as well as largely universal screening in the form of mammography that is generally low-cost, accessible, and efficacious. There have also been great strides among breast cancer treatment including surgery, chemotherapy, radiation, endocrine therapy, and immunotherapy that has evolved tremendously over the past few decades.

Department of Obstetrics and Gynecology, Cancer Genetics & Breast Health Clinic, University of Michigan, 1500 East Medical Center Drive, Ann Arbor, MI 48109, USA
E-mail address: vershap@med.umich.edu

Obstet Gynecol Clin N Am 51 (2024) 69–103
https://doi.org/10.1016/j.ogc.2023.11.001
0889-8545/24/© 2023 Elsevier Inc. All rights reserved.

obgyn.theclinics.com

While breast cancer impacts people of all backgrounds, there are significant disparities experienced by Black communities—from diagnosis to care and treatment to survival. Notably, Black people have a 40% increased risk of dying from breast cancer compared to White people.[3] The disproportionate impact of breast cancer on the Black community is one of national urgency. This article provides a comprehensive overview of the impact of breast cancer among Black people and explores the many potential reasons for poorer outcomes (**Fig. 1**). Suggested strategies to combat these disparities are also outlined.

RISK FACTORS AND PROTECTIVE FACTORS

Among the general population, there are a number of known risk factors for breast cancer. A strong family history of breast cancer (particularly having a first-degree or second-degree affected relative) represents one of the most well-established risk factors for breast cancer. It is estimated that approximately 5% to 10% of all breast cancers involve a hereditary component[4] and there are numerous genes that are known to increase breast cancer risk (such as BRCA1, BRCA2, ATM, BARD1, NF1, PALB2, CHEK2, CDH1, RAD51 C, RAD51D, TP53, STK11, and PTEN).[5] Other risk factors include increasing age (>65 years old), early menses (<12 years old), late menopause (>55 years old), nulliparity or first live birth greater than 30 years old, dense breast tissue, exposure to hormonal therapy, history of high-dose ionizing thoracic radiation in childhood, prior history of high-risk lesions such as atypical hyperplasia or lobular carcinoma in situ, and increasing alcohol intake.[6–14]

Obesity

Obesity is known to increase breast cancer risk and to be correlated with worse survival.[15–17] One retrospective study attributed over 30% of the breast cancer disparity between Blacks and Whites to obesity.[18] Another retrospective study showed a 33% breast cancer risk reduction among Black people compared to White people when controlling for obesity.[19] A prospective cohort study showed that Black postmenopausal patients with body mass index (BMI) greater than 30 had an increased risk of breast cancer including triple-negative breast cancer (TNBC) (hazard ratio [HR] 2.77, 95% confidence interval [CI]: 1.05–7.30).[20]

However, other studies demonstrate conflicting results. The National Cancer Institute (NCI) Black/White Cancer Survival Study demonstrated that no single factor (including increased BMI) explained breast cancer race-stage disparities.[21]

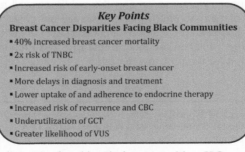

Key Points
Breast Cancer Disparities Facing Black Communities
- 40% increased breast cancer mortality
- 2x risk of TNBC
- Increased risk of early-onset breast cancer
- More delays in diagnosis and treatment
- Lower uptake of and adherence to endocrine therapy
- Increased risk of recurrence and CBC
- Underutilization of GCT
- Greater likelihood of VUS

Fig. 1. Breast cancer disparities faced by Black communities. CBC, contralateral breast cancer; GCT, genetic counseling and testing; TNBC, triple-negative breast cancer; VUS, variant of uncertain significance.

Furthermore, a pooled analysis of 1793 premenopausal and postmenopausal Black people showed no association between obesity and breast cancer subtypes in the Southeastern United States.[22] An evaluation of the effects of obesity on breast cancer survival demonstrated a greater risk of all-cause and breast cancer–related mortality in patients with BMI$\geq$30 compared to BMI 20 to 24.9. However, this was only noted in White patients but not among Black patients.[23] Research regarding obesity as a significant breast cancer risk factor among Blacks should be further explored.

Dense Breasts

Dense breast tissue is an independent risk factor for breast cancer, with data estimating a 1-fold to 6-fold increased risk.[9,24,25] Approximately 40% of AFAB people will have heterogeneously dense breasts and 10% will have extremely dense breasts, accounting for approximately 50% of the total screening population. Compared to White people, one study demonstrated that Blacks were more likely to have extremely dense breasts (odds ratio[OR] 1.31, 95% CI: 1.13–1.52).[26] Another study utilizing the Laboratory for Individualized Breast Radiodensity Assessment software demonstrated that Black people had statistically significantly higher breast area and volume density[27] which could be strong contributors to breast cancer risk.[28]

Breastfeeding

The American College of Obstetricians and Gynecologists and the American Academy of Pediatrics recommend exclusive breastfeeding within the first 6 months of life.[29,30] Along with numerous benefits to parents and infants, breastfeeding is known to provide some protection against breast cancer. Compared to other racial groups, however, Black people have lower overall rates of breastfeeding. With an average estimated initiation rate of 84.1% in the United States across all racial and ethnic groups, Black parents were observed to have a breastfeeding rate of 73.6%,[31] the lowest compared to all other racial groups. Barriers may include lack of familial and social support, lack of lactation spaces, mode of delivery, socioeconomic status (SES), lack of breastfeeding education, and sooner return to work.[32–36] The concept of generational trauma related to Black people forcibly prioritizing the breastfeeding of enslaver's infants over their own has also been hypothesized.[37,38]

Alcohol Intake

Alcohol is another known risk factor for breast cancer.[39–42] There is a paucity of data specifically regarding Black women and breast cancer as it relates to alcohol intake as an independent risk factor. One population-based case-control study did not demonstrate increased breast cancer–related mortality for Black or White patients with various prediagnosis levels of alcohol consumption.[43] However, another study looked at genetic variants in ethanol metabolism in the African American Breast Cancer Epidemiology and Risk Consortium. Black study participants were noted to have statistically significant associations between a specific genomic region in CYP2E1 called rs79865122-C and both estrogen-receptor negative and TNBC.[44] This is an area for which additional research is warranted.

Black Hair Products

Black hair products have garnered significant attention due to studies showing links with increased risk of endometrial cancer.[45] The ingredients found in some hair relaxers, straighteners, and dyes (such as endocrine-disrupting chemicals, formaldehyde-containing and formaldehyde-releasing chemicals, and oxidized paraphenylenediamine) may be implicated in cancer risk.[46–55]

There are limited data showing a strong correlation between Black hair products and breast cancer risk at this time. One national prospective cohort demonstrated that hair dye carried a 45% increased risk of breast cancer among Black people (HR = 1.45, 95% CI: 1.10–1.90).[56] Another nationwide prospective study showed that among a cohort of 50,543 Black people, 2311 incident breast cancers were diagnosed. Multivariate HR for those using chemical relaxers (>7 times per year for at least 15 years, compared to never/light use) was 1.13 (95% CI: 0.96–1.33), with no significant breast cancer association observed with duration, frequency, age at initiation, or number of scalp burns.[57] Data from the Sisters Study showed an increased risk of premenopausal breast cancer with frequent use of hair straighteners and perms (HR = 2.11, 95% CI: 1.26–3.55 and HR = 1.55, 95% CI: 0.96–2.53, respectively), but was not powered enough to fully extrapolate race-specific risk.[58] Additional research is needed to further explore the downstream impact of these products on breast cancer risk.

SCREENING AND EARLY DETECTION
Screening Mammography

Screening mammography currently represents the best tool for the early detection of breast cancer in the general population. Annual screening mammograms from ages 40 to 84 have demonstrated an approximately 40% decreased mortality when compared to no screening.[59] Furthermore, screening-detected breast cancers demonstrate a survival advantage compared to symptomatic breast cancers, likely due to tumor size and node status.[60]

There are conflicting opinions across professional societies regarding the optimal age of initiation and frequency of screening mammography.[61–64] More recently evolving is the unique consideration of increased mortality and high incidence of early-onset breast cancer among the Black community, along with some data demonstrating that Black people are more likely than White people to be diagnosed with breast cancer at their first mammogram ($P < .001$).[65] One model showed a 57% reduction in Black-White mortality disparities when Black patients started screening mammography 10 years earlier, thereby concluding that screening mammography should be started at age 40 for Black people.[66] A nationwide population-based cross-sectional study argued that due to increased breast cancer mortality among Black people between ages 40 to 49, an earlier threshold should be considered in which Black people should begin screening at age 42 (8 years prior than recommended screening for the general population by some professional groups).[67]

Data regarding uptake of mammography have been conflicting longitudinally. Some previous research has suggested a lower uptake of screening mammogram in Black people compared to White people[68–70]—for which barriers included lack of insurance coverage and cost, inconvenience, beliefs that undergoing mammogram could cause breast cancer, perceptions that treatment for breast cancer would be worse than a breast cancer diagnosis, other medical comorbidities, and pain.[71] Conversely, more recent data from the 2023 to 2024 Cancer Prevention and Early Detection Screening from the American Cancer Society suggest that Black, non-Hispanic White, and Hispanic people are more likely to undergo screening mammogram than those of other races and ethnic groups (such as American Indian/Alaskan Native and Asian).[72] Furthermore, tomosynthesis (also known as digital breast tomosynthesis (DBT) or 3-dimensional (3-D) mammography) has been US Food and Drug Administration–approved and has largely replaced 2-dimensional mammography resulting in fewer callbacks. Research suggests that Black people are less likely to undergo 3-D mammography compared to White people.[73] These findings were reiterated by another retrospective cohort study demonstrating that Black and Asian people were less likely to undergo DBT compared to White people. In this cohort, those who underwent DBT had a lower recall rate (9.1% vs 11.2%, $P < .001$) and greater cancer detection (6.0 vs 4.1, $P < .001$) compared to the full-field digital mammogram group.[74] Another study examining uptake of screening mammogram across numerous facilities in Chicago showed that White people (compared to Black and Hispanic people) were more likely to have mammograms performed at academic facilities and centers in which mammograms are read specifically by breast specialists, and ones in which digital mammogram was available ($P < .001$).[75]

The coronavirus disease 2019 (COVID-19) pandemic has also impacted the uptake of screening mammography with mixed results. Yacona and colleagues demonstrated that while screening mammograms and breast cancer detection decreased globally in 2019 and 2020, the percentage change was greater at a study institution that served predominantly Black people (as well as a marked decrease in diagnostic exams and image-guided biopsies at this institution) compared to one that served predominantly non-Black patients.[76] Sprague and colleagues showed a global decrease in screening mammography during the onset of the pandemic across races and ethnicities. However, compared to July 2019 volumes, both White and Black populations rebounded in both the level of screening and diagnostic mammograms by July 2020 compared to Hispanic and Asian populations.[77] A revealing qualitative study titled "Sister, Give Me Your Hand" identified COVID-19–related screening mammography barriers among the Black community which included poverty, insurance coverage, medical mistrust, and fear of diagnosis.[78]

Risk Models

There exists a variety of breast cancer risk models, with some that predict the likelihood of BRCA1/2 pathogenic variants, the eligibility of a patient for tamoxifen use, or the lifetime risk of breast cancer in the setting of negative BRCA1/2 testing. These models include the Breast Cancer Risk Assessment Tool, which is also known as the Gail model, the Claus model, the Tyrer-Cuzick model (also known as the International Breast Cancer Intervention Study or IBIS), the Breast Cancer Surveillance Consortium model, the Rosner-Colditz model, the BRCAPRO model, and the Breast and Ovarian Analysis of Disease Incidence and Carrier Estimation Algorithm (BOADICEA).

These calculators often guide recommendations for genetic testing as well as determine a patient's screening and chemoprevention options (such as tamoxifen or eligibility for supplemental screening with breast magnetic resonance imaging or MRI). Historically, these models have largely been developed utilizing data from European populations.[79] This calls into question their accuracy in predicting risk in patients of the African diaspora. One prospective clinical study demonstrated that Black patients were significantly less likely to have elevated Tyrer-Cuzick scores, which would otherwise qualify them for intensive breast surveillance with MRI.[80]

Certain models have been developed to address this gap. In 2007, Dr Mitchell Gail (creator of the Gail model) and colleagues at the NCI developed an assessment tool specifically for Black people to address the concerns about racial generalizability. This new model—utilizing data extrapolated from the Women's Contraceptive and Reproductive Experiences Study—demonstrated higher risk estimations and is recommended in assessing breast cancer risk among Black people.[81] Palmer and colleagues developed the Black Women's Health Study Breast Cancer Risk Calculator in 2021, which utilizes reproductive and family history to estimate 5-year and 10-year breast cancer risk among Black people ages 30 to 70.[82,83] Another model estimating risk of contralateral breast cancer (CBC) in Black populations (called CBCRisk-Black) focuses on 4 primary risk factors—breast density, family history of breast cancer, tumor size, and age at diagnosis.[84] Data on the accuracy of these models in practice are needed.

DIAGNOSIS

Although the incidence of breast cancer is slightly lower among Black people compared to White people (127.8 cases per 100,000 vs 133.7 cases per 100,000, respectively), breast cancer is still the most commonly diagnosed cancer among Black AFAB people, with 36,260 estimated cases in 2022.[3] Black people have an earlier median age at diagnosis compared to White people (60 and 64 years old, respectively)[85] and are more likely to be diagnosed with early-onset breast cancer before the age of 40 compared to other racial and ethnic groups.[86,87] Black people are also more likely to have the highest risk of no biopsy 90 days after an abnormal mammogram (adjusted risk ratio [RR] = 1.27, 95% CI: 1.12–1.44)[88] and more advanced stages at the time of diagnosis,[85] with a 40% to 70% higher risk of being diagnosed with stage IV breast cancer regardless of subtype compared to White people.[89]

People Assigned Male at Birth and Gender Diverse Populations

While this article primarily focuses on AFAB people, it is important to recognize the possibility of breast cancer in those assigned male at birth (AMAB), who may fall under the care of a gynecologist during their lifetime. While breast cancer among those AMAB is rare (<1%), these patients do have a higher frequency of later-stage diagnoses.[90–92] This may be due to lack of awareness of risk, lack of screening, and stigma. Survival rates are generally lower compared to those AFAB. Risk factors include family history of breast cancer, history of chest wall radiation, germline mutation, Klinefelter syndrome, atrial fibrillation, advanced age, diabetes mellitus, end-stage renal disease, elevated BMI, testicular disorders, and gynecomastia.[93–96]

Compared to other races, Black people AMAB have a higher incidence of breast cancer compared to other racial and ethnic groups,[97–99] along with an incidence ratio of 2.27 for TNBC (95% CI: 1.67–3.03).[99] Reasons for these findings are unclear and risk factors among the Black AMAB population require further investigation.

There is little data that clearly estimate the prevalence of breast cancer among transgender individuals in the United States. However, a 2015 study of transgender veterans in the United States showed a breast cancer incidence rate of 20.0/100,000 person-years (regardless of hormonal therapy use).[100] There are a variety of factors that could impact risk in this community, such as exogenous gender-affirming hormonal therapy and chest surgery. The long term impact of these therapies remains unclear.[101–104] There is a lack of data regarding incidence rates and outcomes of breast cancer among transgender individuals who identify as Black. Additional research in this area is warranted globally on breast cancer in gender-diverse groups, as well as racial differences within those groups.

HISTOLOGIC AND MOLECULAR SUBTYPES

Representing 1 in 6 new cancer diagnoses, ductal carcinoma in situ (DCIS or stage-0 breast cancer or preinvasive cancer) is characterized by cancer cells lining the breast ducts which do not actually invade through the ducts into neighboring tissue. While some data suggest that DCIS rates are largely similar between Black and White people,[105] some data demonstrate that Black people are more likely to be diagnosed with DCIS at older ages.[106,107] Notably, research shows that along with Asian people, Black people are more likely than other races to develop invasive breast cancers after DCIS.[108]

Regarding invasive breast cancer, staging, treatment options, and outcomes are directly correlated to breast tumor pathology as it relates to the presence of estrogen and progesterone receptors (collectively referred to as hormone receptor [HR]-positive), as well as the presence of human epidermal growth factor receptor 2 (HER2). The majority of breast cancer cases (68%) are categorized as HR-positive/HER2-negative, which are slower growing, less aggressive molecular subtypes that generally have a good response to therapy.[85,109] According to the American Cancer Society statistics, White people have a 71% prevalence of HR-positive/HER2-negative breast cancer (compared to Black people at 57%, Asian/Pacific Islander people at 66%, American Indian/Alaskan Native people at 66%, and Hispanic people at 63%). Black people have generally similar prevalence of HR-positive/HER2-positive and HR-negative/HER2-positive breast cancers compared to Whites (10% vs 9%, respectively, and 5% and 4%, respectively).[85]

Furthermore, histologic grade can also impact prognosis, with grade 3 having a worse prognosis than grade 1 breast tumors. While some studies do not show a race difference in regard to tumor grade,[110] other data suggest that Black patients are more likely to be diagnosed with high-grade breast cancer compared to White patients.[111,112]

Triple-Negative Breast Cancer

HR-negative/HER2-negative (also known as TNBC) has the poorest prognosis of all subtypes, more limited treatment options, more aggressive tumor characteristics, and higher likelihood of metastasis.[113,114] While this subtype is seen in 10% of the general population, it represents 20% of breast cancer cases among Black people.[115–117] Risk factors largely overlap with those that increase risk of HR-positive breast cancers, such as early menses, late menopause, and alcohol consumption. Of those with pathogenic variants, there is a particularly increased risk of TNBC with BRCA1 (compared to BRCA2) as well as PABL2 pathogenic variants.[117]

This trend is also seen among the African diaspora but displays some variation depending on region of origin. In regard to TNBC, one particular study demonstrated a prevalence rate ratio of 0.92 among West African–born Blacks compared to 0.87 and 0.53 among Caribbean-born and East African–born Blacks, respectively.[118] This phenotypic link may be reflective of the history of the transatlantic slave trade for which 12.5 million Blacks were forcibly displaced between the 16th and 19th centuries primarily from Western Africa.[119]

Inflammatory Breast Cancer

Inflammatory breast cancer (IBC) represents approximately 0.3% of all invasive breast cancer diagnoses.[85] It is a rare subtype that carries a poor prognosis, largely due to its high propensity to metastasize. Black race is a known risk factor for IBC,[120] with a statistically significantly higher prevalence in Black people of 3.1/100,000 woman-years compared to White people at 2.2/100,000 woman-years ($P < .001$).[121] Black race is also linked to higher mortality with IBC.[3,122] The reasons for this are not entirely clear. Some data suggest that patients with IBC may be more likely to have higher BMI[123] and greater number and severity of medical comorbidities, along with research showing a higher association with Black patients on Medicaid, living in poverty, or residing in urban areas.[124]

CARE AND TREATMENT

Breast cancer care and treatment may differ across patients based on various factors such as breast cancer subtype, tumor grade, HR status, surgical approach, patient age, lymph node involvement, tumor oncotype score, a known germline mutation, and patient preferences. Generally, there are 4 major pillars of breast cancer treatment: surgery, chemotherapy, radiation, and endocrine therapy. Based on the aforementioned variables, a patient may receive one, some, or all elements of treatment.

Unfortunately, Black people continue to experience barriers to care and treatment that impact their breast cancer outcomes. Numerous studies suggest greater treatment delays in Black patients. An analysis of Medicare beneficiaries demonstrated that Black people had significantly higher risk of delays between biopsy and initiation of treatment (HR = 1.42, P = .003), as well as between abnormal mammogram and initiation of treatment (HR = 1.26, P = .015).[125] Another study showed that Black people had higher frequency of treatment delays (>60 days after diagnosis) than White people (adjusted relative frequency difference = 5.5% [95% CI: 3.2%-7.8%]), a finding that was noted across all socioeconomic levels in Black patients.[126] Another retrospective study demonstrated that Black patients were more likely than Whites to experience delays in treatment when seeking a second opinion for breast cancer care, with Black patients averaging 56 days from diagnosis to surgery compared to 42 days for White patients (RR = 1.37, P < .01).[127] Another study showed delays of greater than 90 days from the time of diagnosis to surgery of Black breast cancer patients compared to their White counterparts (OR 1.93, 95% CI: 1.76–2.11, P < .001), regardless of residence in lower education versus higher income areas.[128]

Delays in surgery are multifactorial, for which barriers to care, provider bias, and systemic racism may explain such disparities.[129] The culmination of these factors may impact a patient's acceptance or refusal of care and treatment. One 2022 retrospective study examined the Surveillance, Epidemiology, and End Results Program (SEER) data of 113,987 patients with nonmetastatic breast cancer. Black race was found to be an independent risk factor for surgery refusal (with 562 of the total 799 patients who refused surgery being non-Hispanic Black). Refusal was noted to be more likely in those who were greater than 81 years old, unmarried, and uninsured or on Medicaid.[130]

Data regarding the uptake of chemotherapy and radiation specifically among Black people are limited. A systematic review and meta-analysis evaluating the impact of race on chemotherapy treatment among breast cancer patients demonstrated that Blacks were significantly more likely to have delays in initiation of chemotherapy of 90 days or more (OR = 1.41, 95% CI: 1.06–1.87, P < .00001).[131] While Blacks were significantly more likely to discontinue chemotherapy, this was no longer statistically significant in Black patients with more advanced-stage disease.

Postsurgical radiation therapy has been shown to decrease the risk of locoregional recurrence and lower breast cancer–related mortality.[132,133] Data on the uptake of radiation therapy among the Black community are generally limited. Contrary to data suggesting lower uptake of radiation among Black people,[134] Snead and colleagues demonstrated that Black breast cancer patients were more likely to receive radiation compared to their White counterparts. This prospective study also identified provider communication and trust as factors influencing uptake of radiation therapy.[135]

Endocrine therapy represents another important aspect of breast cancer care for those patients who have HR-positive breast cancer, with data suggesting that the long-term use of agents such as tamoxifen and aromatase inhibitors may reduce the risk of breast cancer recurrence and improve survival.[136–138] While this endocrine therapy has become a standard component of breast cancer care, research suggests that up to 31% of all breast cancer patients are nonadherent to therapy.[139] Specifically regarding Black patients, one study examined factors such as race, sociocultural factors, and process-of-care factors. The lowest initiation of endocrine therapy was among Black women aged≤50 years (59.7%) compared to Black women greater than 50 years (87.1%), white women≤50 years (73.7%), or white women greater than 50 years (72.0%). Issues such as financial access, medical comorbidities, and provider communication all played a role in uptake.[140] Numerous other studies have demonstrated low adherence of endocrine therapy among Black patients.[141–144] Much of this data suggest that medication side effects may be implicated.

Trastuzumab (also known as Herceptin) is a monoclonal antibody that binds and blocks HER2 and is a key component of treatment in those with HER2-positive breast cancer. With data demonstrating an overall improved survival of 37%,[145] trastuzumab has long since been adopted as standard therapy. However, there are still inconsistencies in care nationwide. A national cohort of Medicare recipients with HER2-positive breast cancer demonstrated that 50% of White people and 40% of Black people who were eligible for treatment received some trastuzumab therapy. However, among those with more advanced disease (stage III), 74% of White people and 56% of Black people received trastuzumab. Even when adjusting for factors such as poverty, medical comorbidities, and tumor specifications, Black people were 25% less likely to receive the treatment within 1 year of diagnosis compared to White people (RR = 0.745, 95% CI:0.60–0.93).[146]

Finally, some data suggest that Black people may be less likely to receive standard treatments for breast cancer. A retrospective study examining SEER data demonstrated that Black and Hispanic people were 30% to 40% more likely to undergo non–guideline-concordant treatment for invasive breast cancer across breast cancer subtypes.[89] However, another retrospective study utilizing data from the Georgia Cancer Registry found that Black people were just as likely to receive guideline-concordant care (GCC) compared to White patients (65% vs 63%, respectively) and that failure to receive GCC led to increased mortality. Despite these findings, racial disparities in breast cancer mortality were still observed even in the setting of GCC.[147]

OUTCOMES
Overall Survival

Breast cancer has a largely favorable prognosis of 90% over 5 years, as it is generally identified at stage I.[85] However, Black people have lower overall survival at each stage of diagnosis. SEER data from 2012 to 2018 demonstrate that Black people have an 83% 5-year relative survival rate compared to 92% among White people. From 2016 to 2020, breast cancer deaths were reported to be 27.6 per 100,000 for Black people versus 19.7 per 100,000 for White people. Currently, the American Cancer Society reports that Black people have a 40% increased breast cancer–related mortality compared to non-Hispanic White people.[3] These statistics are both alarming and unacceptable.

It is commonly believed that this breast cancer–related mortality among the Black community is in large part due to higher rates of aggressive histologic subtypes such as TNBC. Notably, population-based mortality rates were largely similar until the 1980s, where tamoxifen (a selective-estrogen receptor modulator) emerged as the first effective adjuvant endocrine treatment. Due to the higher rates of TNBC observed among Black populations, it was theorized that the mortality discrepancy was largely due to this community's ineligibility for tamoxifen.[148]

While this is an important discrepancy, it does not entirely explain the health disparities observed. A population-based, retrospective cohort examining both Black and White people with TNBC showed that even after adjusting for sociodemographic, clinicopathologic, and county-level factors, Blacks still had higher mortality (HR = 1.28, 95% CI: 1.18–1.38). This could be partially explained by Black people having lower odds of undergoing surgery or receiving chemotherapy compared to White patients in this cohort (OR 0.69, 95% CI:0.60–0.79 and OR 0.89, 95% CI:0.81–0.99, respectively).[149] Carbajal-Ochoa and colleagues evaluated SEER data by race for patients diagnosed with IBC between 2010 and 2016. This study demonstrated that although the odds of receiving chemotherapy and radiation were comparable between races, the outcomes were dramatically different. At 39-month follow-up, Black people had an overall survival of 40 months (compared to 81 months for non-Hispanic White people) and a higher death rate of 51% (compared to 35% for non-Hispanic White people), both of which were statistically significant ($P < .0001$).[150]

While some data suggest no improvement in survival of Black patients when given treatments such as cyclin-dependent kinase 4/6 inhibitors (CDK4/6i),[151] there is generally a dearth of data on racial differences in outcomes with treatments such as CDK4/6i and Poly(ADP-ribose) polymerase (PARP) inhibitors for metastatic breast cancer. Black communities are generally underrepresented in these clinical trials,[152–155] despite representing the group that carries the highest breast cancer–related mortality burden.

Recurrence and Second Primary Breast Cancer

Locoregional recurrence of breast cancer is associated with increased mortality.[132,156,157] Some data suggest that there are racial disparities to this occurrence. A retrospective analysis evaluating HR-positive/HER2-negative, node-negative breast cancer patients enrolled in the Trial Assigning Individualized Options for Treatment (TAILORx) demonstrated that following Asian patients, Black patients showed the next highest odds of having locoregional recurrence of breast cancer (HR = 1.78, 95% CI: 1.15–2.77) even after adjusting for patient, tumor, and treatment factors. Furthermore, this locoregional recurrence did show an association with breast cancer mortality (HR = 5.71, 95% CI: 3.50–9.31).[158] Terman and colleagues demonstrated that early-onset Black breast cancer patients had the highest risk of recurrence (22% higher risk than White patients, $P = .434$) after neoadjuvant chemotherapy (NAC), with subsequently worse survival outcomes.[159]

The most commonly used prognostic genomic indicator estimating the risk of recurrence and informing possible benefit from chemotherapy is the 21-gene recurrence score of the Oncotype DX Breast Recurrence Score Test.[160] This algorithm for determining recurrence scores was extrapolated using data from the National Surgical Adjuvant Breast and Bowel Project B-20 trial, for which only 6% of participants from the original study and 5% from the subset validated study were Black.[161–163] Given the lack of racial diversity in these trials, there is concern about prognostic accuracy among Black patients with breast cancer.[164]

Black people are also more likely to be diagnosed with a CBC compared to other racial groups. One retrospective study demonstrated that the risk of CBC was increased among Black patients (HR 1.44, 95% CI: 1.35–1.54) compared to non-Hispanic White patients.[165] According to researchers, these data were not explained by clinical or socioeconomic factors, and the disparity was most profound in younger breast cancer survivors. Another SEER-based analysis demonstrated that people with unilateral breast cancer have an approximately 0.4% annual risk of CBC over a period of 25 years. This risk was higher for Black people (12.7%) than for White people (9.7%) in the cohort.[166]

Treatment-Related Complications

Some data suggest that Black patients experience significant side effects from treatment which lead to distress and can impact adherence.[167] For instance, one of the painful treatment side effects—chemotherapy-induced neuropathy—is more prevalent among Black patients compared to White patients.[168,169] Breast cancer patients are also at higher risk of cardiovascular (CV) toxicity from treatments including trastuzumab and chemotherapy. Some studies suggest a 2-fold higher risk of CV toxicity among Black people compared to White people as a result of these treatments.[170,171] In addition, Black patients may enter breast cancer treatments with preexisting CV risk factors.[172] Furthermore, lymphedema impacts 1 in 5 breast cancer survivors, representing one of the most bothersome and oftentimes debilitating side effects of breast cancer treatment.[173] The risk of lymphedema in Black patients is found to be 1.5-fold to 3.5-fold higher than that in White patients[174] and is more likely to have a severe presentation.[175] These are important findings that can impact functional status and quality of life.

Psychosocial Impact

Survivorship may involve a host of issues including mental health challenges that may impact identity, self-worth, and self-determination—particularly among Black breast cancer survivors.[176] Black populations remain underrepresented in research evaluating the short-term and long-term psychological impact of breast cancer. Some research demonstrates that Black breast cancer survivors have worse psychological functioning compared to White patients[177]; however, one particular cross-sectional study showed overall low anxiety and depression posttreatment (although a subset reported clinically significant psychological symptoms).[178] Additionally, Black patients in this study who had better provider communication and greater self-efficacy were observed to experience overall less anxiety and depression.

Perceptions of body image may also be affected. Due to the higher incidence of aggressive cancer subtypes, Black patients are more likely to require neoadjuvant chemotherapy (NAC)[120,179–181] which puts them at higher risk of diffuse, permanent alopecia.[182] Hair carries incredible sociocultural meaning among Black communities and more research should be performed regarding treatment options.[183] Black patients are also historically less likely to undergo breast reconstruction after mastectomy[184–186] due to factors such as health literacy, lack of physician referral, comorbidities, spiritual and cultural beliefs, and insurance.[187–189] These are just some factors that can impact mental health and self-esteem, for which longer term impacts on care and outcomes necessitate further research.

Reproductive Considerations

There is a paucity of data regarding birthing outcomes and family planning decision-making among Black patients of reproductive age impacted by invasive breast cancer. The small volume of data that exist on Black people and the use of assisted reproductive technology (ART) demonstrate that they are less likely to utilize these services overall.[190,191] ART becomes particularly relevant for Black patients, as they are more likely to experience early-onset breast cancer during childbearing years and are more likely to require NAC (some of which can be gonadotoxic).[192] Reproductive endocrinology and infertility services are a key component to care in early-onset breast cancer patients. This represents a disparity for which there must be increased referrals but also greater subsidies to cover costs, as this may be a significant barrier for patients.

GENETIC COUNSELING AND TESTING

In light of the disparate statistics regarding breast cancer mortality among the Black community, prevention could play a key role. Genetic counseling and testing (GCT) represents the cutting edge of precision medicine and offers promise in the areas of early detection, cancer prevention, and risk reduction. The National Comprehensive Cancer Network (NCCN) has set forth specific criteria for genetic testing for breast cancer risk assessment,[5] although the American Society of Breast Surgeons has recommended universal testing for all breast cancer patients.[193]

Unfortunately, research demonstrates that GCT is largely underutilized in Black communities.[154,194,195] This gap is multifactorial and likely represents a combination of patient, clinician, and system-level factors. One study in Michigan evaluating utilization of preventive services among early onset breast cancer survivors demonstrated that only 26% of Blacks reported receiving genetic counseling and only 17% underwent genetic testing (compared to 37% and 33% of White and other races, respectively). This study noted that one of the barriers Black patients encountered was that some were not offered GCT services by their health care providers even when they met criteria for genetic testing.[196] Another study reflected this same phenomena, demonstrating lower physician referral rates to genetic counseling to Black breast cancer survivors (75.7%) compared to White survivors (92.7%), but interestingly with no significant difference in subsequent uptake of genetic counseling by race (non-Hispanic Black = 95.4% vs non-Hispanic White = 97.6%, P = .25).[197] Another study similarly demonstrated that Black breast cancer survivors were less likely to receive a recommendation from their doctor to undergo BRCA1/2 testing.[195]

In addition, medical mistrust stemming from a history of racialized medical mistreatment and systemic racism throughout the health care system remains a challenge. Research demonstrates that Blacks may have hesitancy and medical mistrust regarding GCT.[198–200] There is also the issue of lack of information regarding GCT, with one qualitative study showing an information gap among Blacks relating to the GCT process and related costs. Fear of having a germline mutation and concerns about genetic discrimination were also barriers.[201]

In regard to germline mutations, the prevalence of BRCA1/2 in the general population is estimated to be 1 in 400 individuals (0.2%–0.3%), with a higher prevalence among those of Ashkenazi Jewish ancestry (2.0%–2.5%).[202] Some research suggests that there are largely similar rates of BRCA1/2 pathogenic variants among Black people compared to White people,[203] along with other breast cancer–associated pathogenic variants.[204] However, a BRCA1 pathogenic variant called c.815_824dup has been identified in Black communities in the Bahamas, South Carolina, Florida, and Washington, DC, suggesting that it may represent a founder mutation of West African origin.[205,206] Additionally, one particular population-based study from Florida demonstrated a BRCA prevalence that was double that of the non-Hispanic White population,[207] similar to another study that showed a higher prevalence among Black people.[208]

Aside from genetic testing itself, the interpretation of genetic testing results among Black people may pose certain challenges. Data overwhelmingly demonstrate that Blacks are more likely than Whites to have variants of unknown or uncertain significance (VUSs),[209–212] which are equivocal nonactionable results. Among recent studies, a multicenter study showed that one-third of patients in a cohort of 488 Blacks with invasive breast cancer had variants that could not be classified.[213] A population-based retrospective cohort using SEER data from breast cancer patients demonstrated 44.5% VUS among Blacks versus 23.7% VUS among Whites.[214] Finally, a study examining racial and ethnic differences with multigene panel testing demonstrated again that Blacks were again less likely to have pathogenic variants but more likely to have VUSs (OR = 1.53, 95% CI: 1.18–1.98, P = .001).[215]

These findings are not entirely but largely rooted in underlying bias in genome-wide association studies (GWAS), from which these genomic classifications are primarily extrapolated. An analysis by Popejoy and Fullerton demonstrated that in 2016, approximately 81% of the makeup of GWAS consisted of individuals of European descent (only a moderate decrease from 2009 data that demonstrated 96% of groups in GWAS were of European ancestry).[216] Another study demonstrated that 71.8% of GWAS participants have been recruited from either the United States, Europe, or Iceland.[217] This lack of diversity raises concern about the racial and ethnic translatability of genomic research.[218] While some data suggest that most VUSs reclassify to benign,[219,220] it is unclear if this is generalizable to the Black community as their genetics continue to be grossly ignored in the global genomics landscape.

Racial Health Duplicity

In contrast to these glaring omissions of Black communities in both genomic research and breast cancer clinical trials, America unfortunately has a tortured history regarding the harmful involvement of Black people in medical science. The Tuskegee Syphilis Study represents only one example, where the goal was to observe the natural progression of syphilis in Black people, even after treatment became widely available.[221,222] Henrietta Lacks, a Black woman from Virginia, underwent the removal of her immortal cells (HeLa cells) while undergoing treatment for cervical cancer in the 1950s at Johns Hopkins University. Collected and distributed without her awareness or consent, her cells have been the basis for over 110,000 scientific publications and have revolutionized the field of medicine from the polio vaccine to human immunodeficiency virus drug therapy to space research.[223] J. Marion Sims, often referred to as the "Father of Modern Gynecology," perfected the repair of the vesicovaginal fistula through repeated public surgeries on 3 Black enslaved people. Lucy, Betsy, and Anarca each underwent numerous unanesthetized surgeries until successful repair was achieved using silver sutures, for which Sims then proceeded to perform the surgery on White people utilizing anesthesia.[224] The Virginia and North Carolina Sterilization programs represented a larger eugenics movement in the United States in which individuals who were deemed 'unfit' to procreate were forcibly sterilized, a significant portion of whom were Black and some of whom are still alive today.[225] The commonality of these events involve the inclusion of Black people in studies, interventions, and research for which they did not achieve any direct medical benefit or, even worse, they were explicitly and seriously harmed.

Medical history has trended in one of two ways—either the harmful *inclusion* or the detrimental *exclusion* of Blacks in medical discovery. This concept is best described as racial health duplicity: the intentional inclusion of Black people with the goal of advancing science primarily for the benefit or curiosity of non-Black people, with the simultaneous (intentional or unconscious) exclusion of Blacks in medical research that may indirectly contribute to poor health outcomes (**Fig. 2**). It represents the problematic duality of scientific research and medical care in America toward Black people. While Tuskegee represents the active mistreatment of Blacks and genomic science has simply excluded those of the African diaspora in GWAS, both situations cause harm and conflict with the pillars of medical ethics. Breast cancer genetics is a direct product of racial health duplicity, for which the noninclusion of Black communities in GWAS impacts the interpretability of genetic variants which then has

> ### Racial Health Duplicity:
>
> The intentional **inclusion** of Black people with the goal of advancing science primarily for the benefit or curiosity of non-Black people, with the simultaneous (intentional or unconscious) **exclusion** of Black people in medical research that may indirectly contribute to poor health outcomes.

Fig. 2. Racial health duplicity definition.

downstream health implications on Black communities. Rather than precision medicine, there is only medical inertia.

THE WAY FORWARD: STEPS TOWARD IMPROVING BREAST CANCER-RELATED RACIAL DISPARITIES

Breast cancer–related racial disparities represent an urgent public health issue. As discussed throughout this article, breast cancer is complex and involves many contributing risk factors. Similarly, care and treatment is also layered. The complex nature of these racial health disparities requires an equally intricate, multifaceted, and multidisciplinary approach (**Fig. 3**).

Enhancing Breast Cancer Education and Awareness

One of the first and most important steps in reducing disparities is education. The use of peer education has proven to be a key tool in this effort. One particular study examined the efficacy of peer education in increasing breast cancer knowledge among

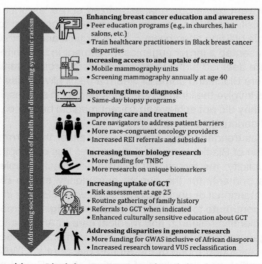

Fig. 3. Strategies to address Black breast cancer–related disparities. GCT, genetic counseling and testing; GWAS, genome-wide association study; REI, reproductive endocrinology and infertility; TNBC, triple-negative breast cancer; VUS, variant of uncertain significance.

Black communities, titled Community Empowerment Partners. Twelve peer educators were trained, who then trained 121 community members (94 of whom were Black). Results demonstrated that both peer educators and community members had comparable levels of understanding of breast cancer etiology and screening. Additionally, the majority of community members expressed intentions to share the information they learned with family and friends.[226] Another peer education initiative utilized Breast Care Champions (BCC) to implement breast cancer awareness and screening events, as well as direct outreach in the form of check-in calls to community members. Haynes and colleagues demonstrated that after the implementation of over 245 outreach events, more Black people underwent screening in the BCC-covered area over a period of 15 months compared to prior historical values.[227]

The effectiveness of peer-to-peer communication highlights the fact that for some communities, health information may not always be obtained within a doctor's office. There is a need for increased involvement of community-based and faith-based organizations for which Black communities may have a greater sense of safety and trust, and may consist of members who reflect their racial and cultural backgrounds. Innumerous Black churches across the country are engaged in breast cancer education efforts among their congregations. Brown and colleagues evaluated culturally appropriate messaging from pastoral leadership through the Breast Cancer Awareness and Education Program, with participants demonstrating an increased knowledge of breast cancer, heightened awareness of the disproportionate mortality impacting Black people, clinical signs and symptoms, and available screening resources.[228] The Susan G. Komen Organization launched "Worship in Pink," a volunteer-based initiative that trains ambassadors to spark conversations about breast cancer and supply breast cancer education resources to their respective congregations.[229] Furthermore, hair stylists often represent pillars of trust in the Black community. Some studies have created partnerships with Black stylists as peer educators to increase awareness of breast cancer. One randomized control trial utilized hair stylists as breast cancer peer educators, with clients showing greater breast self-examination rates and increased plans to have a clinical breast examination (OR = 1.6, 95% CI: 1.2–2.1, and OR = 1.9, 95% CI: 1.1–3.3, respectively).[230]

Standardizing Screening Mammography

In light of historically conflicting recommendations by various professional societies, many societies are recognizing the increasing incidence of breast cancer among younger people as well as the increased mortality and higher likelihood of early-onset breast cancer among Black communities. While shared decision-making with patients and competing mortality are important, there is a need for more standardized and universal language across medical societies regarding age at initiation and frequency of screening mammography. While data are still evolving, there is consensus among some professional societies for which annual screening at age 40 is recommended.[63,231] This recommendation is particularly relevant for Black individuals given the disparate outcomes.[231] There needs to be enhanced nationwide efforts to increase knowledge both among the general population and the medical community regarding the importance of timely screening and its possible role in addressing the disproportionate impact of breast cancer on Black people.

Increasing Access to Screening

In 1990, Congress passed the Breast and Cervical Cancer Mortality Prevention Act which prompted the formation of the National Breast and Cervical Cancer Early Detection Program (NBCCEDP). In 2021, the NBCCEDP provided over 263,651 people with breast cancer screening and diagnostic services, for which there were subsequently 2221 invasive breast cancers diagnosed.[232] This nationwide initiative has been critical in reaching low-income, underinsured and uninsured populations.

However, insurance coverage is not the only barrier. Access to facilities that have a radiology suite can present a challenge for certain communities, particularly those of lower income or racially underserved populations. Mobile mammography represents another tool to increase access to screening mammography. First established in the 1960s, mobile mammography has demonstrated decreased mortality over an 18-year follow-up.[233] One retrospective study demonstrated that more Black people were screened at a mobile unit (cancer center = 49.30% vs mobile unit = 54.15%) compared to White people screened in a cancer facility (cancer center = 47.28% vs mobile unit = 33.30%) ($P < .001$).[234] The data also demonstrated greater racial diversity in those that visited the mobile unit. Mobile units are widespread across the United States particularly following the COVID-19 pandemic and should be employed more frequently to provide convenient access to racial minority groups such as Black communities.[235]

Shortening Time to Diagnosis

As previously mentioned, Black patients experience greater delays in care. One possible solution to this challenge is same-day biopsy programs. One particular study by Dontchos and colleagues demonstrated that same-day biopsy decreased time from imaging to biopsy from 9.6 to 3.6 days, and that there was no evidence of racial disparities after implementation of the program.[236] However, other studies show conflicting data. A retrospective study showed that while wait times decreased overall with same-day biopsy, there was a significant reduction for White people ($P < .001$) but not for Black people ($P = .527$) in regard to time from diagnostic mammogram to biopsy.[237] While it appears as if same-day biopsy programs could offer shortened times in identifying patients with breast cancer, more research could illuminate how this service could be maximized to create significant change in the Black community.

Addressing Social Determinants of Health

The repercussions of a longstanding history of racial oppression in the United States rooted in slavery and Jim Crow have had a profound impact on all aspects of society, including health care. The permeating impact of systemic racism must be addressed and dismantled in order to fully and comprehensively eliminate breast cancer–related racial disparities. "Weathering," characterized by the culmination of societal insults that is rooted in systemic racism, may translate to physiologic changes in areas like cell signaling, inflammation, and other metabolic pathways, leading to illness and disability.[238,239] Furthermore, allostatic load refers to a chronically activated stress response due to weathering.[240] Early life stressors (such as abuse, neglect, and childhood adversity) as well as stressors in adulthood (such as unemployment, living in areas of high poverty and crime, less purchasing power, and less income at a given educational level) can all play a role in breast cancer–related racial health disparities.[241] Dismantling these systemic structures is a gargantuan task but one that is equally necessary and urgent. While there are innumerable levels at which social determinants of health influence breast cancer outcomes, certain areas can be prioritized.

While SES is linked in part to poorer breast cancer outcomes,[87,242,243] studies still show that Black Americans have higher allostatic loads than White Americans (even after adjusting for poverty).[244] Higher allostatic loads are also linked to the development of larger, higher grade breast cancers and lower quality of life.[245–247] Some studies exploring ways to alleviate allostatic load—such as case managers and nurse navigators to address logistic barriers like transportation and housing, and access to services such as cancer screening and exercise programs—have been successful in creating a positive impact on breast cancer risk.[248–250] Health care systems should work to systematically and proactively identify social determinants of health when patients initially present to care in order to preemptively address barriers that may impact outcomes.

Creating environments where Black patients feel welcome and have increased trust in their care team is critical. On a macro level, data suggest that the larger environment of living in disadvantaged neighborhoods may portend worse breast cancer survival.[251] This concept is reinforced by data demonstrating that redlining impacts breast cancer outcomes on both a physical and molecular level.[252–254] On a micro level, Black breast cancer patients may have overall poor communication with their health care providers.[255] Medication adherence for Black patients, for instance, may be linked to not feeling cared for or having good communication with their medical team.[256] Factors which could explain this include not only racial bias in the health care system but also medical mistrust rooted in a longstanding history of mistreatment.[257–259] Antiracism trainings have become more widespread throughout the nation. It is important that health care providers are educated and trained in delivering culturally sensitive care and creating safe, equitable spaces for Black patients. Furthermore, another intervention which could improve patient-physician communication and potentially outcomes includes increasing the volume of racially and ethnically congruent health care providers[260–263]; this is an approach that should also be considered to address breast cancer disparities.

Increasing Tumor Biology Research

Research surrounding TNBC is particularly important, especially regarding how it may be molecularly distinct in Black individuals. One study evaluated 8 biomarkers in Blacks with breast cancer, noting that 90% of TNBC tested positive for cyclin A2 and Ki-67 and that these markers carried a poorer breast cancer prognosis.[264] Various other proteins have been overexpressed among Black communities and may play a role in tumorogenesis.[112,265,266] A better understanding of the molecular distinctions in tumor biology—coupled with appropriate treatments—could have long-term implications for Black breast cancer patients.

Increasing Risk Assessment and Referrals to Genetic Counseling and Testing

General obstetrics and gynecology practitioners—as well as family medicine and internal medicine physicians—play a critical role in identifying patients who may be at increased risk for breast cancer. The American College of Radiology recently released new breast cancer screening guidelines to address high-risk populations. This includes recommendations that all AFAB people, especially Black people, undergo risk assessment by age 25 to determine if earlier breast cancer screening is indicated.[231] This recommendation represents a crucial step toward addressing breast cancer disparities impacting Black communities.

One critical approach involves the routine gathering of a family cancer history for all patients presenting to primary care and subsequently providing referrals to genetic counselors to those who meet NCCN criteria (such as those with family histories significant for multiple breast cancers, early onset breast cancer, TNBC, male breast cancer, ovarian cancer, and pancreatic cancer).[5] While there are some online tools for health care workers as they relate to breast cancer and family cancer history (such as continuing medical education courses), the data overwhelmingly suggest that genetics is a rapidly evolving field for which physicians are not adequately trained.[267] Along with greater awareness of training tools (such as those made available by the

Centers for Disease Control and Prevention[268]), there is a need for increased training efforts among health care providers at all levels in regard to breast cancer disparities, the importance of routinely collecting family cancer history, and periodic review of the evolving national genetic testing guidelines.

In regard to genetic testing criteria, future considerations should include offering universal genetic testing to Black communities (as is the case of those of Ashkenazi Jewish ancestry) given the higher risk TNBC (which is currently an NCCN testing criterion itself), higher likelihood of early-onset breast cancer, and higher breast cancer–related mortality. Furthermore, with some data suggesting that Black patients may present with a germline mutation in the absence of a family cancer history,[207] these patients could theoretically be missed based on current genetic testing criteria.

Addressing Disparities in Genetics Research

The work that is currently being done to address genomic disparities is hopeful. Initiatives such as the 1000 Genomes Project, the African Genome Variation Project, the Human Heredity and Health in Africa (H3Africa) Initiative, and efforts by the National Human Genome Research Institute (NHGRI) all aim to increase ethnic representation in genomic research.[269–271] In 2016, the NCI spearheaded the largest study of breast cancer genetics in Black people to date, with the goal of assessing genetic variations in breast cancer to address racial disparities.[272]

Despite these accomplishments, there remains much work to be done. In light of the mandate from the National Institutes of Health calling for the inclusion of more diverse populations in genomic research,[273] these efforts must prioritize the inclusion of Black communities in GWAS by defining clear language in funding mechanisms that includes communities of the African diaspora. This effort must be coupled with candidly acknowledging the dark history of medical mistreatment, drawing near to Black communities to reestablish trust, appreciating the legacy of generational trauma, and actively listening and responding to concerns raised by its members. It is also imperative to address issues of hesitancy of genetic testing among Black people through education and tailored community outreach initiatives that stress the importance of their participation to increase prediction accuracy and potentially identify private variants. Ultimately, all efforts need to be characterized by a thoughtful inclusion of Blacks in research that directly improves medical outcomes in this very same community.

SUMMARY

Breast cancer represents a major cancer burden in the United States but remains a largely treatable cancer due to early detection and robust treatment options. Black people, however, have a higher likelihood of dying from breast cancer compared to all other racial groups. This racial mortality gap is unacceptable and represents a national emergency in our country. Clinical care as well as research efforts must be intentional and persistent in addressing these racial disparities affecting Black communities through an equitable, multidisciplinary, compassionate, and holistic approach.

CLINICS CARE POINTS

- Black people have a similar incidence rate of breast cancer compared to White people but a 40% increased risk of dying from breast cancer.
- Breast cancer–related mortality among Black communities is likely multifactorial, with higher rates of more aggressive breast cancer subtypes such as triple-negative breast cancer.

- Black breast cancer patients are more likely to experience delays in care and barriers to treatment.
- Black communities have lower uptake of genetic testing and higher rates of equivocal genetic testing results.
- There is a need for greater inclusion of the African diaspora in oncologic and genomic research to address racial and ethnic health disparities.
- Health care practitioners should be aware of how breast cancer disproportionately impacts the Black community.

ACKNOWLEDGMENTS

The author would like to acknowledge Dr Mark Pearlman for his assistance and expertise.

DISCLOSURE

The author has no disclosures. Dr V. Pleasant is the recipient of a MICHR K12 research grant through the University of Michigan (UM1TR004404; K12TR004374; and T32TR004371).

REFERENCES

1. Cancer facts & figures 2023. American Cancer Society. Available at: https://www.cancer.org/content/dam/cancer-org/research/cancer-facts-and-statistics/annual-cancer-facts-and-figures/2023/2023-cancer-facts-and-figures.pdf. Accessed January 23, 2023.
2. Survival Rates for Breast Cancer. American cancer society. Available at: https://www.cancer.org/cancer/breast-cancer/understanding-a-breast-cancer-diagnosis/breast-cancer-survival-rates.html. Accessed January 29, 2023.
3. Cancer facts & figures for African Americans 2022-2024. American Cancer Society. Available at: https://www.cancer.org/content/dam/cancer-org/research/cancer-facts-and-statistics/cancer-facts-and-figures-for-african-americans/2022-2024-cff-aa.pdf. Accessed July 16, 2023.
4. Bray F, Ferlay J, Soerjomataram I, et al. Global cancer statistics 2018: GLOBOCAN estimates of incidence and mortality worldwide for 36 cancers in 185 countries. CA Cancer J Clin 2018;68(6):394–424.
5. Genetic/Familial High-Risk Assessment: Breast, Ovarian, and Pancreatic, Version 2.2024. National Comprehensive Cancer Network (NCCN). Published September 27, 2023. Available at: https://www.nccn.org/professionals/physician_gls/pdf/genetics_bop.pdf. Accessed October 15, 2023.
6. Pleasant V. Management of breast complaints and high-risk lesions. Best Pract Res Clin Obstet Gynaecol 2022;83:46–59.
7. Bhatia S, Yasui Y, Robison LL, et al. High risk of subsequent neoplasms continues with extended follow-up of childhood Hodgkin's disease: report from the Late Effects Study Group. J Clin Oncol 2003;21(23):4386–94.
8. Collaborative Group on Hormonal Factors in Breast Cancer. Menarche, menopause, and breast cancer risk: individual participant meta-analysis, including 118 964 women with breast cancer from 117 epidemiological studies. Lancet Oncol 2012;13(11):1141–51.

9. McCormack VA, dos Santos Silva I. Breast density and parenchymal patterns as markers of breast cancer risk: a meta-analysis. Cancer Epidemiol Biomarkers Prev 2006;15(6):1159–69.

10. Morrow M, Schnitt SJ, Norton L. Current management of lesions associated with an increased risk of breast cancer. Nat Rev Clin Oncol 2015;12(4):227–38.

11. Pharoah PD, Day NE, Duffy S, et al. Family history and the risk of breast cancer: a systematic review and meta-analysis. Int J Cancer 1997;71(5):800–9.

12. Trichopoulos D, MacMahon B, Cole P. Menopause and breast cancer risk. J Natl Cancer Inst 1972;48(3):605–13.

13. White E. Projected changes in breast cancer incidence due to the trend toward delayed childbearing. Am J Public Health 1987;77(4):495–7.

14. McDonald JA, Goyal A, Terry MB. Alcohol Intake and Breast Cancer Risk: Weighing the Overall Evidence. Curr Breast Cancer Rep 2013;5(3). https://doi.org/10.1007/s12609-013-0114-z.

15. Lee K, Kruper L, Dieli-Conwright CM, et al. The Impact of Obesity on Breast Cancer Diagnosis and Treatment. Curr Oncol Rep 2019;21(5):41.

16. Abe R, Kumagai N, Kimura M, et al. Biological characteristics of breast cancer in obesity. Tohoku J Exp Med 1976;120(4):351–9.

17. Protani M, Coory M, Martin JH. Effect of obesity on survival of women with breast cancer: systematic review and meta-analysis. Breast Cancer Res Treat 2010; 123(3):627–35.

18. Cui Y, Whiteman MK, Langenberg P, et al. Can obesity explain the racial difference in stage of breast cancer at diagnosis between black and white women? J Womens Health Gend Based Med 2002;11(6):527–36.

19. Jones BA, Kasi SV, Curnen MG, et al. Severe obesity as an explanatory factor for the black/white difference in stage at diagnosis of breast cancer. Am J Epidemiol 1997;146(5):394–404.

20. Friebel-Klingner TM, Ehsan S, Conant EF, et al. Risk factors for breast cancer subtypes among Black women undergoing screening mammography. Breast Cancer Res Treat 2021;189(3):827–35.

21. Hunter CP, Redmond CK, Chen VW, et al. Breast cancer: factors associated with stage at diagnosis in black and white women. Black/White Cancer Survival Study Group. J Natl Cancer Inst 1993;85(14):1129–37.

22. Moore J, Pal T, Beeghly-Fadiel A, et al. A pooled case-only analysis of obesity and breast cancer subtype among Black women in the southeastern United States. Cancer Causes Control 2022;33(4):515–24.

23. Lu Y, Ma H, Malone KE, et al. Obesity and survival among black women and white women 35 to 64 years of age at diagnosis with invasive breast cancer. J Clin Oncol 2011;29(25):3358–65.

24. Boyd NF, Guo H, Martin LJ, et al. Mammographic density and the risk and detection of breast cancer. N Engl J Med 2007;356(3):227–36.

25. Bodewes FTH, van Asselt AA, Dorrius MD, et al. Mammographic breast density and the risk of breast cancer: A systematic review and meta-analysis. Breast 2022;66:62–8.

26. Moore JX, Han Y, Appleton C, et al. Determinants of Mammographic Breast Density by Race Among a Large Screening Population. JNCI Cancer Spectr 2020;4(2):kaa010.

27. McCarthy AM, Keller BM, Pantalone LM, et al. Racial Differences in Quantitative Measures of Area and Volumetric Breast Density. J Natl Cancer Inst 2016; 108(10). https://doi.org/10.1093/jnci/djw104.

28. Pettersson A, Graff RE, Ursin G, et al. Mammographic density phenotypes and risk of breast cancer: a meta-analysis. J Natl Cancer Inst 2014;106(5). https://doi.org/10.1093/jnci/dju078.
29. Challenges Breastfeeding, ACOG Committee Opinion. Number 820. Obstet Gynecol 2021;137(2):e42–53.
30. Meek JY, Noble L, Breastfeeding. S on. Policy Statement: Breastfeeding and the Use of Human Milk. Pediatrics 2022;150(1).
31. Chiang KV, Li R, Anstey EH, et al. Racial and Ethnic Disparities in Breastfeeding Initiation – United States, 2019. MMWR Morb Mortal Wkly Rep 2021;70(21):769–74.
32. Snyder K, Hulse E, Dingman H, et al. Examining supports and barriers to breastfeeding through a socio-ecological lens: a qualitative study. Int Breastfeed J 2021;16(1):52.
33. Quintero SM, Strassle PD, Londoño Tobón A, et al. Race/ethnicity-specific associations between breastfeeding information source and breastfeeding rates among U.S. women. BMC Publ Health 2023;23(1):520.
34. Sayres S, Visentin L. Breastfeeding: uncovering barriers and offering solutions. Curr Opin Pediatr 2018;30(4):591–6.
35. Wallenborn JT, Ihongbe T, Rozario S, et al. Knowledge of Breastfeeding Recommendations and Breastfeeding Duration: A Survival Analysis on Infant Feeding Practices II. Breastfeed Med 2017;12:156–62.
36. Marshall NA, Cook CS. Trust Black Women: Using Photovoice to Amplify the Voices of Black Women to Identify and Address Barriers to Breastfeeding in Southeast Georgia. Health Promot Pract 2023;24(1_suppl):128S–39S.
37. Mieso BR, Burrow H, Lam SK. Beyond Statistics: Uncovering the Roots of Racial Disparities in Breastfeeding. Pediatrics 2021;147(5). https://doi.org/10.1542/peds.2020-037887.
38. Green VL, Killings NL, Clare CA. The Historical, Psychosocial, and Cultural Context of Breastfeeding in the African American Community. Breastfeed Med 2021;16(2):116–20.
39. Terry MB, Zhang FF, Kabat G, et al. Lifetime alcohol intake and breast cancer risk. Ann Epidemiol 2006;16(3):230–40.
40. Chen WY, Rosner B, Hankinson SE, et al. Moderate alcohol consumption during adult life, drinking patterns, and breast cancer risk. JAMA 2011;306(17):1884–90.
41. Smith-Warner SA, Spiegelman D, Yaun SS, et al. Alcohol and breast cancer in women: a pooled analysis of cohort studies. JAMA 1998;279(7):535–40.
42. Hamajima N, Hirose K, Tajima K, et al. Alcohol, tobacco and breast cancer–collaborative reanalysis of individual data from 53 epidemiological studies, including 58,515 women with breast cancer and 95,067 women without the disease. Br J Cancer 2002;87(11):1234–45.
43. Ma H, Malone KE, McDonald JA, et al. Pre-diagnosis alcohol consumption and mortality risk among black women and white women with invasive breast cancer. BMC Cancer 2019;19(1):800.
44. Young KL, Olshan AF, Lunetta K, et al. Influence of alcohol consumption and alcohol metabolism variants on breast cancer risk among Black women: results from the AMBER consortium. Breast Cancer Res 2023;25(1):66.
45. Chang CJ, O'Brien KM, Keil AP, et al. Use of Straighteners and Other Hair Products and Incident Uterine Cancer. J Natl Cancer Inst 2022;114(12):1636–45.
46. Crews D, McLachlan JA. Epigenetics, evolution, endocrine disruption, health, and disease. Endocrinology 2006;147(6 Suppl):S4–10.

47. Leung YK, Biesiada J, Govindarajah V, et al. Low-Dose Bisphenol A in a Rat Model of Endometrial Cancer: A CLARITY-BPA Study. Environ Health Perspect 2020;128(12):127005.

48. Mallozzi M, Leone C, Manurita F, et al. Endocrine Disrupting Chemicals and Endometrial Cancer: An Overview of Recent Laboratory Evidence and Epidemiological Studies. Int J Environ Res Publ Health 2017;14(3). https://doi.org/10.3390/ijerph14030334.

49. Weathersby C, McMichael A. Brazilian keratin hair treatment: a review. J Cosmet Dermatol 2013;12(2):144–8.

50. Aglan MA, Mansour GN. Hair straightening products and the risk of occupational formaldehyde exposure in hairstylists. Drug Chem Toxicol 2020;43(5):488–95.

51. Flyvholm MA, Andersen P. Identification of formaldehyde releasers and occurrence of formaldehyde and formaldehyde releasers in registered chemical products. Am J Ind Med 1993;24(5):533–52.

52. Malinauskiene L, Blaziene A, Chomiciene A, et al. Formaldehyde may be found in cosmetic products even when unlabelled. Open Med 2015;10(1):323–8.

53. Rojanapo W, Kupradinun P, Tepsuwan A, et al. Carcinogenicity of an oxidation product of p-phenylenediamine. Carcinogenesis 1986;7(12):1997–2002.

54. Turesky RJ, Freeman JP, Holland RD, et al. Identification of aminobiphenyl derivatives in commercial hair dyes. Chem Res Toxicol 2003;16(9):1162–73.

55. Stiel L, Adkins-Jackson PB, Clark P, et al. A review of hair product use on breast cancer risk in African American women. Cancer Med 2016;5(3):597–604.

56. Eberle CE, Sandler DP, Taylor KW, et al. Hair dye and chemical straightener use and breast cancer risk in a large US population of black and white women. Int J Cancer 2020;147(2):383–91.

57. Coogan PF, Rosenberg L, Palmer JR, et al. Hair product use and breast cancer incidence in the Black Women's Health Study. Carcinogenesis 2021;42(7):924–30.

58. White AJ, Gregoire AM, Taylor KW, et al. Adolescent use of hair dyes, straighteners and perms in relation to breast cancer risk. Int J Cancer 2021;148(9):2255–63.

59. Hendrick RE, Helvie MA. United States Preventive Services Task Force screening mammography recommendations: science ignored. AJR Am J Roentgenol 2011;196(2):W112–6.

60. Allgood PC, Duffy SW, Kearins O, et al. Explaining the difference in prognosis between screen-detected and symptomatic breast cancers. Br J Cancer 2011;104(11):1680–5.

61. American cancer society recommendations for the early detection of breast cancer. American Cancer Society. Available at: https://www.cancer.org/cancer/types/breast-cancer/screening-tests-and-early-detection/american-cancer-society-recommendations-for-the-early-detection-of-breast-cancer.html. Accessed September 1, 2023.

62. Practice Bulletin Number 179: Breast Cancer Risk Assessment and Screening in Average-Risk Women. Obstet Gynecol 2017;130(1):e1–16.

63. Breast cancer screening and diagnosis. National Comprehensive Cancer Network. Published Version 1.2023. June 19 2023. Available at: https://www.nccn.org/professionals/physician_gls/pdf/breast-screening.pdf.   Accessed September 21, 2023.

64. Breast Cancer: Screening. U.S. Preventive Services Task Force. Published May 9, 2023. Available at: https://www.uspreventiveservicestaskforce.org/uspstf/

document/draft-evidence-review/breast-cancer-screening-adults.   Accessed October 7, 2023.

65. Wilkerson AD, Obi M, Ortega C, et al. Young Black Women May be More Likely to Have First Mammogram Cancers: A New Perspective in Breast Cancer Disparities. Ann Surg Oncol 2023;30(5):2856–69.

66. Chapman CH, Schechter CB, Cadham CJ, et al. Identifying Equitable Screening Mammography Strategies for Black Women in the United States Using Simulation Modeling. Ann Intern Med 2021;174(12):1637–46.

67. Chen T, Kharazmi E, Fallah M. Race and Ethnicity-Adjusted Age Recommendation for Initiating Breast Cancer Screening. JAMA Netw Open 2023;6(4): e238893.

68. Centers for Disease Control (CDC). Use of mammography–United States, 1990. MMWR Morb Mortal Wkly Rep 1990;39(36):627–30, 621.

69. Ahmed AT, Welch BT, Brinjikji W, et al. Racial Disparities in Screening Mammography in the United States: A Systematic Review and Meta-analysis. J Am Coll Radiol 2017;14(2):157–65.e9.

70. Purc-Stephenson RJ, Gorey KM. Lower adherence to screening mammography guidelines among ethnic minority women in America: a meta-analytic review. Prev Med 2008;46(6):479–88.

71. Jones T, Wisdom-Chambers K, Freeman K, et al. Barriers to Mammography Screening among Black Women at a Community Health Center in South Florida, USA. Med Res Arch 2023;11(4). https://doi.org/10.18103/mra.v11i4.3814.

72. Cancer prevention and early detection facts & figures 2023-2024. American Cancer Society. Published 2023. Available at: https://www.cancer.org/content/dam/cancer-org/research/cancer-facts-and-statistics/cancer-prevention-and-early-detection-facts-and-figures/2023-cped-files/2023-cancer-prevention-and-early-detection.pdf. Accessed August 9, 2023.

73. Alsheik N, Blount L, Qiong Q, et al. Outcomes by Race in Breast Cancer Screening With Digital Breast Tomosynthesis Versus Digital Mammography. J Am Coll Radiol 2021;18(7):906–18.

74. Ambinder EB, Oluyemi E, Kong X, et al. Disparities in the uptake of digital breast tomosynthesis for breast cancer screening: A retrospective cohort study. Breast J 2021;27(12):872–6.

75. Rauscher GH, Allgood KL, Whitman S, et al. Disparities in screening mammography services by race/ethnicity and health insurance. J Womens Health 2012; 21(2):154–60.

76. Yacona K, Hanna MW, Niyazi S, et al. Can COVID-19 worsen racial disparities in breast cancer screening and diagnosis? J Clin Imaging Sci 2022;12:35.

77. Sprague BL, Lowry KP, Miglioretti DL, et al. Changes in Mammography Use by Women's Characteristics During the First 5 Months of the COVID-19 Pandemic. J Natl Cancer Inst 2021;113(9):1161–7.

78. Bea VJ, Jerome-D'Emilia B, Antoine F, et al. Sister, Give Me Your Hand: a Qualitative Focus Group Study on Beliefs and Barriers to Mammography Screening in Black Women During the COVID-19 Era. J Racial Ethn Health Disparities 2023;10(3):1466–77.

79. Anderson H, Bladström A, Olsson H, et al. Familial breast and ovarian cancer: a Swedish population-based register study. Am J Epidemiol 2000;152(12): 1154–63.

80. Porterhouse MD, Paul S, Lieberenz JL, et al. Black Women Are Less Likely to Be Classified as High-Risk for Breast Cancer Using the Tyrer-Cuzick 8 Model. Ann Surg Oncol 2022;29(10):6419–25.

81. Gail MH, Costantino JP, Pee D, et al. Projecting individualized absolute invasive breast cancer risk in African American women. J Natl Cancer Inst 2007;99(23): 1782–92.
82. BWHS breast cancer risk calculator. Boston University Slone Epidemiology Center. Available at: https://www.bu.edu/slone/bwhs-brcarisk-calculator/. Accessed September 7, 2023.
83. Palmer JR, Zirpoli G, Bertrand KA, et al. A Validated Risk Prediction Model for Breast Cancer in US Black Women. J Clin Oncol 2021;39(34):3866–77.
84. Sajal IH, Chowdhury M, Wang T, et al. CBCRisk-Black: a personalized contralateral breast cancer risk prediction model for black women. Breast Cancer Res Treat 2022;194(1):179–86.
85. Breast cancer facts & figures 2022-2024. American Cancer Society. Published 2022. Available at: https://www.cancer.org/content/dam/cancer-org/research/cancer-facts-and-statistics/breast-cancer-facts-and-figures/2022-2024-breast-cancer-fact-figures-acs.pdf. Accessed September 7, 2023.
86. Dunn BK, Agurs-Collins T, Browne D, et al. Health disparities in breast cancer: biology meets socioeconomic status. Breast Cancer Res Treat 2010;121(2): 281–92.
87. Stringer-Reasor EM, Elkhanany A, Khoury K, et al. Disparities in breast cancer associated with African American identity. American Society of Clinical Oncology Educational Book 2021;(41):e29–46.
88. Lawson MB, Bissell MCS, Miglioretti DL, et al. Multilevel Factors Associated With Time to Biopsy After Abnormal Screening Mammography Results by Race and Ethnicity. JAMA Oncol 2022;8(8):1115–26.
89. Chen L, Li CI. Racial disparities in breast cancer diagnosis and treatment by hormone receptor and HER2 status. Cancer Epidemiol Biomarkers Prev 2015; 24(11):1666–72.
90. Giordano SH. A review of the diagnosis and management of male breast cancer. Oncol 2005;10(7):471–9.
91. Mathew J, Perkins GH, Stephens T, et al. Primary breast cancer in men: clinical, imaging, and pathologic findings in 57 patients. AJR Am J Roentgenol 2008; 191(6):1631–9.
92. Fentiman IS, Fourquet A, Hortobagyi GN. Male breast cancer. Lancet 2006; 367(9510):595–604.
93. Brinton LA, Cook MB, McCormack V, et al. Anthropometric and hormonal risk factors for male breast cancer: male breast cancer pooling project results. J Natl Cancer Inst 2014;106(3):djt465.
94. Ruddy KJ, Winer EP. Male breast cancer: risk factors, biology, diagnosis, treatment, and survivorship. Ann Oncol 2013;24(6):1434–43.
95. Sogunro OA, Maini M, Deldar R, et al. Prognostic Predictors of Mortality in Male Breast Cancer: Outcomes in an Urban Population. J Surg Res 2023;281:192–9.
96. Gucalp A, Traina TA, Eisner JR, et al. Male breast cancer: a disease distinct from female breast cancer. Breast Cancer Res Treat 2019;173(1):37–48.
97. DeSantis CE, Miller KD, Goding Sauer A, et al. Cancer statistics for African Americans. CA Cancer J Clin 2019;69(3):211–33.
98. Goodman MT, Tung KH, Wilkens LR. Comparative epidemiology of breast cancer among men and women in the US, 1996 to 2000. Cancer Causes Control 2006;17(2):127–36.
99. Sung H, DeSantis C, Jemal A. Subtype-Specific Breast Cancer Incidence Rates in Black versus White Men in the United States. JNCI Cancer Spectr 2020;4(1): kz091.

100. Brown GR, Jones KT. Incidence of breast cancer in a cohort of 5,135 transgender veterans. Breast Cancer Res Treat 2015;149(1):191–8.
101. Bedrick BS, Fruhauf TF, Martin SJ, et al. Creating Breast and Gynecologic Cancer Guidelines for Transgender Patients With BRCA Mutations. Obstet Gynecol 2021;138(6):911–7.
102. Gooren LJ, van Trotsenburg MAA, Giltay EJ, et al. Breast cancer development in transsexual subjects receiving cross-sex hormone treatment. J Sex Med 2013; 10(12):3129–34.
103. Jaber C, Ralph O, Hamidian Jahromi A. BRCA Mutations and the Implications in Transgender Individuals Undergoing Top Surgery: An Operative Dilemma. Plast Reconstr Surg Glob Open 2022;10(1):e4012.
104. American College of Obstetrics & Gynecology. Health care for transgender and gender diverse individuals. ACOG Committee Opinion Number 823. Available at: https://www.acog.org/-/media/project/acog/acogorg/clinical/files/committee-opinion/articles/2021/03/health-care-for-transgender-and-gender-diverse-individuals.pdf.
105. Oseni TO, Zhang B, Coopey SB, et al. Twenty-Five Year Trends in the Incidence of Ductal Carcinoma in Situ in US Women. J Am Coll Surg 2019;228(6):932–9.
106. Nassar H, Sharafaldeen B, Visvanathan K, et al. Ductal carcinoma in situ in African American versus Caucasian American women: analysis of clinicopathologic features and outcome. Cancer 2009;115(14):3181–8.
107. Bailes AA, Kuerer HM, Lari SA, et al. Impact of race and ethnicity on features and outcome of ductal carcinoma in situ of the breast. Cancer 2013;119(1): 150–7.
108. Liu Y, West R, Weber JD, et al. Race and risk of subsequent aggressive breast cancer following ductal carcinoma in situ. Cancer 2019;125(18):3225–33.
109. Parise CA, Caggiano V. Risk of mortality of node-negative, ER/PR/HER2 breast cancer subtypes in T1, T2, and T3 tumors. Breast Cancer Res Treat 2017; 165(3):743–50.
110. Foy KC, Fisher JL, Lustberg MB, et al. Disparities in breast cancer tumor characteristics, treatment, time to treatment, and survival probability among African American and white women. npj Breast Cancer 2018;4(1):1–6.
111. Miller BA, Hankey BF, Thomas TL. Impact of sociodemographic factors, hormone receptor status, and tumor grade on ethnic differences in tumor stage and size for breast cancer in US women. Am J Epidemiol 2002;155(6):534–45.
112. Chen VW, Correa P, Kurman RJ, et al. Histological characteristics of breast carcinoma in blacks and whites. Cancer Epidemiol Biomarkers Prev 1994;3(2): 127–35.
113. O'Reilly D, Sendi MA, Kelly CM. Overview of recent advances in metastatic triple negative breast cancer. World J Clin Oncol 2021;12(3):164–82.
114. Aysola K, Desai A, Welch C, et al. Triple Negative Breast Cancer - An Overview. Hered Genet 2013;2013(Suppl 2). https://doi.org/10.4172/2161-1041.S2-001.
115. Prat A, Adamo B, Cheang MCU, et al. Molecular characterization of basal-like and non-basal-like triple-negative breast cancer. Oncol 2013;18(2):123–33.
116. Yin L, Duan JJ, Bian XW, et al. Triple-negative breast cancer molecular subtyping and treatment progress. Breast Cancer Res 2020;22(1):61.
117. Howard FM, Olopade OI. Epidemiology of Triple-Negative Breast Cancer: A Review. Cancer J 2021;27(1):8–16.
118. Sung H, DeSantis CE, Fedewa SA, et al. Breast cancer subtypes among Eastern-African-born black women and other black women in the United States. Cancer 2019;125(19):3401–11.

119. Micheletti SJ, Bryc K, Ancona Esselmann SG, et al. Genetic Consequences of the Transatlantic Slave Trade in the Americas. Am J Hum Genet 2020;107(2): 265–77.
120. Hester RH, Hortobagyi GN, Lim B. Inflammatory breast cancer: early recognition and diagnosis is critical. Am J Obstet Gynecol 2021;225(4):392–6.
121. Hance KW, Anderson WF, Devesa SS, et al. Trends in inflammatory breast carcinoma incidence and survival: the surveillance, epidemiology, and end results program at the National Cancer Institute. J Natl Cancer Inst 2005;97(13): 966–75.
122. Gudina AT, Copeland G, Soliman AS, et al. Racial/ethnic disparities in inflammatory breast cancer survival in the Michigan Cancer Surveillance Program. Breast Cancer Res Treat 2019;173(3):693–9.
123. Chang S, Buzdar AU, Hursting SD. Inflammatory breast cancer and body mass index. J Clin Oncol 1998;16(12):3731–5.
124. Denu RA, Hampton JM, Currey A, et al. Racial and Socioeconomic Disparities Are More Pronounced in Inflammatory Breast Cancer Than Other Breast Cancers. J Cancer Epidemiol 2017;2017:7574946.
125. Selove R, Kilbourne B, Fadden MK, et al. Time from Screening Mammography to Biopsy and from Biopsy to Breast Cancer Treatment among Black and White, Women Medicare Beneficiaries Not Participating in a Health Maintenance Organization. Wom Health Issues 2016;26(6):642–7.
126. Emerson MA, Golightly YM, Aiello AE, et al. Breast cancer treatment delays by socioeconomic and health care access latent classes in Black and White women. Cancer 2020;126(22):4957–66.
127. Blazek A, O'Donoghue C, Terranella S, et al. Impact of Inequities on Delay in Breast Cancer Management in Women Undergoing Second Opinions. J Surg Res 2021;268:445–51.
128. Jain U, Jain B, Fayanju OM, et al. Disparities in timely treatment among young women with breast cancer. Am J Surg 2022;224(2):811–5.
129. Khubchandani JA, Greenup RA. Time to surgery delays: Barriers to care for black women with breast cancer. Am J Surg 2022;224(2):809–10.
130. Relation T, Ndumele A, Bhattacharyya O, et al. Surgery Refusal Among Black and Hispanic Women with Non-Metastatic Breast Cancer. Ann Surg Oncol 2022;29(11):6634–43.
131. Green AK, Aviki EM, Matsoukas K, et al. Racial disparities in chemotherapy administration for early-stage breast cancer: a systematic review and meta-analysis. Breast Cancer Res Treat 2018;172(2):247–63.
132. EBCTCG (Early Breast Cancer Trialists' Collaborative Group), McGale P, Taylor C, Correa C, et al. Effect of radiotherapy after mastectomy and axillary surgery on 10-year recurrence and 20-year breast cancer mortality: meta-analysis of individual patient data for 8135 women in 22 randomised trials. Lancet 2014;383(9935):2127–35.
133. Overgaard M, Jensen MB, Overgaard J, et al. Postoperative radiotherapy in high-risk postmenopausal breast-cancer patients given adjuvant tamoxifen: Danish Breast Cancer Cooperative Group DBCG 82c randomised trial. Lancet 1999;353(9165):1641–8.
134. Smith GL, Shih YCT, Xu Y, et al. Racial disparities in the use of radiotherapy after breast-conserving surgery: a national Medicare study. Cancer 2010;116(3): 734–41.

135. Snead F, Slade AN, Oppong BA, et al. Narrowing Racial Gaps in Breast Cancer: Factors Affecting Probability of Adjuvant Radiation Therapy. Adv Radiat Oncol 2020;5(1):17–26.
136. Davies C, Pan H, Godwin J, et al. Long-term effects of continuing adjuvant tamoxifen to 10 years versus stopping at 5 years after diagnosis of oestrogen receptor-positive breast cancer: ATLAS, a randomised trial. Lancet 2013; 381(9869):805–16.
137. Francis PA, Pagani O, Fleming GF, et al. Tailoring Adjuvant Endocrine Therapy for Premenopausal Breast Cancer. N Engl J Med 2018;379(2):122–37.
138. Collin LJ, Cronin-Fenton DP, Ahern TP, et al. Early Discontinuation of Endocrine Therapy and Recurrence of Breast Cancer among Premenopausal Women. Clin Cancer Res 2021;27(5):1421–8.
139. Wigertz A, Ahlgren J, Holmqvist M, et al. Adherence and discontinuation of adjuvant hormonal therapy in breast cancer patients: a population-based study. Breast Cancer Res Treat 2012;133(1):367–73.
140. Sheppard VB, de Mendoza AH, He J, et al. Initiation of Adjuvant Endocrine Therapy in Black and White Women With Breast Cancer. Clin Breast Cancer 2018; 18(5):337–46.e1.
141. Hu X, Walker MS, Stepanski E, et al. Racial Differences in Patient-Reported Symptoms and Adherence to Adjuvant Endocrine Therapy Among Women With Early-Stage, Hormone Receptor-Positive Breast Cancer. JAMA Netw Open 2022;5(8):e2225485.
142. Heiney SP, Truman S, Babatunde OA, et al. Racial and Geographic Disparities in Endocrine Therapy Adherence Among Younger Breast Cancer Survivors. Am J Clin Oncol 2020;43(7):504–9.
143. Farias AJ, Wu WH, Du XL. Racial differences in long-term adjuvant endocrine therapy adherence and mortality among Medicaid-insured breast cancer patients in Texas: Findings from TCR-Medicaid linked data. BMC Cancer 2018; 18(1):1214.
144. Wheeler SB, Spencer J, Pinheiro LC, et al. Endocrine Therapy Nonadherence and Discontinuation in Black and White Women. J Natl Cancer Inst 2019; 111(5):498–508.
145. Perez EA, Romond EH, Suman VJ, et al. Trastuzumab plus adjuvant chemotherapy for human epidermal growth factor receptor 2-positive breast cancer: planned joint analysis of overall survival from NSABP B-31 and NCCTG N9831. J Clin Oncol 2014;32(33):3744–52.
146. Reeder-Hayes K, Peacock Hinton S, Meng K, et al. Disparities in Use of Human Epidermal Growth Hormone Receptor 2-Targeted Therapy for Early-Stage Breast Cancer. J Clin Oncol 2016;34(17):2003–9.
147. Collin LJ, Yan M, Jiang R, et al. Receipt of Guideline-Concordant Care Does Not Explain Breast Cancer Mortality Disparities by Race in Metropolitan Atlanta. J Natl Compr Cancer Netw 2021;19(11):1242–51.
148. Newman LA. Parsing the Etiology of Breast Cancer Disparities. J Clin Oncol 2016;34(9):1013–4.
149. Cho B, Han Y, Lian M, et al. Evaluation of Racial/Ethnic Differences in Treatment and Mortality Among Women With Triple-Negative Breast Cancer. JAMA Oncol 2021;7(7):1016–23.
150. Carbajal-Ochoa WH, Johnson D, Alvarez A, et al. Racial disparities in treatment and outcomes between non-Hispanic Black and non-Hispanic White women with nonmetastatic inflammatory breast cancer. Breast Cancer Res Treat 2023;201(2):275–87.

151. Alvarez A, Bernal AM, Anampa J. Racial disparities in overall survival after the introduction of cyclin-dependent kinase 4/6 inhibitors for patients with hormone receptor-positive, HER2-negative metastatic breast cancer. Breast Cancer Res Treat 2023;198(1):75–88.

152. Robson M, Im SA, Senkus E, et al. Olaparib for Metastatic Breast Cancer in Patients with a Germline BRCA Mutation. N Engl J Med 2017;377(6):523–33.

153. Litton JK, Rugo HS, Ettl J, et al. Talazoparib in Patients with Advanced Breast Cancer and a Germline BRCA Mutation. N Engl J Med 2018;379(8):753–63.

154. Reid S, Cadiz S, Pal T. Disparities in Genetic Testing and Care among Black women with Hereditary Breast Cancer. Curr Breast Cancer Rep 2020;12(3): 125–31.

155. Wagar MK, Mojdehbakhsh RP, Godecker A, et al. Racial and ethnic enrollment disparities in clinical trials of poly(ADP-ribose) polymerase inhibitors for gynecologic cancers. Gynecol Oncol 2022;165(1):49–52.

156. Anderson SJ, Wapnir I, Dignam JJ, et al. Prognosis after ipsilateral breast tumor recurrence and locoregional recurrences in patients treated by breast-conserving therapy in five National Surgical Adjuvant Breast and Bowel Project protocols of node-negative breast cancer. J Clin Oncol 2009;27(15):2466–73.

157. Early Breast Cancer Trialists' Collaborative Group (EBCTCG), Darby S, McGale P, Correa C, et al. Effect of radiotherapy after breast-conserving surgery on 10-year recurrence and 15-year breast cancer death: meta-analysis of individual patient data for 10,801 women in 17 randomised trials. Lancet 2011; 378(9804):1707–16.

158. Kantor O, King TA, Freedman RA, et al. Racial and Ethnic Disparities in Locoregional Recurrence Among Patients With Hormone Receptor-Positive, Node-Negative Breast Cancer: A Post Hoc Analysis of the TAILORx Randomized Clinical Trial. JAMA Surg 2023;158(6):583–91.

159. Terman E, Sheade J, Zhao F, et al. The impact of race and age on response to neoadjuvant therapy and long-term outcomes in Black and White women with early-stage breast cancer. Breast Cancer Res Treat 2023;200(1):75–83.

160. Ibraheem A, Olopade OI, Huo D. Propensity score analysis of the prognostic value of genomic assays for breast cancer in diverse populations using the National Cancer Data Base. Cancer 2020;126(17):4013–22.

161. Petkov VI, Miller DP, Howlader N, et al. Breast-cancer-specific mortality in patients treated based on the 21-gene assay: a SEER population-based study. NPJ Breast Cancer 2016;2:16017.

162. Paik S, Shak S, Tang G, et al. A multigene assay to predict recurrence of tamoxifen-treated, node-negative breast cancer. N Engl J Med 2004;351(27): 2817–26.

163. Fisher B, Dignam J, Wolmark N, et al. Tamoxifen and chemotherapy for lymph node-negative, estrogen receptor-positive breast cancer. J Natl Cancer Inst 1997;89(22):1673–82.

164. Hoskins KF, Danciu OC, Ko NY, et al. Association of Race/Ethnicity and the 21-Gene Recurrence Score With Breast Cancer-Specific Mortality Among US Women. JAMA Oncol 2021;7(3):370–8.

165. Watt GP, John EM, Bandera EV, et al. Race, ethnicity and risk of second primary contralateral breast cancer in the United States. Int J Cancer 2021;148(11): 2748–58.

166. Giannakeas V, Lim DW, Narod SA. The risk of contralateral breast cancer: a SEER-based analysis. Br J Cancer 2021;125(4):601–10.

167. Yee MK, Sereika SM, Bender CM, et al. Symptom incidence, distress, cancer-related distress, and adherence to chemotherapy among African American women with breast cancer. Cancer 2017;123(11):2061–9.

168. Jordache P, Danahey K, Reizine NM, et al. Investigating the prevalence and risk of chemotherapy-induced neuropathy among cancer patients. J Clin Orthod 2021;39(15_suppl):12078.

169. Sreeram K, Seaton R, Greenwald MK, et al. Chemotherapy-induced peripheral neuropathy in the detroit research on cancer survivors (ROCS) cohort. Cancer Causes Control 2023;34(5):459–68.

170. Al-Sadawi M, Hussain Y, Copeland-Halperin RS, et al. Racial and Socioeconomic Disparities in Cardiotoxicity Among Women With HER2-Positive Breast Cancer. Am J Cardiol 2021;147:116–21.

171. Sutton AL, Felix AS, Wahl S, et al. Racial disparities in treatment-related cardiovascular toxicities amongst women with breast cancer: a scoping review. J Cancer Surviv 2022. https://doi.org/10.1007/s11764-022-01210-2.

172. Collin LJ, Troeschel AN, Liu Y, et al. A balancing act: racial disparities in cardiovascular disease mortality among women diagnosed with breast cancer. Ann Cancer Epidemiol 2020;4. https://doi.org/10.21037/ace.2020.01.02.

173. Gillespie TC, Sayegh HE, Brunelle CL, et al. Breast cancer-related lymphedema: risk factors, precautionary measures, and treatments. Gland Surg 2018;7(4):379–403.

174. Ren Y, Kebede MA, Ogunleye AA, et al. Burden of lymphedema in long-term breast cancer survivors by race and age. Cancer 2022;128(23):4119–28.

175. Shakir A, Coalson E, Beederman M, et al. Health Disparities in Patients Seeking Physiological Surgical Treatment for Lymphedema. Plast Reconstr Surg 2023;151(1):217–24.

176. Ko NY, Fikre TG, Buck AK, et al. Breast cancer survivorship experiences among Black women. Cancer 2023;129(S19):3087–101.

177. Calhoun C, Helzlsouer KJ, Gallicchio L. Racial differences in depressive symptoms and self-rated health among breast cancer survivors on aromatase inhibitor therapy. J Psychosoc Oncol 2015;33(3):263–77.

178. Lake PW, Conley CC, Pal T, et al. Anxiety and depression among Black breast cancer survivors: Examining the role of patient-provider communication and cultural values. Patient Educ Counsel 2022;105(7):2391–6.

179. Newman LA, Kaljee LM. Health Disparities and Triple-Negative Breast Cancer in African American Women: A Review. JAMA Surg 2017;152(5):485–93.

180. Killelea BK, Yang VQ, Wang SY, et al. Racial Differences in the Use and Outcome of Neoadjuvant Chemotherapy for Breast Cancer: Results From the National Cancer Data Base. J Clin Oncol 2015;33(36):4267–76.

181. Pastoriza JM, Karagiannis GS, Lin J, et al. Black race and distant recurrence after neoadjuvant or adjuvant chemotherapy in breast cancer. Clin Exp Metastasis 2018;35(7):613–23.

182. Hrin ML, McMichael AJ. Chemotherapy-induced alopecia in African American women: A literature review demonstrates a knowledge gap. J Am Acad Dermatol 2022;86(6):1434–5.

183. Pleasant VA, Purkiss AS, Merjaver SD. Redefining the "crown": Approaching chemotherapy-induced alopecia among Black patients with breast cancer. Cancer 2023;129(11):1629–33.

184. Soni SE, Lee MC, Gwede CK. Disparities in Use and Access to Postmastectomy Breast Reconstruction Among African American Women: A Targeted Review of the Literature. Cancer Control 2017;24(4). 1073274817729053.

185. Tseng JF, Kronowitz SJ, Sun CC, et al. The effect of ethnicity on immediate reconstruction rates after mastectomy for breast cancer. Cancer 2004;101(7): 1514–23.

186. Morrow M, Mujahid M, Lantz PM, et al. Correlates of breast reconstruction: results from a population-based study. Cancer 2005;104(11):2340–6.

187. Rubin LR, Chavez J, Alderman A, et al. "Use what God has given me": difference and disparity in breast reconstruction. Psychol Health 2013;28(10): 1099–120.

188. Yang RL, Newman AS, Reinke CE, et al. Racial disparities in immediate breast reconstruction after mastectomy: impact of state and federal health policy changes. Ann Surg Oncol 2013;20(2):399–406.

189. Stacey DH, Spring MA, Breslin TM, et al. Exploring the effect of the referring general surgeon's attitudes on breast reconstruction utilization. Wis Med J 2008;107(6):292–7.

190. Jackson-Bey T, Morris J, Jasper E, et al. Systematic review of racial and ethnic disparities in reproductive endocrinology and infertility: where do we stand today? F&S Reviews 2021;2(3):169–88.

191. Meernik C, Jorgensen K, Wu CF, et al. Disparities in the use of assisted reproductive technologies after breast cancer: a population-based study. Breast Cancer Res Treat 2023;198(1):149–58.

192. Pleasant V, Ulrich N, Pearlman MD, et al. Reproductive Considerations for Patients with Early-Onset Breast Cancer. Curr Breast Cancer Rep 2022. https://doi.org/10.1007/s12609-022-00445-3.

193. Consensus guideline on genetic testing for hereditary breast cancer. The American Society of Breast Surgeons. Published 2019. Available at: https://www.breastsurgeons.org/docs/statements/Consensus-Guideline-on-Genetic-Testing-for-Hereditary-Breast-Cancer.pdf. Accessed October 15, 2023.

194. Halbert CH, Kessler L, Stopfer JE, et al. Low rates of acceptance of BRCA1 and BRCA2 test results among African American women at increased risk for hereditary breast-ovarian cancer. Genet Med 2006;8(9):576–82.

195. McCarthy AM, Bristol M, Domchek SM, et al. Health Care Segregation, Physician Recommendation, and Racial Disparities in BRCA1/2 Testing Among Women With Breast Cancer. J Clin Oncol 2016;34(22):2610–8.

196. Nikolaidis C, Duquette D, Mendelsohn-Victor KE, et al. Disparities in genetic services utilization in a random sample of young breast cancer survivors. Genet Med 2019;21(6):1363–70.

197. Peterson JM, Pepin A, Thomas R, et al. Racial disparities in breast cancer hereditary risk assessment referrals. J Genet Counsel 2020;29(4):587–93.

198. McCall MK, Ibikunle S, Murphy Y, et al. Knowledge and Attitudes About Genetic Testing Among Black and White Women with Breast Cancer. J Racial Ethn Health Disparities 2021;8(5):1208–16.

199. Sheppard VB, Mays D, Tercyak KP, et al. Medical Mistrust Influences Black Women's Level of Engagement in BRCA1/2 Genetic Counseling and Testing. J Natl Med Assoc 2013;105(1):17–22.

200. Ademuyiwa FO, Salyer P, Tao Y, et al. Genetic Counseling and Testing in African American Patients With Breast Cancer: A Nationwide Survey of US Breast Oncologists. J Clin Oncol 2021;39(36):4020–8.

201. Sheppard VB, Graves KD, Christopher J, et al. African American women's limited knowledge and experiences with genetic counseling for hereditary breast cancer. J Genet Counsel 2014;23(3):311–22.

202. Warner E, Foulkes W, Goodwin P, et al. Prevalence and Penetrance of BRCA1 and BRCA2 Gene Mutations in Unselected Ashkenazi Jewish Women With Breast Cancer. J Natl Cancer Inst 1999;91(14):1241–7.
203. Malone KE, Daling JR, Doody DR, et al. Prevalence and predictors of BRCA1 and BRCA2 mutations in a population-based study of breast cancer in white and black American women ages 35 to 64 years. Cancer Res 2006;66(16): 8297–308.
204. Domchek SM, Yao S, Chen F, et al. Comparison of the Prevalence of Pathogenic Variants in Cancer Susceptibility Genes in Black Women and Non-Hispanic White Women With Breast Cancer in the United States. JAMA Oncol 2021; 7(7):1045–50.
205. Diop JPD, Sène ARG, Dia Y, et al. New Insights Into c.815_824dup Pathogenic Variant of BRCA1 in Inherited Breast Cancer: A Founder Mutation of West African Origin. Front Oncol 2021;11:810060.
206. Mefford HC, Baumbach L, Panguluri RC, et al. Evidence for a BRCA1 founder mutation in families of West African ancestry. Am J Hum Genet 1999;65(2): 575–8.
207. Pal T, Bonner D, Cragun D, et al. A high frequency of BRCA mutations in young black women with breast cancer residing in Florida. Cancer 2015;121(23): 4173–80.
208. John EM, Miron A, Gong G, et al. Prevalence of pathogenic BRCA1 mutation carriers in 5 US racial/ethnic groups. JAMA 2007;298(24):2869–76.
209. Haffty BG, Silber A, Matloff E, et al. Racial differences in the incidence of BRCA1 and BRCA2 mutations in a cohort of early onset breast cancer patients: African American compared to white women. J Med Genet 2006;43(2):133–7.
210. Haffty BG, Choi DH, Goyal S, et al. Breast cancer in young women (YBC): prevalence of BRCA1/2 mutations and risk of secondary malignancies across diverse racial groups. Ann Oncol 2009;20(10):1653–9.
211. Nanda R, Schumm LP, Cummings S, et al. Genetic testing in an ethnically diverse cohort of high-risk women: a comparative analysis of BRCA1 and BRCA2 mutations in American families of European and African ancestry. JAMA 2005;294(15):1925–33.
212. Ricker C, Culver JO, Lowstuter K, et al. Increased yield of actionable mutations using multi-gene panels to assess hereditary cancer susceptibility in an ethnically diverse clinical cohort. Cancer Genet 2016;209(4):130–7.
213. Lovejoy LA, Rummel SK, Turner CE, et al. Frequency and spectrum of mutations across 94 cancer predisposition genes in African American women with invasive breast cancer. Fam Cancer 2021;20(3):181–7.
214. Kurian AW, Ward KC, Hamilton AS, et al. Uptake, Results, and Outcomes of Germline Multiple-Gene Sequencing After Diagnosis of Breast Cancer. JAMA Oncol 2018;4(8):1066–72.
215. Tatineni S, Tarockoff M, Abdallah N, et al. Racial and ethnic variation in multi-gene panel testing in a cohort of BRCA1/2-negative individuals who had genetic testing in a large urban comprehensive cancer center. Cancer Med 2022;11(6): 1465–73.
216. Popejoy AB, Fullerton SM. Genomics is failing on diversity. Nature 2016; 538(7624):161–4.
217. Mills MC, Rahal C. A scientometric review of genome-wide association studies. Commun Biol 2019;2:9.
218. Sirugo G, Williams SM, Tishkoff SA. The Missing Diversity in Human Genetic Studies. Cell 2019;177(1):26–31.

219. Slavin TP, Manjarrez S, Pritchard CC, et al. The effects of genomic germline variant reclassification on clinical cancer care. Oncotarget 2019;10(4):417–23.
220. Macklin S, Durand N, Atwal P, et al. Observed frequency and challenges of variant reclassification in a hereditary cancer clinic. Genet Med 2018;20(3): 346–50.
221. The U.S. Public Health Service Untreated Syphilis Study at Tuskegee. Centers for Disease Control and Prevention. Available at: https://www.cdc.gov/tuskegee/index.html. Accessed October 8, 2023.
222. Gamble VN. Under the shadow of Tuskegee: African Americans and health care. Am J Public Health 1997;87(11):1773–8.
223. Significant Research Advances Enabled by HeLa Cells. National institutes of Health, Office of Science Policy. Available at: https://osp.od.nih.gov/scientific-sharing/hela-cells-timeline/. Accessed April 23, 2022.
224. McGregor DK. From midwives to medicine: the birth of American Gynecology. Rutgers University Press; 1998.
225. Begos Kevin, Deaver Danielle, Railey John, et al. Against their will: North Carolina's sterilization program and the campaign for reparations. Gray Oak Books; 2012.
226. Hempstead B, Green C, Briant KJ, et al. Community Empowerment Partners (CEPs): A Breast Health Education Program for African-American Women. J Community Health 2018;43(5):833–41.
227. Haynes D, Hughes K, Haas M, et al. Breast Cancer Champions: a peer-to-peer education and mobile mammography program improving breast cancer screening rates for women of African heritage. Cancer Causes Control 2023; 34(7):625–33.
228. Brown MT, Cowart LW. Evaluating the effectiveness of faith-based breast health education. Health Educ J 2018;77(5):571–85.
229. Susan G. Komen. Susan G. Komen: Worship in Pink. Available at: https://www.komen.org/how-to-help/programs/worship-in-pink/. Accessed September 18, 2023.
230. Wilson TE, Fraser-White M, Feldman J, et al. Hair salon stylists as breast cancer prevention lay health advisors for African American and Afro-Caribbean women. J Health Care Poor Underserved 2008;19(1):216–26.
231. New ACR Breast Cancer Screening Guidelines call for earlier and more-intensive screening for high-risk women. American College of Radiology. Published May 3, 2023. Available at: https://www.acr.org/Media-Center/ACR-News-Releases/2023/New-ACR-Breast-Cancer-Screening-Guidelines-call-for-earlier-screening-for-high-risk-women. Accessed October 8, 2023.
232. Centers for Disease Control and Prevention. National Breast and Cervical Cancer Early Detection Program (NBCCEDP). Available at: https://www.cdc.gov/cancer/nbccedp/about.htm. Accessed September 18, 2023.
233. Gold RH, Bassett LW, Widoff BE. Highlights from the history of mammography. Radiographics 1990;10(6):1111–31.
234. Stanley E, Lewis MC, Irshad A, et al. Effectiveness of a Mobile Mammography Program. AJR Am J Roentgenol 2017;209(6):1426–9.
235. Trivedi U, Omofoye TS, Marquez C, et al. Mobile Mammography Services and Underserved Women. Diagnostics 2022;12(4). https://doi.org/10.3390/diagnostics12040902.
236. Dontchos BN, Narayan AK, Seidler M, et al. Impact of a Same-Day Breast Biopsy Program on Disparities in Time to Biopsy. J Am Coll Radiol 2019;16(11): 1554–60.

237. Yoon SC, Taylor-Cho MW, Charles MG, et al. Racial Disparities in Breast Imaging Wait Times Before and After the Implementation of a Same-Day Biopsy Program. J Breast Imaging 2023;5(2):159–66.

238. Geronimus AT, Phillip Thompson J. TO DENIGRATE, IGNORE, OR DISRUPT: Racial Inequality in Health and the Impact of a Policy-induced Breakdown of African American Communities. Du Bois Rev 2004;1(2):247–79.

239. Geronimus AT, James SA, Destin M, et al. Jedi Public Health: Co-creating an Identity-Safe Culture to Promote Health Equity. SSM Popul Health 2016;2: 105–16.

240. Obeng-Gyasi S, Tarver W, Carlos RC, et al. Allostatic load: a framework to understand breast cancer outcomes in Black women. NPJ Breast Cancer 2021; 7(1):100.

241. Williams DR, Mohammed SA, Shields AE. Understanding and effectively addressing breast cancer in African American women: Unpacking the social context. Cancer 2016;122(14):2138–49.

242. Singh GK, Jemal A. Socioeconomic and Racial/Ethnic Disparities in Cancer Mortality, Incidence, and Survival in the United States, 1950-2014: Over Six Decades of Changing Patterns and Widening Inequalities. J Environ Public Health 2017;2017:2819372.

243. Mudaranthakam DP, Nollen N, Wick J, et al. Evaluating Work Impairment as a Source of Financial Toxicity in Cancer Healthcare and Negative Impacts on Health Status. Cancer Res Commun 2023;3(7):1166–72.

244. Geronimus AT, Hicken M, Keene D, et al. "Weathering" and age patterns of allostatic load scores among blacks and whites in the United States. Am J Public Health 2006;96(5):826–33.

245. Xing CY, Doose M, Qin B, et al. Prediagnostic Allostatic Load as a Predictor of Poorly Differentiated and Larger Sized Breast Cancers among Black Women in the Women's Circle of Health Follow-Up Study. Cancer Epidemiol Biomarkers Prev 2020;29(1):216–24.

246. Xing CY, Doose M, Qin B, et al. Pre-diagnostic allostatic load and health-related quality of life in a cohort of Black breast cancer survivors. Breast Cancer Res Treat 2020;184(3):901–14.

247. Zhao H, Song R, Ye Y, et al. Allostatic score and its associations with demographics, healthy behaviors, tumor characteristics, and mitochondrial DNA among breast cancer patients. Breast Cancer Res Treat 2021;187(2):587–96.

248. Adams-Campbell LL, Taylor T, Hicks J, et al. The Effect of a 6-Month Exercise Intervention Trial on Allostatic Load in Black Women at Increased Risk for Breast Cancer: the FIERCE Study. J Racial Ethn Health Disparities 2022;9(5):2063–9.

249. Clark CR, Baril N, Kunicki M, et al. Addressing Social Determinants of Health to Improve Access to Early Breast Cancer Detection: Results of the Boston REACH 2010 Breast and Cervical Cancer Coalition Women's Health Demonstration Project. J Womens Health 2009;18(5):677–90.

250. Nelson HD, Cantor A, Wagner J, et al. Effectiveness of Patient Navigation to Increase Cancer Screening in Populations Adversely Affected by Health Disparities: a Meta-analysis. J Gen Intern Med 2020;35(10):3026–35.

251. Goel N, Hernandez A, Thompson C, et al. Neighborhood Disadvantage and Breast Cancer-Specific Survival. JAMA Netw Open 2023;6(4):e238908.

252. Beyer KMM, Zhou Y, Laud PW, et al. Mortgage Lending Bias and Breast Cancer Survival Among Older Women in the United States. J Clin Oncol 2021;39(25): 2749–57.

253. Pleasant VA, Griggs JJ. Contemporary Residential Segregation and Cancer Disparities. J Clin Oncol 2021;39(25):2739–41.
254. Miller-Kleinhenz JM, Moubadder L, Beyer KM, et al. Redlining-associated methylation in breast tumors: the impact of contemporary structural racism on the tumor epigenome. Front Oncol 2023;13:1154554.
255. White-Means SI, Osmani AR. Racial and Ethnic Disparities in Patient-Provider Communication With Breast Cancer Patients: Evidence From 2011 MEPS and Experiences With Cancer Supplement. Inquiry 2017;54. 46958017727104.
256. Bigatti SM, Weathers T, Hayes L, et al. Challenges Experienced by Black Women with Breast Cancer During Active Treatment: Relationship to Treatment Adherence. J Racial Ethn Health Disparities 2023;1–12.
257. Bickell NA, Weidmann J, Fei K, et al. Underuse of breast cancer adjuvant treatment: patient knowledge, beliefs, and medical mistrust. J Clin Oncol 2009; 27(31):5160–7.
258. Sheppard VB, Hurtado-de-Mendoza A, Talley CH, et al. Reducing Racial Disparities in Breast Cancer Survivors' Ratings of Quality Cancer Care: The Enduring Impact of Trust. J Healthc Qual 2016;38(3):143–63.
259. Sutton AL, He J, Edmonds MC, et al. Medical Mistrust in Black Breast Cancer Patients: Acknowledging the Roles of the Trustor and the Trustee. J Cancer Educ 2019;34(3):600–7.
260. Jetty A, Jabbarpour Y, Pollack J, et al. Patient-Physician Racial Concordance Associated with Improved Healthcare Use and Lower Healthcare Expenditures in Minority Populations. J Racial Ethn Health Disparities 2022;9(1):68–81.
261. Shen MJ, Peterson EB, Costas-Muñiz R, et al. The Effects of Race and Racial Concordance on Patient-Physician Communication: A Systematic Review of the Literature. J Racial Ethn Health Disparities 2018;5(1):117–40.
262. Greenwood BN, Hardeman RR, Huang L, et al. Physician-patient racial concordance and disparities in birthing mortality for newborns. Proc Natl Acad Sci U S A 2020;117(35):21194–200.
263. Snyder JE, Upton RD, Hassett TC, et al. Black Representation in the Primary Care Physician Workforce and Its Association With Population Life Expectancy and Mortality Rates in the US. JAMA Netw Open 2023;6(4):e236687.
264. Beyene D, Naab T, Apprey V, et al. Cyclin A2 and Ki-67 proliferation markers could be used to identify tumors with poor prognosis in African American women with breast cancer. J Cancer Biol 2023;4(1):3–16.
265. Barrow MA, Martin ME, Coffey A, et al. A functional role for the cancer disparity-linked genes, CRYβB2 and CRYβB2P1, in the promotion of breast cancer. Breast Cancer Res 2019;21(1):105.
266. Porter PL, Lund MJ, Lin MG, et al. Racial differences in the expression of cell cycle-regulatory proteins in breast carcinoma. Cancer 2004;100(12):2533–42.
267. Schaibley VM, Ramos IN, Woosley RL, et al. Limited Genomics Training Among Physicians Remains a Barrier to Genomics-Based Implementation of Precision Medicine. Front Med 2022;9:757212.
268. Resources for Healthcare Providers. Centers for Disease Control and Prevention. Available at: https://www.cdc.gov/cancer/health-care-providers/index.htm. Accessed September 19, 2023.
269. H3Africa Human Heredity & Health in Africa. Available at: https://h3africa.org/. Accessed September 18, 2023.
270. National Human Genome Research Institute. Center for Research on Genomics and Global Health. Available at: https://www.genome.gov/about-nhgri/Center-for-Research-on-Genomics-and-Global-Health. Accessed September 18, 2023.

271. Gurdasani D, Carstensen T, Tekola-Ayele F, et al. The African Genome Variation Project shapes medical genetics in Africa. Nature 2014;517(7534):327–32.
272. NIH launches largest-ever study of breast cancer genetics in black women. National Institutes of Health. Published July 6, 2016. Available at: https://www.nih.gov/news-events/news-releases/nih-launches-largest-ever-study-breast-cancer-genetics-black-women. Accessed September 18, 2023.
273. NIH Policy and Guidelines on The Inclusion of Women and Minorities as Subjects in Clinical Research. NIH Grants & Funding. Available at: https://grants.nih.gov/policy/inclusion/women-and-minorities/guidelines.htm#:~:text=It%20is%20the%20policy%20of,that%20inclusion%20is%20inappropriate%20with. Accessed April 26, 2022.

Obstetrics and Gynecology Care in Latinx Communities

Felicia L. Hamilton, MD[a],*, Versha Pleasant, MD, MPH[b]

KEYWORDS

- Latinx • Hispanic • Health disparities • OB/GYN health care
- Cultural considerations • Policy implications

KEY POINTS

- Latinx people represent a diverse community that comprises the largest minority population in the United States.
- Social determinants of health—such as cultural differences, language barriers, and insurance coverage—can affect obstetrics and gynecology care among this community.
- Practitioners should engage in care that is culturally sensitive, as well as serve as health advocates in policy and legislation that can facilitate positive change in the Latinx community.

INTRODUCTION

Latinos are not a monolithic culture. It's impossible to have a 'one size fits all' Latinx character, and because of that, our well of stories is endless.

—Sonia Manzano[1]

Definition and Significance of Latinx Communities in Health Care

Latinx is the nonbinary form for Latino or Latina that describes any person with ancestry from anywhere in Latin America.[2] The term Hispanic was created by the US government in the 1970s and typically referred to people in the Americas and Spain who speak Spanish or descended from Spanish-speaking populations.[2] This large and diverse community was initially marked as White on national census counts before this designation.[2] Recognizing the incredible diversity within this community, we will use the term Latinx throughout this article.

---

[a] Department of Obstetrics & Gynecology, OB/Gyn Practice Committee, MedStar Washington Hospital Center, Georgetown University Medical Center, 110 Irving Street, Northwest Room 5B-45A, Washington, DC 20010, USA; [b] Department of Obstetrics and Gynecology, Cancer Genetics & Breast Health Clinic, University of Michigan, 1500 East Medical Center Drive, Ann Arbor, MI 48109, USA
* Corresponding author.
E-mail address: Felicia.l.hamilton@medstar.net

Obstet Gynecol Clin N Am 51 (2024) 105–124
https://doi.org/10.1016/j.ogc.2023.11.007
0889-8545/24/© 2023 Elsevier Inc. All rights reserved.

obgyn.theclinics.com

According to the 2020 Census data, there are 62.1 million Latinx people living in the United States, which represents a 23% increase from the 2010 census. According to the Pew Research Center, there was a significant undercount of the Latinx community due to the coronavirus pandemic as well as the fact that this group may be historically less likely to complete census forms due to feelings of distrust of the government.[3] However, more recent data have demonstrated growth in states that did not have a historically large Latinx population.[4] The Latinx community grew in every region of the United States but most significantly in South and Midwest,[3] for which the South saw a 57% increase in its Latinx population.[4] This group now comprises the second largest racial/ethnic group behind non-Hispanic Whites.[5] **Figs. 1** and **2** demonstrate the incredible diversity of this community.

Purpose of the Article

Although health disparities affect all people of color, the focus of this article is primarily on Latinx communities with respect to obstetrics and gynecology (OB/GYN) care. In order to best serve this community and address racial health disparities, it is critical to gain a deeper sociocultural awareness. We will first review cultural considerations and barriers to care to gain a deeper understanding of cultural context. We will then explore how these differences can affect OB/GYN care. We will discuss reproductive health issues, strategies to improve OB/GYN care, best practices, and future directions for this very diverse and prolific community that deserves quality care despite perceived cultural differences, language, and socioeconomic barriers.

CULTURAL CONSIDERATIONS IN LATINX COMMUNITIES
Understanding Cultural Beliefs, Values, and Traditions

Although it is important to avoid broad categorizations among this large and diverse community, there are some common shared beliefs and practices that should be acknowledged. Research has indicated that Latinx communities may share some

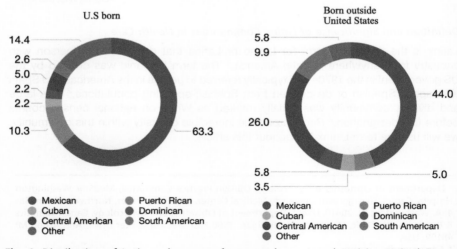

Fig. 1. Distribution of Latinx subgroups of women, by maternal nativity: United States, 2021. (*Adapted from* Driscoll AK. Maternal characteristics and infant outcomes by Hispanic subgroup and nativity: United States, 2021. National Vital Statistics Reports; vol 72 no 2. Hyattsville, MD: National Center for Health Statistics. 2023. DOI: https://dx.doi.org/10.15620/cdc:122515.)

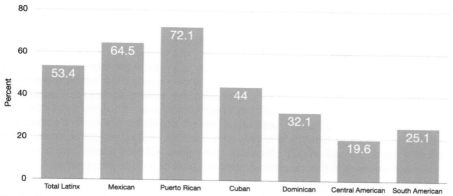

Fig. 2. Percentage of women born in the United States, by Latinx subgroup: United States, 2021. (*Adapted from* Driscoll AK. Maternal characteristics and infant outcomes by Hispanic subgroup and nativity: United States, 2021. National Vital Statistics Reports; vol 72 no 2. Hyattsville, MD: National Center for Health Statistics. 2023. DOI: https://dx.doi.org/10. 15620/cdc:122515.)

major values that include (but are not limited to): *familismo*, *respeto*, and *fatalismo*.[6–8] These values may play a critical role in the way an individual perceives the health-care system and engages within it.

Familismo refers to the importance of the family unit. Decision-making, therefore, becomes a collective one and is not just the sole responsibility of the patient. This is incredibly relevant in health care because this dynamic may be confusing or perceived as a hindrance by providers who may not understand the expectation of family involvement in medical decision-making. The sense of family belonging and consultation is very strong, and hierarchy within the family setting is prevalent. Although there have been some shifts concerning American acculturation, this family dynamic may be common among many new immigrants.[6,7] The father or oldest man in the family may hold the greatest power and may be designated to make the health decisions for the family.[6,7]

Respeto involves placing a high value on persons perceived to be of greater authority. In Latin American cultures, there may be an appreciation for and respect of status differences compared with American culture in which individuals may interact more informally.[6] Health-care providers, for instance, are seen as authority figures and respeto is expected in all encounters.[6,7] Many traditional cultures will not appreciate informality despite the best intentions.[6]

Fatalismo is described as a belief that life is uncertain and an individual can do little to affect the future.[6,7] This leads to the belief that one can do little to control their own health, which can translate to delayed preventive screening and treatment until symptoms become severe.[6] This cultural belief—in which uncertainty is not only tolerated but accepted—could translate to more relaxed attitudes about time and tardiness being viewed as a socially acceptable behavior.[6] Health-care providers can see this as being disrespectful of their time and can lead to miscommunication. If this leads to a hurried visit, patients could perceive it as disrespectful. Church and religious faith are also a large part of Latinx communities because they may provide sources of hope and strength.[7] This may also explain some of the *fatalismo* regarding perceptions of God's will or divine punishment.[7] There are many illnesses for which people may seek care and advice from folk healers, for which a patient may perceive disease as being attributed to an imbalance between the person and their environment.[8] Folk healers, known as *curanderos*, are lay healers that use home remedies to treat various pathologic conditions. Some examples include a *yerbatero* (herbalist), *sobador* (massage therapist) and *partera* (midwife who can also treat children).[8] **Fig. 3** outlines some common cultural beliefs and remedies.

Developing trust among the Latinx community is a critical component to providing quality care.[9] Providers must be intentional about developing trust, which is based on an understanding of cultural differences. Furthermore, several studies have suggested that the dissemination of community health workers who are from the same community, speak the same language, and share similar beliefs as the patient population could be beneficial to facilitating health care and discussions on culturally sensitive topics.[8] Embracing certain cultural beliefs and values will help health-care providers to promote wellness in this community with the goal of reducing disparities.

Language and Communication Barriers

According to the Pew Research Center in 2013, 6 in 10 US adults in the Latinx community speak English or are bilingual.[10] However, language barriers can pose challenges to quality of health care, patient safety, and patient/provider satisfaction.[11] Although Spanish is the primary language of many Latinx communities, reading and writing are not always a common means of communication among those from lower socioeconomic backgrounds.[7] Patients and families with limited English proficiency can face barriers to care, experience a lower quality of care, and subsequently have poorer health outcomes.[12] Having access to translators—whether in person or virtually—can greatly facilitate communication for both providers and patients.[11] It is also mandated by federal and state regulations.[11,13] However, translator use can also increase the length of health-care visits. Given universal staffing shortages and pressures on providers to manage increasing patient volume, this can create challenges for patients who may have to wait longer times and for providers who feel like they are unable to provide care in a timely fashion. Using family members for translation should be avoided due to potential bias or inaccurate translation of medical terminology. Using providers as translators is also not ideal because interpreters must remain neutral in direct patient care.[14] In the absence of medically approved language

Illness	Definition	Belief
Mal de Ojo	The "Evil Eye" that may affect infants or women	It is caused by a person with a "strong eye" (especially green or blue) looking with admiration or jealousy at another person. Mal de Ojo is avoided by touching an infant when admiring or complimenting them.
Nerviosimo	"Sickness of the nerves"	Is common and may be treated spiritually and/or medicinally
Pasmo	Paralysis or paresis of extremities or face	Is treated with massage
Susto	Fright resulting in "soul loss"	Susto may be acute or chronic and includes a variety of vague complaints, woman are are affected more than men
Antojos	Cravings in a pregnant woman	Failure to satisfy the cravings may lead to injury to the baby, including genetic defects
Ataque de nervios	Episodic, dramatic outbursts of negative emotion	Usually in response to a current stressor
Bilis	Thought to be bile flowing into the blood stream after a traumatic event	With the end result of nervousness
Caida de la mollera	Presence of a sunken fontanelle in an infant	Is explained to occur as a result of a bump or fall to the head of the infant, or due to quickly taking a baby away from the breast during breastfeeding
Empacho	Intestinal obstruction and is characterized by abdominal pain, vomiting, constipation, anorexia, or gas and bloating	Post-partum women and infants and children pain are most susceptible

Fig. 3. Folk illness in Latinx community. (Medina, Claudia, MD, MHA, MPH. Beliefs and Traditions that impact the Latino Healthcare. Delta Region AETC. Accessed June 17, 2023.)

translators, some health-care organizations use online translation platforms such as Google Translate or MediBabble to address these language challenges because they are free, easy to access, and have increased patient satisfaction.[11]

HEALTH DISPARITIES IN LATINX COMMUNITIES
Disparities in Access to Health-Care Services

The health of a population is affected by both social and economic factors.[15] Among Latinx communities, language and cultural barriers, access to health care, higher likelihood of being uninsured, and higher levels of poverty (particularly among recent immigrants) can lead to disparate outcomes.[16] Lower average income and educational attainment can present obstacles and can be prohibitive to quality health care. Inability to navigate a complex health system and lack of health insurance are important barriers to receiving adequate health care. Recent immigration status can affect access to health care along with degree of acculturation and English language proficiency.[15,16] In 2020, the US Census Bureau reported that 17% of Hispanics in comparison to 8.2% of non-Hispanic Whites were living at the poverty level.[17] All of these socioeconomic factors contribute to health-care access in Latinx communities and can increase disparities. The Pew Research Center surveyed this population as to their beliefs about factors contributing to health risks, with data demonstrating concern for job-related health risk, less access to quality medical care, and language barriers being the areas of major concern.[16]

Health insurance is a huge component of access. It is not typically offered in jobs that recent immigrants may obtain, differing from US-born Latinx people.[15] Before the implementation of the Affordable Care Act in 2010, more in the Latinx community were uninsured (approximately 33% in 2010 vs 20% in 2019).[18] However, several states have reversed some elements of Medicaid expansion following the onset of the coronavirus disease 2019 (COVID-19) pandemic. This will likely affect Latinx communities by potentially increasing uninsured rates. Inability to obtain insurance coverage through an employer may make accessing health care unaffordable, for which people may subsequently forgo much needed care. Limits on new immigrants' eligibility for Medicaid and the time limits can be confusing and difficult to navigate.[15] According to the 2019 Census bureau statistics for educational attainment, Hispanics were lower in comparison to non-Hispanic Whites in high school diploma, bachelor's degree, and graduate or advanced professional degrees.[19–21] They were also the highest in uninsured rates of any racial or ethnic group.[20]

Higher Rate of Medical Comorbidities

The existence of prior health conditions was also an important factor to the survey population by the Pew Research Center.[16] Health conditions that can lead to significant medical sequelae including obesity, hypertension, and diabetes. According to 2019 data from the Centers for Disease Control and Prevention (CDC), some of the leading causes of death among Hispanics included cancer, heart disease, unintentional injuries (accidents), stroke and other cerebrovascular diseases, diabetes, and Alzheimer disease.[18,22] In 2020, the leading cause of death among Hispanics was COVID-19, with preexisting medical conditions likely playing a role in increased mortality.[18] Some other causes of mortality that significantly affect Hispanics include chronic lower respiratory diseases (including asthma and chronic obstructive pulmonary disease), liver disease, influenza and pneumonia, suicide, and kidney disease.[19] Preventing and/or addressing chronic disease requires access to preventive medical care visits. As previously mentioned, there are numerous barriers in the form of language, cultural differences, and insurance coverage.

Importance of Cultural Awareness and Sensitivity in Obstetrics and Gynecology Care

In regard to general medical care, Roncoroni and colleagues found that providers were rated higher in competence than in respect and sensitivity.[23] This is important when addressing care in the context of sociocultural values and beliefs. Given the sensitive nature of the care that is provided in OB/GYN, cultural awareness is essential. This involves understanding cultural norms for which the provider may not be innately familiar, addressing language barriers for improved communication, and providing sensitive care during physical examinations that can be very invasive. Patient-centered culturally sensitive health care has been reviewed as best practice toward to eliminating disparities.[23] This involves cultural awareness training for providers to understand when adaptions may be warranted and needed for patient satisfaction and adherence to medical treatments. Latinx communities value provider sensitivity because they already have high respect for those in authority and wish for more time and appropriate care. The American College of Obstetricians and Gynecologist (ACOG) prefers to address cultural respect versus competency given culture is not a skill to master but rather a provider recognizing their own limitations about a patient circumstance, avoiding generalizations based on a culture, being aware of patient and provider biases, and being respectful through patient-centered communication.[24]

OBSTETRIC CARE IN LATINX COMMUNITIES

Preconception and prenatal care is care before and during a pregnancy. According to the 2018 Latina Maternal & Child Health Review, access to maternal health-care services is low, with lack of insurance being a major contributor.[19,25] Social determinants of health—income, education, health-care access, health literacy, and acculturation—all play a part in maternal health. Latinx people can have complications in the pregnancy because of preexisting conditions. Preventive care is best if used to optimize health before pregnancy to decrease risks during pregnancy and delivery. Preconception counseling may facilitate optimization of health, risk assessment, and intervention before a pregnancy.

Gestational Diabetes

Gestational diabetes mellitus (GDM) is an example of a common disorder of pregnancy that can have significant short-term and long-term implications. Although some studies demonstrate increasing trends overall of GDM across races and ethnicities, some data suggest that Hispanic people may be at an increased risk.[26,27] One cross-sectional analysis using National Center for Health statistics data to evaluate gestational diabetes trends by race and ethnicity from 2011 to 2019 found that although Indian Asian people demonstrated the highest risk (2019 gestational diabetes rate = 129.1 per 1000 live births), Hispanic people had a 2019 gestational diabetes rate of 66.6 (95% CI, 65.6–67.7; RR, 1.15 [95% CI, 1.13–1.18]).[28] This is elevated compared with non-Hispanic Blacks and non-Hispanic Whites (2019 gestational diabetes rate, 55.7 [95% CI, 54.5–57.0]; RR, 0.97 [95% CI, 0.94–0.99], and 2019 gestational diabetes rate, 57.7 [95% CI, 57.2–58.3], respectively).[28] Within the Hispanic community, the rate was highest among Puerto Rican individuals (2019 gestational diabetes rate, 75.8 [95% CI, 71.8–79.9]; RR, 1.31 [95% CI, 1.24–1.39]).[28]

This disorder can be associated with various maternal and fetal complications.[29] Several studies have demonstrated an increased risk of macrosomia among Hispanic birthing people compared with other racial groups with GDM.[30,31] Fetal macrosomia can increase the risk of fetal nerve injury. Some data also suggest that there may be an increased risk of brachial plexus birth injury as a result among infants delivered from Hispanic birthing people.[32,33] There may also be an increased risk of cesarean section. A retrospective analysis using data from the National Inpatient Sample database evaluated 932,431 deliveries complicated by GDM from 2000 to 2015.[34] Among the total study population, 26.7% were Hispanic people (compared with 44.5% White and 14.0% Black). Irrespective of race, cesarean section rates were highest among those who had private insurance (White OR = 1.21 [1.17–1.25], Black OR = 1.33 [1.26–1.41], and Hispanic OR = 1.12 [1.06–1.18]).[34] Those undergoing cesarean section were also less likely to experience postpartum hemorrhage compared with vaginal delivery (OR = 0.67 [0.63–0.71]).[34] Other data also suggest higher rates of postpartum hemorrhage in general with increasing rates of GDM.[35]

Furthermore, the long-term implications of GDM can also be significant. Data suggest that those with GDM have an increased risk of developing type 2 diabetes later in life (up to 70% increased risk within 22–28 years after pregnancy).[36–38] One study from 1995 demonstrated a diabetes cumulative incidence of 47% among Latinx people 5 years after a pregnancy complicated by gestational diabetes.[39] A more recent probability sample and community-based cohort study evaluated patients self-identifying as Hispanic/Latino from 18 to 74 year old in 4 major US cities.[40] Those participants with a history of GDM in a prior pregnancy were 4 times more likely to have prevalent diabetes compared with those without a history (adjusted OR [aOR] = 3.94, 95% CI 2.75–5.64), even after adjusting for various factors such as sociodemographics and cardiovascular risk.[40] The study also identified that people with a history of GDM who were of Cuban or Puerto Rican ancestry were significantly more likely to have incident diabetes compared with people of Mexican ancestry (aOR = 2.15, 95% CI 1.17–3.95; aOR = 1.95, 95% CI 1.07–3.55, respectively).[40] This has significant implications on how Latinx people should be counseled and monitored during pregnancy but also necessitates enhanced preventive care interventions after pregnancy due to the potential morbidity and mortality related to diabetes.

Preeclampsia

Although birthing people can develop preeclampsia independently, those with GDM have a higher risk of developing preeclampsia.[29] Regarding preeclampsia among Latinx communities, the data are conflicting, with some research suggesting an increased risk[41] and other data showing lower (or equal) risk compared with non-Hispanic White people.[42,43] One cross-sectional analysis from the Boston Birth Cohort demonstrated that non-Hispanic Black people had higher rates of chronic hypertension, obesity, and preeclampsia compared with Hispanic and non-Hispanic White people. Although nativity and duration of residence in the United States were associated with lower likelihood of preeclampsia in Black patients, this trend was not seen in Hispanic patients (aOR = 1.07 [95% CI, 0.72–1.60] and aOR <10 years = 1.04 [95% CI, 0.67–1.59], respectively).[44] Another retrospective cohort study using 2007 to 2018 data from the CDC natality database demonstrated that although non-Hispanic Black people had the highest prevalence of hypertensive disorders of pregnancy and Hispanic people consistently had the lowest rates, Hispanic people demonstrated the greatest increase in prevalence over time compared with Black and White people (OR 2.23, 95% CI 2.2–2.26, P<.001).[45] This same trend was observed with chronic hypertension among Hispanic people.[45]

Maternal Mortality

Maternal mortality represents a huge issue in the United States and has recently garnered significant attention from both the medical community and the media. Of all racial groups, Black birthing people have demonstrated the highest maternal mortality compared with all other racial and ethnic groups. Although there are still persistent disparities in prenatal care and outcomes for Latinx communities, mortality data in this population is more favorable compared with other races.[46] The CDC estimated that maternal mortality rates from 2018 in the United States were 11.8 per 100,000 live births for Hispanic people (compared with 37.3 for non-Hispanic Blacks and 13.9 for non-Hispanic Whites per 100,000).[47] However, more recent data from 2020 from the CDC demonstrate that this rate increased to 18.2 per 100,000 live births among Hispanics.[47] The reason for this increase is unclear, although it may speak to a larger universal trend of worse maternity outcomes among all people of color.

Cultural Considerations in Labor and Delivery/Postpartum

Awareness of cultural beliefs can be helpful during labor and postpartum periods for providers. It is important to remember that beliefs can vary within this population. For instance, a belief that is held by someone from rural Mexico may differ from someone from urban Mexico. Maternidad Latina reviewed some pregnancy beliefs that can be helpful.[48] Pregnancy is considered a normal life event and not an illness.[48] As such, women may seek care later in the pregnancy.[48] Some women will visit a partera (unlicensed midwife) with pregnancy complications, such as if a baby is breech or at the time of labor.[48] Many fear epidurals and perceive them as life threatening. As such, some among the Latinx community may labor with the intention of having an unmedicated vaginal delivery.[48] Many Latinx individuals will observe the cuarentena— 40 days of rest and recuperation after birth. As a result, postpartum visits may be missed.[48] All of these beliefs are important to better understand and provide optimal care to this community.

Social Determinants of Health in Obstetrics

The concern is that given preexisting conditions (hypertension, obesity, and diabetes), postpartum maternal health has implications across the life course.[49] Nativity is an important factor as well. As characterized by a concept referred to as the "Latina paradox," despite worse health-care access and other social disadvantages, foreign-born Latinx individuals may have better health outcomes. It is thought that some of the cultural beliefs and values previously reviewed contribute to this phenomenon and are protective.[50,51] However, when people from the Latinx global community acculturate to the United States, data suggest that they may have poorer outcomes.[46] Barriers to prenatal care in the Latinx community have included lack of childcare, inadequate access to transportation, language barriers, work constraints, and health literacy.[25]

Another social determinant of health may be related to weathering regarding citizenship barriers. Stress and immigration status can affect early prenatal care initiation. US-born Latinx birthing people were more likely than their non-US-born counterparts to get prenatal care in the first trimester.[5] Gutierrez and colleagues reported that rates of preterm birth and low birth weight infants increased during the Trump administration, given possible chronic stress among Latinx birthing people, particularly due to targeting of people from Mexico and Central America during that time.[52]

Ultimately, prenatal care can reduce adverse downstream fetal and maternal outcomes. Higher risk pregnancies require closer monitoring, more frequent visits, and increased high-risk obstetric consultation to maintain health of the patient. Having access to critical care obstetrics is essential for maternal and child health. This is particularly crucial in rural and frontier areas in decreasing morbidity and mortality of birthing people.[53] Early prenatal care is important for reasons reviewed but also for review of genetic testing options offered early on in pregnancy. Garza and colleagues found that immigrant Latinx people desired this option of testing and were perhaps mostly limited by early access to prenatal care given intermittent insurance coverage and gaps.[25,51] Many states offer Medicaid once a person is pregnant but many may have challenges in access, language barriers, and navigating a complicated health system.

GYNECOLOGIC CARE IN LATINX COMMUNITIES

Quality, compassionate, and culturally sensitive gynecologic care is critical for the Latinx community. It is important for the provider to recognize disparities that exist as well as cultural nuances that may affect care. Although this section is not meant to serve as an exhaustive review of all gynecologic conditions affecting the Latinx community, we will focus on several key topics.

Cervical Cancer Screening

Pap smears represent a highly specific screening tool for cervical dysplasia and cancer. Cotesting for human papillomavirus further increases the sensitivity of this intervention. However, barriers such as limited access due to insurance coverage can have serious sequelae such as delayed diagnosis and resulting treatment challenges. The CDC reports that Latinx people are less likely to be screened for cervical cancer than non-Hispanic Whites.[54] Some studies cite various possible contributing factors, such as fear, embarrassment, pain, gender of the physician, insensitivity to patient needs, fatalism, and cost.[55,56] Language barriers and lack of knowledge are additional potential barriers.[57] One study by Rauh-Hain and colleagues found that there are significant racial disparities with both Latinx and Black communities in evidence-based care with gynecologic cancers as a whole, which leads to greater mortality in these communities.[58] Specifically, Latinx communities have the highest rate of cervical cancer compared with people of other racial and ethnic groups in the United States. In 2020, the CDC estimated a cervical cancer rate of 8.4 per 100,000 people among Hispanics (compared with non-Hispanic White and non-Hispanic Black at 6.5 and 7.3, respectively).[59] The high incidence of cervical cancer among Hispanics is only comparable to those of the American Indian/Alaskan Native community, who are also disproportionately affected by this disease.[59]

As a result, outreach programs have been initiated to promote cervical cancer screening and prevention among Latinx communities. AMIGAS (which stands for *Ayudando a las Mujeres con Información, Guía y Amor para su Salud*) is a bilingual education program launched by the CDC aimed at promoting cervical cancer awareness and screening among the Latinx community. Through the utilization of community health workers, AMIGAS has demonstrated an up to 33% increase in cervical cancer screening in areas of implementation.[54] There is a need for more culturally tailored, language-concordant community-based programs to improve awareness, access, and service utilization in this community.

Abnormal Uterine Bleeding

Abnormal uterine bleeding (AUB) is a common symptom that can present at any age in life and can affect quality of life, constituting 18% of all gynecologic visits in the United States.[60] The prevalence of AUB among the Latinx community is unclear. One descriptive cross-sectional analysis evaluating AUB among a medically underserved community in New York demonstrated that the highest minority group in this cohort was Hispanic and that the most common cause of AUB was due to leiomyoma.[61]

Although etiology of some AUB is benign, symptoms have the potential to significantly affect the quality of life.

In addition to optimizing quality of life, it is critical for OB/GYN providers to differentiate benign AUB from precancerous or malignant pathologic condition. According to the American Cancer Society, approximately 66,200 new cases of endometrial cancer will be diagnosed in 2023, resulting in 13,030 deaths.[62] One study used data from the United States Cancer Statistics database and the Behavioral Risk Factors Surveillance System survey from 2001 to 2018 to further characterize rates of endometrial cancer among Hispanics. Results demonstrated that in 2018, Hispanic people aged 35 to 39 years had the highest rate of endometrial cancer among those of reproductive age at 13.9 per 100,000 (compared with non-Hispanic White people at 9.3 per 100,000). This represented a 49% higher incidence, with Hispanic people demonstrating the highest interval annual increases of endometrial cancer.[63] It is hypothesized that a major contributor to this disparity is the increasing incidence of obesity, which is a known risk factor for endometrial cancer. Hispanic people from the aforementioned study had a 30.1% obesity rate in 2018, with a 1.4% demonstrated annual increase.[63] Another analysis demonstrated a global increase in uterine cancer mortality rates from 1997 to 2018. However, the most rapid increase in mortality rate was observed among non-Hispanic Black and Hispanic people aged 30 to 39 years (3.3% and 3.8%, respectively) compared with non-Hispanic White people (2.2%).[64] Other studies similarly demonstrate increasing endometrial cancer mortality among Hispanic people.[65,66]

These disparities are alarming. Social determinants of health—such as access to care, language barriers, and cultural differences—can all influence the delivery of timely and appropriate care and treatment. Providers should be aware of these disparities and maintain a heightened awareness when Latinx patients present with AUB. There must be recognition of cultural considerations, recognizing that some Latinx people may turn to medicinal treatments to address AUB.[67] Although there should be sensitivity toward cultural preferences, it is imperative that OB/GYN providers engage in shared decision-making with patients to rule out malignancy given the increasing endometrial cancer trends. In definitively treating AUB, some studies have found racial disparities in route of hysterectomy, with Latinx people undergoing more open surgery versus minimally invasive methods.[68–70] Practitioners must evaluate factors affecting disparate care and how these can be mitigated.

Sexual Health Education and Sexually Transmitted Infection Prevention

Sexually transmitted infections (STIs) can have a significant influence on overall health as well as reproductive health. The CDC has recommended universal screening in sexually active people aged younger than 25 years, as well as older people who may be at increased risk or who are pregnant. Human immunodeficiency virus (HIV) testing should also be offered to those who present for STI testing and to all people aged 13 to 64 years on an opt-out basis.[71] In 2018, the CDC reported that Latinx people accounted for 27% of all new HIV diagnoses.[48,72] Rates of other STIs are also higher among the Latinx community compared with non-Hispanic Whites.[48]

This reinforces the fact that sexual health education and prevention are essential because these can have serious consequences and sequelae. Some concerns surrounding perinatal HIV testing among Latinx birthing people included fear of a positive diagnosis and possible associated social isolation, although these concerns may not necessarily impede testing.[73] A study of an immigrant Latinx group in southeastern United States revealed lack of knowledge about sexual health, along with shame and embarrassment related to clinical examinations and discussions about sex.[74]

Despite the pervasive stigma of STIs, early and adequate sexual health education is essential for prevention.[75–77] Another study found that implementation of culturally sensitive education sessions addressing a range of sexual health topics was beneficial to ethnically and racially diverse participants, highlighting a particular need for recent Latinx immigrants as they navigate new systems and policies.[74] It is essential for providers to discuss STI screening and prevention with patients from the Latinx community.

Contraceptive Options and Usage Patterns

Access to contraception is important for the prevention of unintended pregnancy. It is also at the core of the reproductive justice framework for care. Latinx people are less likely to use contraception than White people, with greater than 50% of pregnancies being unintended.[25,78] Cost is a known barrier.[78] Long-acting reversible methods, such as intrauterine device and implants, have higher upfront costs. However, removing these cost barriers could be highly effective in increasing reproductive autonomy among this community.[78] Increasing access to health insurance can increase likelihood of access to comprehensive family planning options.[78]

In understanding reproductive justice, it is important for providers to acknowledge the historical legacy of abuse and medical mistreatment of people of color in the United States that may influence their current perceptions and medical decision-making. The enslavement of Black individuals in the United States was deeply linked to racism and the disregard for the value of Black bodily autonomy. As such, Black enslaved people were often the focus of medical experimentation. Nearly 70,000 people were sterilized in more than 30 states throughout the twentieth century—with Black, Latinx, and Native American people being specifically targeted and many sterilized without their consent.[72] Another example includes birth control trials performed in Puerto Rico in the 1950s that were criticized as being exploitative and experimental.[79] These atrocities have led to medical distrust among these communities.[72,80] Furthermore, some of these unethical practices perpetrated against people of color are still occurring in modern times. In 2020, allegations of numerous involuntary hysterectomies being performed on detained immigrant people raised awareness of the persistence of racism and ethical misconduct among the gynecologic community.[72] Understanding the historical context facilitates improved shared decision-making with patients and represents an essential component in contraceptive counseling.

STRATEGIES TO IMPROVE OBSTETRICS AND GYNECOLOGY CARE IN LATINX COMMUNITIES
Enhancing Cultural Awareness Among Health-Care Providers

Although it is important to acknowledge social determinants of health, it is equally important to recognize that the causes of these racial and ethnic disparities are deeply rooted in systemic racism.[81] ACOG in conjunction with multiple other societies released a joint statement in August 2020 addressing racism within the profession of OB/GYN.[82] This statement acknowledged bias and racism within the history of the profession, and promised to promote better health care through education and improve delivery of women's health care.[82] The patient-centered care model has been shown to be effective in training health-care teams about delivery of respectful and responsive care across different cultural communities.[83] Being able to identify cultural barriers and respond appropriately to cultural cues without stereotyping is important to quality patient care.[83]

One study used the Healthcare Provider Cultural Competence Instrument to measure 5 dimensions of cultural competence in an OB/GYN department using a presurvey and postsurvey instrument following grand rounds presentation.[84] The 5 dimensions included awareness/sensitivity, behavior, patient-centered communication, practice orientation, and self-assessment.[84] This study demonstrated improvement in levels of awareness across the entire health-care team.[84] Exploring one's own beliefs and biases is essential to providing fair, safe, and evidenced-based medical care. Effective communication, trust building, and improved patient–provider relationships can help to build opportunities for better health.[85] This can be accomplished through interventions such as implicit bias training, cultural sensitivity training, and routine presentations on racial health disparities to spark self-reflection and discussion among team members. OB/GYN departments must also constantly reassess their commitment and impact about addressing racial health disparities.

Promoting Access to Interpretation Services

Effective communication is essential for providing quality health care. As previously discussed, language could present a barrier to care for some in the Latinx community. The Centers for Medicare and Medicaid Services (CMS) have a step-by-step guide to setting up a language access plan that includes a needs assessment, language services, notices, training, and evaluation as outlined in later discussion.[86] This allows organizations to better understand how to access necessary language services and use for best care practices.[86] It is also recommended that hospital systems make a strong commitment to ensuring that translation services (either in-person or virtually) is universally available. This must be implemented not only at the level of direct patient–physician interaction but also at the level of scheduling, nursing care, and case management.

Community Engagement, Collaborations, and Outreach Programs

Having culture-concordant and/or language-concordant community health workers (CHWs) can be a helpful resource.[87] However, some data suggest that poor confidentiality and trust concerns may cause patients to be guarded with CHWs in their community.[87] Nonetheless, CHWs could serve as a tool to bridge the language and cultural gap. Adequate training, support, and supervision are required.[87] CHWs would also be helpful to providers in explaining different cultural beliefs and practices among the Latinx community that could affect care.

Similarly, community-based doula programs have been shown to be beneficial in perinatal outcomes in racial and ethnic minority communities.[88] Doulas are trusted individuals often from the local community who are trained to provide emotional, psychosocial, and educational support during pregnancy, childbirth, and the postpartum period.[88,89] Access to this service for lower socioeconomic groups may be limited but one study did demonstrate some improvements in persistent inequities with access to free doula support.[90] Midwives also provide reproductive health care and attend births in the home, at birthing centers, and at hospitals. Although some states have limitations to the scope of midwifery care, the positive impact of midwifery on maternity outcomes is well documented.[91,92] There is less evidence of success of midwifery on reducing racial inequities but more data on this area is warranted.[88]

Other community partnerships, such as free-standing birthing centers, have been shown to develop trust within their catchment neighborhoods and may be effective alternatives for some patients.[88] The great majority of these centers, however, are not led by people of color. Limited access may also pose a barrier to care.[88] Other models such as group prenatal care have demonstrated benefit and allow for individualized care along with group-facilitated discussions on multiple prenatal topics.[93] One particular cohort study demonstrated the positive influence of group prenatal care for Hispanic people by increased rates of breastfeeding and greater completion of postpartum diabetes screening, suggesting improved outcomes with this intervention.[94] This model also allows for the development of social support and can be tailored to different cultural backgrounds for increased understanding. These groups can facilitate enhanced knowledge and education among patients on variety of topics such as pregnancy symptoms and breastfeeding. In addition, pregnancy medical homes provide comprehensive perinatal health care to include behavioral health and social needs.[88] The National Partnership for Women & Families has called attention to the increased maternal morbidity and mortality during the COVID-19 pandemic and has recommended increasing funding and access for clinical-based and policy-based interventions.[95]

Policy Implications for Addressing Health Disparities

Policy and legislation plays a significant role in OB/GYN care and subsequent outcomes for Latinx communities. In June of 2022, the Biden administration released the Blueprint for Addressing the Maternal Health Crisis. This document outlined goals of increasing access to and coverage of comprehensive high-quality maternal health services by strengthening economic and social supports before, during, and after pregnancy. It also included components of behavioral health services, as well as expanding and diversifying the perinatal workforce.[96] Several federal agencies have plans and actions to support this Blueprint including the CMS, the Health Resources and Services Administration, and the Office of the Assistant Secretary.[81] Each of these organizations have committed to strengthening maternal and child health, and reducing pregnancy-related deaths that disproportionately affect people of color.[81]

Furthermore, Medicaid expansion was implemented in 2014 and has implications for increased service provision for underserved communities. The Kaiser Family Foundation found that the continuous enrollment provision that was adopted during the COVID-19 pandemic increased Medicaid enrollment, with the rate of uninsured individuals dropping as a result.[97] However, this continuous enrollment provision ended March 31, 2023, for which millions of people have been expected to lose Medicaid and face barriers to obtaining health insurance without the Medicaid expansion.[81,97] Ten states (primarily in the south) have not applied for this expanded Medicaid coverage.[97] Medical eligibility for adults is low in regions where programs have no expanded, with the largest coverage gaps in Texas, Florida, and Georgia.[97] Unfortunately, this coverage gap primarily influences people of color.[97]

In particular, due to the high rates of maternal mortality in the United States, healthcare coverage during pregnancy and in the postpartum period is critical. This is particularly relevant for underserved communities as Medicaid covers almost half of births nationally.[81] Historically, many patients would be at risk of loosing their coverage after 60 days postpartum due to Medicaid instability. However, more recently, states that implemented Medicaid expansion have received temporary fiscal incentives under the American Rescue Plan Act passed in 2021. This allows extended postpartum coverage to a full year.[81,97] Federal legislation has expanded access and helped stabilize Medicaid coverage during the postpartum period.[81] Federal and state legislation are imperative for assisting with health-care coverage for those who are uninsured, particularly people of color who are at an increased risk of maternal mortality.

Reproductive Justice

The Kaiser Family Foundation reviewed that when seeking reproductive health care, multiple factors could create barriers to access. This included cultural and social determinants of health, insurance coverage, provider supply and distribution, sex education, and the political landscape concerning abortion.[98] One approach to addressing these challenges involves increasing the involvement of the larger family unit, including partners. Data demonstrate decreased understanding of contraception among male partners and suggests that broadening education efforts to partners (on issues ranging from sexual health to health screenings) are needed.[99,100]

Given the overturning of Roe v Wade and different state legislative efforts to restrict abortion, worsening disparities in maternal and infant health for people of color are expected. One study reviewed effects following the Texas (HB2) law and demonstrated a disproportionate reduction in the abortion rate for Latinx people, with clinic closures and long travel distances to access care emerging as key barriers.[101] Restrictive policies place already disadvantaged groups at a greater risk for potentially worse outcomes.[101] Continued research is essential to assess the scope of this issue moving forward, particularly given the downstream maternal mortality impact on communities of color. Legislation that is developed and implemented with a reproductive justice lens is critical to providing ethical and antiracist care to minority groups, including the Latinx community.

Promoting Diversity and Inclusivity in the Obstetrics and Gynecology Work Force

According to the Pew Research Center only about 7% of all physicians are Hispanic and only 9% of all health-care practitioners are Hispanic.[5] The Biden Administration's Blueprint includes efforts to increase scholarships to students from underrepresented communities in health professions and nursing schools to diversify the workforce.[81,96] Research demonstrates improved patient outcomes with a more diverse health-care workforce.[81,88] Morgan and colleagues reviewed issues with recruiting, selecting, and supporting a diverse physician workforce that can be applicable across underrepresented backgrounds in health care.[102] Some of those proposals included addressing racial differences in assessments and grading, having intentional curriculum development pertaining to OB/GYN inequities, holistic review implementation in residency program priorities, unconscious and implicit bias training for health-care providers at all levels, increased number of faculty of color in interview and ranking committees, universal virtual interviews, and intentional support through mentorship and residency learning communities.[102]

Although it should not be assumed that Spanish language fluency is universal among all Latinx individuals, there is an increasing need for language-congruent providers with a growing Latinx community in the United States. Although data suggest that patients would prioritize access to quality, affordable health care irrespective of language proficiency of providers,[5] preference for Spanish-speaking providers is becoming more widespread and underscores the need for more multilingual health-care workers.

SUMMARY

Although the Latinx community is richly diverse, there are some shared cultural beliefs, practices, and values for which OB/GYN providers should be aware. These cultural considerations could have implications on care, treatment, and overall health outcomes. Providers should practice cultural sensitivity when navigating clinical scenarios that may be affected by cultural differences. Language may also represent barrier to care for some patients and should be addressed through increased availability of interpreter services. Linkages to community-based programs should also be considered to provide more cultural-concordant and language-concordant care. The Latinx community represents the largest minority group in the United States that has the highest likelihood of being uninsured. Lack of health insurance coverage presents a huge barrier to adequate and timely OB/GYN care. There is a need for enhanced legislation that addresses the needs of this community and allows for expanded coverage for OB/GYN care. Policy implications for addressing health disparities are imperative. Addressing social and economic factors that contribute to poorer health outcomes, the role of racism and discrimination within the health-care system, and diversifying the health-care workforce are also elements needed to improve health and advance equity among Latinx communities. Despite these challenges, OB/GYN providers have the capacity to play a significant role in positive change. Health-care providers must recognize the needs in this community and address them through quality, culturally sensitive care, and advocacy.

CLINICS CARE POINTS

- Latinx communities represent the second largest racial group behind non-Hispanic Whites in the United States.
- Understanding cultural considerations in Latinx communities is essential to excellent care.
- Awareness of health disparities and reproductive health issues is important in addressing disease in Latinx communities.
- Strategies to improve OB/GYN care in Latinx communities include enhancing cultural awareness, addressing language barriers, and increasing community involvement.
- Policy reform could have implications that improve health in Latinx communities, particularly to ensure greater health insurance coverage.

DISCLOSURE

The authors have no disclosures.

REFERENCES

1. Manzano, Sonia, Huffpost, @latinovoices.
2. Campos, Antonio. What's the difference between Hispanic, Latino and Latinx? Universityofcalifornia.edu/news/choosing-the-right-word-hispanic-latino-and-latinx. Accessed June 17,2023.
3. Cohn D, Passel J. Key facts about the quality of the 2020 census. Available at: https://pewresearch.org/short-reads/2022/06/08/key-facts-about-the-quality-of-the-2020-census/. Accessed June 17, 2023.
4. Passel, Jeffery S. U.S. Hispanic population continued its geographic spread in the 2010s. https://pewrsr.ch/3J2802s. Accessed June 17, 2023.
5. U.S. Census. 2020 Decennial census, table PL 94–171: hispanic or Latino, and not hispanic or Latino by race. 2011. Available from: https://data.census.gov/cedsci/table?q=Hispanics%20in%20US%202020. Accessed June 17, 2023.
6. Carteret, Marcia, M. Ed., Cultural Values of Latino patients and families, Mar 15, 2011.
7. Medina C, Beliefs and Traditions that impact the Latino Healthcare. Available at: https://coursehero.com. Accessed June 17, 2023.
8. Available at: https://outreach-partners.org/blog-post/familismo-fatalismo-how-cultural-beliefs-affect-health-care/. Accessed June 17, 2023.
9. Moreira T, Hernandez DC, Scott CW, et al. Susto, Coraje, y Fatalismo: cultural-bound beliefs and the treatment of diabetes among socioeconomically disadvantaged hispanics. Am J Lifestyle Med 2018;12(1):30–3.

10. Available at: http://pewrsr.ch/1Hvx3jh. Accessed June 17, 2023.
11. Al Shamsi H, Almutairi AG, Al Mashrafi S, et al. Implications of language barriers for healthcare: a systematic review. Oman Med J 2020;35(2):e122.
12. Espinoza J, Derrington S. How Should Clinicians Respond to Language Barriers That Exacerbate Health Inequity? AMA J Ethics 2021;23(2):E109–16.
13. Chen AH, Youdelman MK, Brooks J. The legal framework for language access in healthcare settings: Title VI and beyond. J Gen Intern Med 2007;22(suppl 2): 362–7.
14. Language is not a barrier—it is an opportunity to improve health equity through education. Health Affairs Blog 2021. https://doi.org/10.1377/hblog20210726. 579549.
15. Escarce JJ and Kapur K. Access to and Quality of Health Care, In: Tienda M. and Mitchell F., *National research council (US) panel on Hispanics in the United States, Hispanics and the future of America*, 2006, National Academies Press (US); Washington (DC), 10, Available at: https://www.ncbi.nlm.nih.gov/books/NBK19910/. Accessed June 17, 2023.
16. Funk C, Hugo Lopez M. Hispanic Americans' experiences with health care, 2022 Available at: https://www.pewresearch.org/science/2022/06/14/hispanic-americans-experiences-with-health-care/. Accessed June 17, 2023.
17. Available at: census.gov/content/dam/Census/library/publications/2021/demo/p620-273.pdf. Accessed June 17, 2023.
18. Artiga S., Hill L., Damico A., Health coverage by race and ethnicity, 2010-2021, 12/20/2022 Available at: https://www.kff.org/racial-equity-and-health-policy/issue-brief/health-coverage-by-race-and-ethnicity/. Accessed June 17, 2023.
19. Available at: cdc.gov/nchs/fastats/ispanic-health.htm. Accessed June 17, 2023.
20. Available at: https://minority health.hhs.gov/omh/browse.aspx?lvl=3&lvlid=64, Accessed June 17, 2023.
21. Available at: census.gov.data/tables/2019/demo/ispanic-origin/2019-cps.html, Accessed June 17, 2023.
22. Available at: cdc.gov/vitalsigns/ispanic-health/, Accessed June 17, 2023.
23. Roncoroni J, Frank M, Hudson A, et al. Latinx Patients' Perceptions of Culturally Sensitive Health Care and their Association with Patient Satisfaction, Patient-Provider Communication, and Therapeutic Alliance. J Racial Ethn Health Disparities 2022 Apr;9(2):620–9. Epub 2021 Mar 15. PMID: 33721290.
24. Committee on Health Care for Underserved Women. Importance of social determinants of health and cultural awareness in the delivery of reproductive health care. ACOG Committee Opinion No. 729. American College of Obstetricians and Gynecologists. Obstet Gynecol 2018;131:e43–8.
25. Derige D., 2018 Latina maternal & child health review Available at: https://www.healthconnectone.org/wp-content/uploads/bsk-pdf-manager/2018_Latina_Maternal_and_Child_Health_Review. Accessed June 17, 2023.
26. Hedderson MM, Darbinian JA, Ferrara A. Disparities in the risk of gestational diabetes by race-ethnicity and country of birth. Paediatr Perinat Epidemiol 2010;24:441–8.
27. Lawrence JM, Contreras R, Chen W, et al. Trends in the prevalence of preexisting diabetes and gestational diabetes mellitus among a racially/ethnically diverse population of pregnant women, 1999-2005. Diabetes Care 2008;31:899–904.
28. Available at: https://jamanetwork.com/journals/jama/fullarticle/2783070. Accessed June 17, 2023.
29. Gestational diabetes mellitus. ACOG Practice Bulletin No. 190. American College of Obstetricians and Gynecologists. Obstet Gynecol 2018;131:e49–64.

30. Available at: https://pubmed.ncbi.nlm.nih.gov/8722067/#: ~ :text=Conclusions %3A%20We%20have%20demonstrated%20that,well%20as%20underlying%20genetic%20factors. Accessed June 17, 2023.
31. Available at: https://www.ncbi.nlm.nih.gov/pmc/articles/PMC7387181/. Accessed June 17, 2023.
32. Available at: https://pubmed.ncbi.nlm.nih.gov/37216973/. Accessed June 17, 2023.
33. Available at: https://pubmed.ncbi.nlm.nih.gov/32501916/. Accessed June 17, 2023.
34. Available at: https://www.ncbi.nlm.nih.gov/pmc/articles/PMC9585922/. Accessed June 17, 2023.
35. Available at: https://www.ncbi.nlm.nih.gov/pmc/articles/PMC10399637/. Accessed June 17, 2023.
36. England LJ, Dietz PM, Njoroge T, et al. Preventing type 2 diabetes: public health implications for women with a history of gestational diabetes mellitus. Am J Obstet Gynecol 2009;200(4):365, e1-e8.
37. O'Sullivan JB. Body weight and subsequent diabetes mellitus. JAMA 1982; 248(8):949–52.
38. Kim C, Newton KM, Knopp RH. Gestational diabetes and the incidence of type 2 diabetes: a systematic review. Diabetes Care 2002;25(10):1862–8.
39. Available at: https://pubmed.ncbi.nlm.nih.gov/7729620/. Accessed June 17, 2023.
40. Available at: https://www.ncbi.nlm.nih.gov/pmc/articles/PMC9664292/#R7). Accessed June 17, 2023.
41. Wolf M, Shah A, Jimenez-Kimble R, et al. Differential risk of hypertensive disorders of pregnancy among Hispanic women. J Am Soc Nephrol 2004;15(5): 1330–8.
42. Brown HL, Chireau MV, Jallah Y, et al. The "Hispanic paradox": an investigation of racial disparity in pregnancy outcomes at a tertiary care medical center. Am J Obstet Gynecol 2007;197(2):197, e1-e7.
43. Medina-Inojosa J, Jean N, Cortes-Bergoderi M, et al. The Hispanic paradox in cardiovascular disease and total mortality. Prog Cardiovasc Dis 2014;57(3):286–92.
44. Available at: https://jamanetwork.com/journals/jamanetworkopen/fullarticle/ 2787261#: ~ :text=Although%20some%20studies%20have%20found,women%20despite%20poorer%20socioeconomic%20profiles). Accessed June 17, 2023.
45. Available at: https://www.ncbi.nlm.nih.gov/pmc/articles/PMC7290488/). This same trend was observed with chronic hypertension among Hispanic people. Accessed June 17, 2023.
46. Richardson DM, Andrea SB, Ziring A, et al. Pregnancy Outcomes and Documentation Status Among Latina Women: A Systematic Review. Health Equity 2020;4(1):158–82.
47. Available at: https://www.cdc.gov/nchs/data/hestat/maternal-mortality/2020/ maternal-mortality-rates-2020.htm. Accessed June 17, 2023.
48. Available at: cdc.gov/nchhstp/healthdisparities/Hispanics.html, Accessed June 17, 2023.
49. McGlade MS, Saha S, Dahlstrom ME. The Latina paradox: an opportunity for restructuring prenatal care delivery. Am J Publ Health 2004;94(12):2062–5.
50. Abraído-Lanza AF, Mendoza-Grey S, Flórez KR. A commentary on the latin american paradox. JAMA Netw Open 2020;3(2):e1921165.

51. Garza G, Hodges-Delgado P, Hoskovec J, et al. Exploring experiences and expectations of prenatal health care and genetic counseling/testing in immigrant Latinas. J Genet Couns 2020.

52. Gutierrez C, Dollar NT. Birth and prenatal care outcomes of Latina mothers in the Trump era: Analysis by nativity and country/region of origin. PLoS One 2023; 18(3):e0281803.

53. Kroelinger CD, Brantley MD, Fuller TR, et al. Geographic access to critical care obstetrics for women of reproductive age by race and ethnicity. Am J Obstet Gynecol 2021;224:304, e1-11.

54. Available at: https://www.cdc.gov/cancer/cervical/amigas/index.htm, Accessed October 14, 2023.

55. Available at: https://pubmed.ncbi.nlm.nih.gov/17274222/. Accessed October 14, 2023.

56. Available at: https://www.ncbi.nlm.nih.gov/pmc/articles/PMC6326179/). Accessed October 14, 2023.

57. Available at: https://link.springer.com/article/10.1007/s10900-017-0316-9). Accessed October 14, 2023.

58. Rauh-Hain JA, Melamed A, Schaps D, et al. Racial and ethnic disparities over time in the treatment and mortality of women with gynecological malignancies. Gynecol Oncol 2018;149(1):4–11.

59. Available at: https://gis.cdc.gov/Cancer/USCS/?CDC_AA_refVal=https%3A%2F%2Fwww.cdc.gov%2Fcancer%2Fdataviz%2Findex.htm#/Demographics/. Accessed October 14, 2023.

60. Knol HM, Mulder AB, Bogchelman DH, et al. The prevalence of underlying bleeding disorders in patients with heavy menstrual bleeding with and without gynecologic abnormalities. Am J Obstet Gynecol 2013;209(3):202.

61. Available at: https://pubmed.ncbi.nlm.nih.gov/33631875/. Accessed October 14, 2023.

62. Available at: https://www.cancer.org/content/dam/cancer-org/research/cancer-facts-and-statistics/annual-cancer-facts-and-figures/2023/2023-cancer-facts-and-figures.pdf. Accessed October 14, 2023.

63. Available at: https://www.sciencedirect.com/science/article/pii/S0090825822016663. Accessed October 14, 2023.

64. Available at: https://www.ncbi.nlm.nih.gov/pmc/articles/PMC10510793/. Accessed October 14, 2023.

65. Available at: https://jamanetwork.com/journals/jamaoncology/article-abstract/2806705. Accessed October 14, 2023.

66. Available at: https://jamanetwork.com/journals/jamaoncology/fullarticle/2792010. Accessed October 14, 2023.

67. Available at: https://www.sciencedirect.com/science/article/abs/pii/S0378874114004978, Accessed October 14, 2023.

68. Ko JS, Suh CH, Huang H, et al. Association of Race/Ethnicity with Surgical Route and Perioperative Outcomes of Hysterectomy for Leiomyomas. J Minim Invasive Gynecol 2021;28(7):143–1410.e2.

69. Carey ET, Moore KJ, McClurg AB, et al. Racial Disparities in Hysterectomy Route for Benign Disease: Examining Trends and Perioperative Complications from 2007 to 2018 Using the NSQIP Database. J Minim Invasive Gynecol 2023;S1553-S4650(23):00145–000150.

70. Pollack LM, Olsen MA, Gehlert SJ, et al. Racial/Ethnic Disparities/Differences in Hysterectomy Route in Women Likely Eligible for Minimally Invasive Surgery. J Minim Invasive Gynecol 2020;27(5):1167–77.e2.

71. Available at: https://www.cdc.gov/std/treatment-guidelines/screening-recommendations.htm. Accessed October 14, 2023.
72. Available at: https://bpr.berkeley.edu/2020/11/04/americas, Accessed October 14, 2023.
73. Patricia A, Lee K, David JP. Perinatal HIV testing among African American, Caucasian, Hmong and Latina women: exploring the role of health-care services, information sources and perceptions of HIV/AIDS. Health Educ Res 2014;29(Issue 1):109–21.
74. Cashman R, Eng E, Simán F, et al. Exploring the sexual health priorities and needs of immigrant Latinas in the southeastern United States: a community-based participatory research approach. AIDS Educ Prev 2011;23(3):236–48.
75. Cardoza VJ, Documét PI, Fryer CS, et al. Sexual health behavior interventions for U.S. Latino adolescents: a systematic review of the literature. J Pediatr Adolesc Gynecol 2012;25(2):136–49.
76. Available at: https://www.advocatesforyouth.org/wp-content/uploads/storage/advfy/documents/latina.pdf. Accessed October 14, 2023.
77. Available at: https://cms.childtrends.org/wp-content/uploads/2013/03/Child_Trends-2012_08_31_FR_LatinaReproductive.pdf. Accessed October 14, 2023.
78. Sutton MY, Anachebe NF, Lee R, et al. Racial and Ethnic Disparities in Reproductive Health Services and Outcomes, 2020. Obstet Gynecol 2021;137(2):225–33.
79. Available at: https://www.thecrimson.com/article/2017/9/28/the-bitter-pill/. Accessed October 14, 2023.
80. Higgins JA, Kramer RD, Ryder KM. Provider bias in long-acting reversible contraception (LARC) promotion and removal: perceptions of young adult women. Am J Publ Health 2016;106:1932–7.
81. Hill L., Artiga S., Ranji U., Racial Disparties in Maternal and Infant Health: Current Status and Efforts to Address Them, 2022, Available at: https://www.kff.org. Accessed October 14, 2023.
82. Available at: https://www.acog.org/news/news-articles/2020/08/joint-statment-obstetrics-and-gynecology-collective-action-adressing-racism. Accessed October 14, 2023.
83. Elson M. Cultural Sensitivity in OB/GYN: The Ultimate Patient-Centered Care. MedEdPORTAL 2009;5:1658.
84. McDonald Lynn R., Schwarz Joshua L., Martin Stephen J., et al., An Initiative to Improve Cultural Competence among GYN/OB Providers, *Journal of Health Disparities Research and Practice*, 14 (3), 2021, Article 7. Available at: https://digitalscholarship.unlv.edu/jhdrp/vol14/iss3/7. Accessed October 14, 2023.
85. Available at: https://healthcare.rti.org/insights/delivering-culturally-compentent-maternal-care-to-BIPOC-women. Accessed October 14, 2023.
86. Available at: https://www.cms.gov/About-CMS/Agency-information/OMH/Downloads/Language-Access-Plan.pdf. Accessed October 14, 2023.
87. Grant M, Wilford A, Haskins L, et al. Trust of community health workers influences the acceptance of community-based maternal and child health services. Afr J Prim Health Care Fam Med 2017;9(1):e1–8.
88. Zephyrin L, Seervai S, Lewis C, Katon JG. Community-based models to improve maternal health outcomes and promote health equity. Commonwealth Fund 2021.
89. Ellman N. Community-based doulas and Midwives: key to addressing the U.S. Maternal health crisis. Center for American Progress; 2020.

90. Thomas MP, Ammann G, Brazier E, et al. Doula services within a healthy start program: increasing access for an underserved population. Matern Child Health J 2017;21(Suppl 1):59–64.

91. Jane Sandall, Soltani H, Gates S, et al. Midwife-led continuity models versus other models of care for childbearing women. Cochrane Database Syst Rev 2013;8(Aug. 21):CD004667.

92. Attanasio Laura B, Alarid-Escudero Fernando, Kozhimannil Katy B. Midwife-led care and obstetrician-led care for low-risk pregnancies: a cost comparison. Birth 2020;47(1):57–66.

93. ACOG Committee Opinion No. 731. Summary: group prenatal care. Obstet Gynecol 2018;131(3):616–8.

94. Available at: https://link.springer.com/article/10.1007/s10995-016-2114-x. Accessed October 14, 2023.

95. Available at: https://nationalpartnership.org/wp-content/uploads/2023/02/improving-our-maternity-care-now.pdf. Accessed October 14, 2023.

96. Available at: https://www.whitehouse.gov/wp-content/uploads/2022/06/Maternal-Health-Blueprint.pdf. Accessed October 14, 2023.

97. Rudowitz R, Drake P, Tolbert J, et al. How Many Uninsured Are in the Coverage Gap and How Many Could be Eligible if All States Adopted the Medicaid Expansion? 31, 2023.

98. Ranji U, Long M, Salganicoff A. Beyond the Numbers: Access to Reproductive Health Care for Low-Income Women in Five Communities, Nov 14, 2019.

99. Borrero S, Farkas A, Dehlendorf C, et al. Racial and ethnic difference in men's knowledge and attitudes about contraception. Contraception 2013;88(4):532–8.

100. Thiel de Bocanegra H, Trinh-Shevrin C, Herrera AP, et al. Mexican Immigrant Male Knowledge and Support Toward Breast and Cervical Cancer Screening. J Immigrant Minority Health 2009;11:326–33.

101. Goyal V, McLoughlin Brooks I, Powers D. Differences in abortion rates by race-ethnicity after implementation of a restrictive Texas law. Contraception 2020; 102(2):109–14.

102. Morgan HK, Winkel AF, Banks E, et al. Promoting diversity, equity, and inclusion in the selection of obstetrician–gynecologists. Obstet Gynecol 2021;138:272–7.

Cervical Cancer
Preventable Deaths Among American Indian/ Alaska Native Communities

Jessica Buck DiSilvestro, MD (Caddo Nation of Oklahoma)[a,b,*],
Keely K. Ulmer, MD (Oglala Sioux Nation of South Dakota)[c], Madeline Hedges[d],
Kimberly Kardonsky, MD (Jamestown S'Klallam Tribe)[e],
Amanda S. Bruegl, MD, MCR (Oneida, Stockbridge-Munsee Nations)[f]

KEYWORDS

- American indian or Alaska native • Uterine cervical neoplasms
- Healthcare disparities • Health status disparities

KEY POINTS

- AI/AN individuals face significant health disparities, with over twice the mortality rate from cervical cancer.
- High prevalence of risk factors, low screening rates, and higher rates of high-risk human papillomavirus (HPV) not covered by the vaccine all contribute to the greater incidence and mortality rates of cervical cancer among AI/AN individuals.
- Interventions across the cervical cancer screening and treatment continuum need to occur to reverse the course of persistent disparities faced by AI/AN individuals.

INTRODUCTION

According to the 2020 US Census, American Indian and Alaska Native (AI/AN) people comprise approximately 3% of the total US population. There are 574 federally recognized AI/AN tribes with 324 distinct reservations, and the majority (71%) of AI/AN people currently reside in urban areas.[1] AI/AN individuals have widespread social disparities and face worse health outcomes compared to their Non-Hispanic White (NHW) counterparts.[2] Some of these major disparities include unemployment,

[a] Brown University, Providence, RI, USA; [b] Women & Infants Hospital, 101 Dudley Street, Providence, RI 02905, USA; [c] University of Iowa Hospitals and Clinics, 200 Hawkins Drive, Iowa City, IA 52242, USA; [d] University of Arizona, Tucson; [e] Department of Family Medicine, University of Washington School of Medicine, Heath Sciences Center, E-304 Box 356391, Seattle, WA 98195, USA; [f] Division of Gynecologic Oncology, Oregon Health and Science University, 3181 SW Sam Jackson Park Road, Mailstop L466, Portland, OR 97239, USA
* Corresponding author. Women & Infants Hospital, 101 Dudley Street, Providence, RI 02905
E-mail address: jbdisilvestro@gmail.com

Obstet Gynecol Clin N Am 51 (2024) 125–141
https://doi.org/10.1016/j.ogc.2023.11.009
0889-8545/24/© 2023 Elsevier Inc. All rights reserved.

diabetes, obesity, and decreased overall life expectancy, with cancer and cardiovascular disease comprising the 2 leading causes of death.[3,4]

Cervical cancer also represents a disease for which AI/AN populations are disproportionately affected. Death from cervical cancer is preventable through human papillomavirus (HPV) vaccination and participation in cervical cancer screening programs (ie, pap smear screening or high-risk HPV testing).[5–7] In the United States, the burden of cervical cancer occurs in never-screened or under screened populations.[8] This review examines the persistent burden of cervical cancer among AI/AN individuals and provides recommendations for eliminating this health disparity.

BACKGROUND

The history behind the development of health care services to sovereign AI/AN people is a complex narrative, and beyond the scope of this article. Understanding the basic structure and its origins provides insight into the persistence of health disparities today. A summary of key events is displayed in **Fig. 1**. The Indian Self Determination Act of 1975 allowed tribes to take control of their health care and other tribal programs. Despite efforts to improve health care services, the life expectancy of an AI/AN person has increased by only 2 years since 1955 and remains 7 years lower than NHW people.[9] Today, the Indian Health Service (IHS) continues to provide health care services for enrolled tribal citizens through clinics and hospitals, distinguished as either IHS-operated, tribally-operated, or urban-based (I/T/U). IHS is divided into 12 administrative regions with 46 hospitals, 522 health centers, and 82 urban organizations, with the majority of these located on tribal lands. These facilities serve approximately 60% of the nation's AI/AN population.[10] IHS is a service-based organization and does not serve as health insurance or cover fees at outside facilities. IHS has had comparably lower funding allocations per capita than other federal health programs such as Medicare and the US Department of Veterans Affairs (VA) with per capita annual rates of $9,726, $15,727, and $13,500, respectively.[11] These funding disparities parallel the drastic health disparities seen in this population and exacerbate existing health inequities.

Further, the genocidal and assimilationist actions conducted on behalf of the US government have led to mistrust with the health care system, intergenerational

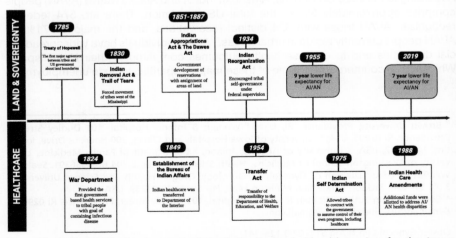

Fig. 1. The chronologic development of the federally-funded health services for the American Indian/Alaska Native population.[9,83–85].

trauma, and has a profound and lasting negative impact on AI/AN people to this day. A full review of acts leading to these inequities cannot be sufficiently addressed in this review.

CERVICAL CANCER
Cervical Cancer Risk Factors

There are several known risk factors that contribute to cervical dysplasia and cancer, including high-risk human papillomavirus (hrHPV) infection, low socioeconomic status, tobacco use, number of lifetime sexual partners, history of sexual infections, sexual trauma, and early sexual debut.[12–15] These variables are all seen at staggering rates within the AI/AN population.[12–15] **Table 1** summarizes the impact of these risk factors on rates of hrHPV and cervical dysplasia as well as their prevalence within the AI/AN and general populations.

Human Papillomavirus Infection

There are numerous oncogenic hrHPV strains of which are identified in the vast majority of genital tract, anal, and oropharyngeal cancers. Over 90% of cervical cancers are caused by hrHPV in the United States, with an estimated 66% of invasive cervical cancer due to either HPV 16 or 18 infection.[16] Acquisition and failure to clear hrHPV are critical components to the development of cervical cancer (**Fig. 2**).[17]

The estimated prevalence of hrHPV in the AI/AN population is 21% to 30%, compared to 20% in the general US population (**Table 2**).[12,13,18,19] Within the AI/AN population, rates of HPV infection decrease with increasing age (42% in 21–24 years to 28% in 50–65 years).[20,21] Although a similar trend is seen amidst the general population with higher rates at younger ages, AI/AN individuals >50 years old are observed to have significantly higher rates of hrHPV than individuals of this age group from all races and ethnicities (general US population: 6.9%).[22]

Table 1
Rates of risk factors for human papillomavirus infection and cervical dysplasia among American Indian/Alaska Native women compared to the general population

Risk Factor (RF)	Rate of RF in General Population	Rate of RF in AI/AN Population	Demonstrated Impact of RF on Rates of HPV/ cervical Dysplasia within the American Indian/Alaska Native (AI/AN) Population
Low socioeconomic status	13%[88]	21%[88]	3 × rate of high-grade cervical dysplasia[14]
Tobacco use	19%[89]	35%[89]	Higher rates of hrHPV infection[13]
History of a sexually transmitted infection	14%[13]	51%[13]	2 × the rate of cervical dysplasia and cancer[14]
Number of sexual partners	≥10 lifetime partners: 12%[13]	≥10 lifetime partners: 24%[13]	Higher rates of hrHPV infection[13]
Earlier age at sexual debut	First intercourse <13 y: 3.9%[90]	First intercourse <13 y: 8.3%[90]	Higher rates of hrHPV infection[13]
History of sexual trauma	Youth: 8%[91] Adult: 50%[92]	Youth: 18%[91] Adult: 56%[92]	2 × the rate of invasive cervical cancer[15]

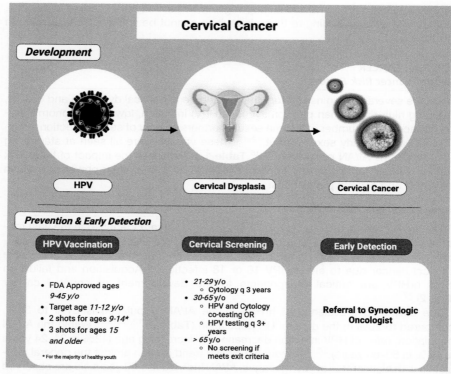

Fig. 2. Primary and secondary prevention interventions to reduce cervical cancer.[86,87].

Human Papillomavirus Vaccination

The 9-valent HPV vaccine comprises the oncogenic variants 16, 18, 31, 33, 45, 52, 58 as well as genital wart-causing variants 6 and 11. The 9-valent vaccine prevents approximately 90% of all cervical cancer cases worldwide.[23] Several hrHPV subtyping studies suggest that the prevalence of non-HPV 16 and 18 subtypes is greater in AI/AN individuals than the general US population, specifically strains that are not included in

Table 2
The prevalence of high-risk human papillomavirus among American Indian/Alaska Native women and the high proportion of HPV strains not included in the 9-valent HPV vaccine

Total Prevalence of hrHPV	
General US population[19]	20%
AI/AN population[12,13,18]	21%–30%
Prevalence of hrHPV excluded from the 9-valent HPV vaccine in the AI/AN population	
Cervical cancer diagnoses in Alaska Native women, 1980–2007 (n = 62)[26]	16%
HPV screening tests in Great Plains AI/AN women, 2014–2015 (n = 698)[21]	17%
Cancer registry of all HPV-associated cancers in AI/AN people, 2013–2017 (n = 1030)[25]	28%
HPV screening tests in South Dakota AI/AN women, 2006–2008 (n = 258)[24]	32%
HPV test in Southwest AI/AN women with cervical dysplasia, 1994–1997 (n = 148)[14]	45%

the 9-valent vaccine.[21,24–26] **Table 2** summarizes the studies assessing the proportion of hrHPV strains not covered by the 9-valent HPV vaccine in the AI/AN community with prevalence rates ranging from 16% to 45%.[12–14,18,19,21,24–27] To date, there are no published efforts to expand vaccine coverage to incorporate hrHPV strains seen at higher proportions in US subpopulations such as the AI/AN community. Despite these higher rates of excluded hrHPV strains, vaccination remains a key component of cervical cancer prevention in the AI/AN population who have up to 1.5 × higher overall rates of hrHPV infection.

Vaccination prior to onset of sexual debut is also a critical factor in risk reduction, and lowers the risk of hrHPV-related cancer and pre-cancers (see **Fig. 2**).[17] HPV vaccination rates have been increasing among AI/AN youth and those aged 13 to 17 years have been found to have higher rates of HPV vaccination than all other racial groups.[28,29] In 2020, the Centers for Disease Control and Prevention (CDC) reported that 85% of AI/AN youth received at least 1 dose and 66% were up-to-date on the HPV vaccine series, with higher rates than NHW youth (71% and 55%, respectively).[28] A 2023 study of IHS services within the Pacific Northwest identified a current vaccination rate of 58.6% for AI/AN youth aged 9 to 26 years with the highest vaccination rates among females[a], all ages, and youth aged 13 to 18 years.[29] Identified facilitators to the rising rates of vaccination include successful funding programs, IHS-based electronic reminders, co-administration of the *tetanus, diphtheria, and pertussis* vaccine, nurse-only visits for vaccine administration, and targeted community educational programs.[30] Despite the increase, these rates remain lower than both the overall national average (73.5%) and the Healthy People 2030 Goal of 80.0%.[29,31]

Knowledge about HPV and its impact is low within AI/AN populations. A survey in the Northern Plains demonstrated less knowledge about HPV and its vaccine among AI/AN individuals compared to NHW.[32] A focus group of AN caregivers found that approximately half of caregivers (56%) knew about the HPV vaccine and 20% knew about its role in cervical cancer prevention.[33] After the focus groups, the majority of these caregivers expressed interest in having their children vaccinated. HPV vaccination initiation was approximately 3 times higher in youth whose caregivers were aware of the HPV vaccine and for those who received a recommendation from their provider.[34]

Parents who declined vaccination listed fear of vaccine side effects and a need for more information as potential barriers to uptake.[33,34] A survey of IHS providers similarly found safety concerns in addition to moral and religious conflicts as barriers to vaccination.[35] Targeted education for AI/AN parents has been effective in increasing HPV vaccine initiation and completion for youth.[36] Culturally tailored education has been developed by organizations such as the American Indian Cancer Foundation (americanindiancancer.org) who have created infographics on cervical cancer screening and HPV vaccination specific to AI/AN populations. Tailoring of HPV vaccination infographics with specific AI/AN culture has proven more appealing and convincing to AI/AN populations.[37]

Cervical Cancer Screening

In 1990, the CDC) established the National Breast and Cervical Cancer Early Detection Program (NBCCEDP) to increase screening for patients who were underinsured or

---

[a] The authors recognize that the term "female" does not fully encompass the breadth of gender diversity but is utilized to refer to gender as it is categorized in published data that are cited. The authors recognize that cervical cancer impacts a variety of gender-diverse communities and try to limit heteronormative terminology.

uninsured.[38] In 1994, the NBCCEDP partnered directly with tribes to develop screening programs. When the program was first instated, less than half of AI/AN participants had ever had a prior pap smear.[39] The first round of screening results demonstrated that AI/AN individuals had the highest rate of abnormal pap smears compared to other racial groups, thereby demonstrating the incredible need for the program.[39] Between 2004 and 2006, the NBCCEDP screened 36% of all the eligible AI/AN individuals aged 18 to 64 years (41,462 of an estimated 115,000). Conversely, of eligible individuals of all racial and ethnic groups, 8.7% were screened during this same time frame.[38] Over half of these individuals were screened at tribally-operative programs, highlighting the importance of the program's direct partnership with tribes.[38]

Assessing current rates of up-to-date cervical cancer screening within the AI/AN population is a challenging task. A study in the 1990s utilized the Behavioral Risk Factor Surveillance System to estimate up-to-date cervical cancer screening with a rate of 82.6%.[40] Although more recent efforts utilize IHS-level data, these estimates omit AI/AN individuals who seek care outside of IHS. Government Performance and Results Act (GPRA) data annually assess cervical cancer screening rates among AI/AN individuals aged 24 to 64 who have received a screening test within the past 3 to 5 years at an IHS facility.[41] There has been a steady decline in screening from 2019 to 2021 (37.1% to 33.6%), which are both significantly below the Healthy People 2030 Goal of 79.2%.[42] IHS regional variation exists with lowest rates seen in Portland (23.7%) and highest in Alaska (43.0%).[41]

A 2023 study exploring the rates of cervical cancer screening of AI/AN individuals receiving care at IHS facilities in the Pacific Northwest from 2010 to 2020 demonstrated higher rates of up-to-date screening (57.1%–65.0%) than previously reported in GPRA.[29] Interestingly, individuals aged 50 to 64 years were identified as a higher risk population due to the significantly lower rates of screening (52.2%) compared to younger ages (66%–67%). Additionally, individuals living in rural areas were more likely to be up-to-date on screening than their urban counterparts.[29]

Colposcopy

Abnormal screening results often require colposcopy for evaluation, a service that may not be available on-site or nearby. In the late 1980s, colposcopy was identified as an area of unmet need among the American College of Obstetricians and Gynecologists Committee of AI/AN Affairs during a site visit to a rural clinic in the Navajo Nation.[38,43] IHS has responded by partnering with Southcentral Foundation and the University of New Mexico to provide IHS, tribal, and urban health care providers with courses in colposcopy through both online platforms and in-person trainings.[44,45] By 2013, 375 health care providers had participated in these trainings.[38] A 1992 study found that rates of follow-up colposcopic evaluation after an abnormal pap smear were similar for AI/AN in the Pacific Northwest (75%) as compared to published data of other racial groups.[46] Unfortunately, there are no data to date on the availability or functionality of colposcopies at IHS facilities. Furthermore, there is a lack of data on treatment availability with ablation or electrosurgical cervical excision equipment at these sites. Despite the dearth of data in this area, there is an obvious and significant gap between an abnormal pap smear and death from cervical cancer, highlighting the disproportionately increased cervical cancer–related mortality among AI/AN people.

Diagnosis

In 2023, an estimated 13,960 individuals will be newly diagnosed with invasive cervical cancer and 4310 will die from cervical cancer in the United States[47] The incidence of cervical cancer has steadily declined since the 1970s due to the uptake in screening. A recent steep decline in incidence was also observed in individuals aged 20 to 24 years, likely due to the rising utilization of the HPV vaccine.[48] Approximately half of new cases (46%) of invasive cervical cancer are diagnosed in individuals between the ages of 35 to 54 years.[49] Furthermore, racial disparities exist in regard to both incidence and mortality rates of cervical cancer.[49,50]

Assessing the status of cancer burden within the AI/AN population has been historically challenging for a multitude of reasons. Proportionately smaller numbers often pose a statistical challenge when making racial comparisons. Racial misclassification for AI/AN people is a well-documented issue; it is a limitation that has been partially addressed by developing linkages between cancer registries and the IHS enrollment records.[51,52] Efforts to overcome these challenges have subsequently revealed higher incidence and mortality rates of cervical cancer within the AI/AN population. Cervical cancer incidence estimates from US cancer registries have demonstrated a 1.5 × higher incidence in AI/AN individuals at 11.5 per 100,000 individuals compared to 7.4 per 100,000 for NHW ($P < .05$).[50,53] Geographic differences exist in the prevalence of invasive cervical cancer, with higher rates seen in the Southern Plain (Texas, Oklahoma, and Kansas) and Northern Plain regions (from Montana and Wyoming to Michigan and Indiana).[54]

Treatment

Treatment for cervical cancer is dependent on the stage of disease determined by tumor size and spread of disease.[55] The majority of newly diagnosed cervical cancers in the United States are diagnosed at an early stage (56%), while 34% and 9% are diagnosed at regional and advanced stages, respectively.[56] Early-stage disease is often managed with surgery alone (cervical conization, hysterectomy with or without lymphadenectomy), with few patients requiring adjuvant radiation therapy. Fertility-sparing options are offered to select candidates. Locally advanced disease is primarily treated with a combination of chemotherapy and pelvic radiation. For those with distant metastatic disease, systemic chemotherapy is used, often in combination with immunotherapy and anti-angiogenic therapy.

AI/AN patients with cancer are less likely to receive guideline-adherent cancer treatments.[57] IHS does not provide gynecologic oncology services and therefore patients with cervical cancer are referred to other facilities outside of IHS for treatment. Due to geographic barriers, AI/AN individuals have to travel significantly farther to receive cancer treatments (including daily radiation therapies) and are more likely to receive their cancer surgery at a rural hospital.[58–60] A retrospective review of AI/AN individuals seeking cervical cancer care at a tertiary hospital in Oklahoma City found that AI/AN individuals on average traveled 93 miles to receive care.[61] Of the 34 patients in the review, mean time to treatment initiation was 35 days and 92% completed the prescribed treatment regimen. Use of care navigation programs has not demonstrated benefit in initiation or completion of treatment for cervical cancer in AI/AN individuals.[61] A 2023 scoping review on the volume of research in cervical cancer among AI/AN populations demonstrated a significant scarcity of data on treatment.[62] Only 3 studies from 1990 to 2018 (3.6% of total studies) published on cervical cancer focused on treatment type or treatment completion in AI/AN individuals.

Survival and Outcomes

In the US population, the 5-year survival rate for cervical cancer is 67% with worse outcomes for those diagnosed at older ages, later stages of disease, and in non-White racial groups.[63] It is well demonstrated in the literature that AI/AN individuals have experienced persistent disparities in cervical cancer mortality rates compared to NHW individuals, with a 2-fold increase in mortality rate.[53,64] The age-adjusted death rate for cervical cancer in the AI/AN population is estimated at 4.2 per 100,000 persons (compared to 2.0 per 100,000 persons for NHW) and ranks 10th in cancer-related deaths for AI/AN communities (compared to 19th for NHW).[53] The American Cancer Society showed that AI/AN individuals have the second highest mortality rate (after Hispanic people) compared to other racial and ethnic groups.[49]

Data specific to AI/AN individuals with cervical cancer are heterogenous (ie, include some but not all AI/AN populations) and are limited in number.[62] However, data that are available show that AI/AN individuals experience higher rates of risk factors for cervical cancer, are less likely to be diagnosed at an early stage of disease, and are more likely to receive their treatment at a rural facility (**Table 1**).[54,64,65]

STRATEGIES FOR ADDRESSING AMERICAN INDIAN/ALASKA NATIVE (AI/AN) CERVICAL CANCER DISPARITIES

Eliminating cervical cancer inequities faced by AI/AN people requires a multimodal approach rooted in cultural humility. In this review, the authors have highlighted several steps along the cervical cancer development continuum that contribute to this disparity. Strategies for addressing these disparities are outlined in **Table 3**. The authors have identified 4 core areas: funding-related barriers, provider-related challenges, patient-facing challenges, and suboptimal uptake of cancer prevention tools (ie, HPV vaccination and participation in cervical cancer screening programs).

Funding-Related Challenges and Solutions

As stated in the background section, the per capita funding for the IHS is $9726, substantially lower than Medicaid ($15,727) or the VA ($13,500).[11] The legal history between the federal government and sovereign tribes is complex, but the Snyder Act and Indian Health Care Improvement Act of 1976 establish the foundations of the right to health care services to AI/AN citizens.[66] The per capita funding is far below what is needed to meet the health care needs of a population that faces greater disparities not only in cervical cancer mortality but also for a multitude of additional health conditions such as maternal mortality, diabetes, and cardiovascular disease.[67–69] The IHS is within the Federal Department of Health and Human Services, and its budget is reviewed by the House and Senate Committees on Appropriations. Lobbying to US Congress and Senate officials on behalf of AI/AN people is the best way to amplify the voices of those testifying on behalf of the IHS.

Cervical cancer research specific to the AI/AN population is sparse compared to the persistent health inequities the authors have described. A recently published scoping review evaluating the volume and nature of publications between 1990 and 2022 identified only 87 publications during this time period.[62] Most studies were found to be a cross-sectional study design, focused on cervical cancer screening, used utilized race as the intervention/exposure for comparisons in outcomes, and were primarily funded through government mechanisms (ie, National Institutes of Health, Centers for Disease Control and Prevention). Increasing funding opportunities and including tribal nations in the development and execution of cervical cancer–related research is necessary to narrow the disparity gap in this population.[70]

Provider-Related Challenges and Solutions

Concordance of race and gender between health care providers and patients is associated with improved patient satisfaction.[71–73] AI/AN individuals make up an estimated 2.5% of the US population, yet represent only 0.3% of the physician workforce.[74,75]

Table 3
Evidence-based recommendations to reduce cervical cancer disparities in American Indian/Alaska Native individuals

Challenge	Possible Solutions	Resources
Non-AI/AN providers are seeing AI/AN patients	Increase number of AI/AN health care providers	AAIP & AAMC "Reshaping the Journey" report on recruitment and retention of AI/AN physicians[77] Practicing Cultural Competence and Cultural Humility in the Care of Diverse Patients[76]
Informational materials and messaging are not tailored to the AI/AN population	Provide AI/AN-specific outreach, advertising, & handouts[93,94] More education during training for non-Native physicians[76] Community-driven health campaigns and partnership with IHS providers and/or traditional healers[79,80]	American Indian Cancer Foundation cervical cancer infographics[95] NIH "Tailored Communication for Cervical Cancer Risk" program[96]
HPV vaccination rates are below Healthy People 2030 Goal	Designate Elder HPV champions for communities Increase access to HPV vaccines at sites that are Native available (schools, powwows, community gatherings)[76,79,80]	American Indian Cancer Foundation HPV vaccination infographics[97]
Participation in Cervical Cancer screening programs is below Healthy People 2030 Goal	Engage with community stakeholders/champions to increase cervical cancer and promote screening[70,80] Standardizing cervical cancer screening to all eligible AI/AN individuals[81] Provide gynecologic trauma- informed care training to all providers caring for AI/AN individuals[82]	Framework for community engagement[80] ACOG "Caring for Patients Who Have Experienced Trauma" Committee Opinion[82]
Colposcopy-trained providers are not on-site at IHS/Tribal/Urban Indian clinics and follow-up requires travel and time	Designate staff to participate in the IHS colposcopy training and provide service on-site[46]	IHS Colposcopy Training Programs[98]
Per capita funding for IHS remains below that of other government sponsored health care	Increase cervical cancer screening and treatment funding[99]	Increasing Funding for IHS to Improve AI/AN Health Outcomes Policy Brief[11]
Research related to AI/AN population and cervical cancer and its prevention remains understudied[62]	Increase NIH designated funding by and with Tribes to identify culturally specific and evidence-based solutions[70,100]	NIH Native American Research Centers for Health programs[101]

Associate of American Indian Physicians (AAIP); Association of American Medical Colleges (AAMC); National Institutes of Health (NIH); American College of Obstetricians and Gynecologists (ACOG).

Concerted efforts must be made to improve the representation of AI/AN individuals in all fields of medicine, but particularly in the areas of cervical cancer care and treatment.[76,77] Increasing AI/AN recruitment to medical school is not enough. Efforts must be made across the training continuum starting prior to college. The Northwest Native American Center of Excellence at Oregon Health and Science University has invested tremendous energy into inspiring AI/AN youth to pursue health care–related fields across a wide span of ages.[78] Programs such as these are a rarity at medical schools with just a handful in existence across the United States Each medical institution should commit to develop programming to inspire and support AI/AN youth to pursue these careers.

In addition to workforce shortages, there are shortages at I/T/U clinics for colposcopy-trained health care providers.[38,43] As stated earlier, IHS co-sponsors a colposcopy training course geared specifically for health care providers at these clinical sites and waives tuition for attendees. I/T/U sites should *designate* at least 1 health care provider in their clinic to attend this training and to provide these services to their patients.[46]

Patient Facing Challenges and Solutions

The discussion of shortages of colposcopy-trained health care providers underscores the greater issue of access to medical care. Patients need access to both trained physicians and to centers with the technology to diagnose (ie, colposcopies) and treat (ie, radiotherapy) cervical cancer. Although there has been a trend in relocation of the AI/AN population to urban centers, a significant portion of AI/AN individuals remain in rural areas with limited access to care.[1] On average, AI/AN individuals travel farther to receive cancer treatments, are more likely to have their cancer surgery performed at a rural hospital, and are less likely to receive guideline-concordant care.[57,58,60] I/T/U sites should designate referral centers to streamline their oncologic care to higher volume hospitals. Furthermore, financial support should be provided with transportation or temporary relocation assistance for patients undergoing treatment at distant sites.

Challenges Related to Uptake of Cancer Prevention Tools

Primary prevention of cervical cancer begins with robust HPV vaccination programs. The Vaccines for Children Program covers the cost of recommended vaccines for all children under age 19 across the nation who qualify for Medicaid, do not have insurance, or cannot afford out-of-pocket costs from insurance co-pays. Thus, all children in the United States are eligible to receive the HPV vaccine at the recommended ages free of charge. Despite this availability, vaccination rates for all populations remain well below the Healthy People 2030 Goal of 80.4%. As previously mentioned, education is a huge barrier. More robust tailored and culturally-sensitive advertising to AI/AN communities should be implemented (ie, brochures, public service announcements, and other marketing materials such as those made available by the American Indian Cancer Foundation).[79] Each community has its own unique and preferred methods of communication. Engaging trusted community sources in these initiatives is the key (such as trusted Elders and community stakeholders, tribally operated radio stations, and other tribally owned and operated venues). Access and education are important tools to increasing vaccination rates. Expanding HPV vaccination opportunities at schools, cultural events such as powwows, and community gatherings could positively impact vaccine awareness.[76,79,80]

Cervical cancer screening—a critical cornerstone to preventing death from cervical cancer—is not fully utilized among AI/AN populations. As described previously, this is likely multifactorial but several interventions could be employed to help reduce barriers to uptake. It is imperative that health care providers are aware of the cervical cancer screening guidelines and *offer* it to patients. Survey data from AI/AN individuals show that 1 recurrent barrier to participating in cervical cancer screening is that it has not been recommended by a provider.[81] Additionally, engaging with community stakeholders and/or respected Elders to urge the importance of cervical cancer screening can be pivotal to increasing patients comfort with participating in programs.[70,80] Furthermore, data suggest that up to 50% of AI/AN women have been the victim of physical or sexual abuse, which may or may not be information shared with the health care provider. Clinics serving this patient population should be aware of this high percentage *and* receive adequate training in gynecologic trauma-informed care.[82] Increasing the comfort and experience each individual has with the gynecologic examination will reduce perpetuating the trauma and has the potential to increase guideline adherent care.[70,80,81]

SUMMARY

Health disparities persist among AI/AN people for a variety of health conditions. This review focused on cervical cancer mortality, a highly preventable cause of death in a well-resourced country. AI/AN people have lower rates of HPV vaccination and up-to-date cervical cancer screening compared to their NHW counterparts that contribute to disproportionate cervical cancer–related mortality that is twice that of the general population. Contributors to these health disparities are vast and include socioeconomic status, geographic barriers, and high rates of medical comorbidities. Efforts to increase uptake and engagement of the AI/AN population in cervical cancer screening and HPV vaccination are essential next steps to address these health disparities.

CLINICS CARE POINTS

- Incidence rates of cervical cancer are higher in AI/AN individuals.
- Individuals from AI/AN communities are more likely to be diagnosed at later stages, and suffer from greater cervical cancer–related mortality compared to other racial and ethnic groups.
- AI/AN individuals have lower rates cervical cancer screening and HPV vaccination initiation, and are more likely to be infected with a hrHPV strain not covered by the 9-valent vaccine.
- Higher rates of health and behavioral risk factors, as well as geographic barriers, contribute to health disparities.

DISCLOSURE

The authors report no conflicts of interest. No funding was utilized in the development of this review.

REFERENCES

1. Urban Indian Health – Urban Indian Health Institute. Accessed August 25, 2022. https://www.uihi.org/urban-indian-health/.
2. Bureau UC. 2020 Census Illuminates Racial and Ethnic Composition of the Country. Accessed July 18, 2023. https://www.census.gov/library/stories/2021/08/improved-race-ethnicity-measures-reveal-united-states-population-much-more-multiracial.html.

3. Health Services I. Indian Health Focus: Injuries 2017 Edition. Published online 2017.

4. Statistics P. Indian Health Focus: Women 2012 Edition. Published online 2012.

5. Hall MT, Simms KT, Lew J Bin, et al. The projected timeframe until cervical cancer elimination in Australia: a modelling study. Lancet Public Health 2019;4(1): e19–27.

6. Sasieni P, Castanon A, Cuzick J, et al. Effectiveness of cervical screening with age: population based case-control study of prospectively recorded data. BMJ 2009;339(7716):328.

7. Moyer VA, U.S. Preventive Services Task Force. Screening for cervical cancer: U.S. preventive services task force recommendation statement. Ann Intern Med 2012;156(12):880–91.

8. Benard VB, Jackson JE, Greek A, et al. A population study of screening history and diagnostic outcomes of women with invasive cervical cancer. Cancer Med 2021;10(12):4127.

9. Arias E, Xu J, Curtin S, et al. Mortality profile of the non-hispanic american indian or alaska native population. Natl Vital Stat Rep 2019. Available at: https://www.cdc.gov/nchs/products/index.htm. Accessed July 13, 2023.

10. Quick Look | Fact Sheets. Accessed July 17, 2023. https://www.ihs.gov/newsroom/factsheets/quicklook/.

11. Lofthouse J. Increasing funding for the Indian health service to improve native American health outcomes. Mercatus Center; 2022. Available at: https://www.mercatus.org/research/policy-briefs/increasing-funding-indian-health-service-improve-native-american-health. Accessed July 13, 2023.

12. Bell MC, Schmidt-Grimminger D, Patrick S, et al. There is a high prevalence of human papillomavirus infection in American Indian women of the Northern Plains. Gynecol Oncol 2007;107(2):236–41.

13. Bell MC, Schmidt-Grimminger D, Jacobsen C, et al. Risk Factors for HPV Infection among American Indian and White Women in the Northern Plains. Gynecol Oncol 2011;121(3):532.

14. Schiff M, Becker TM, Masuk M, et al. Risk factors for cervical intraepithelial neoplasia in southwestern American Indian women. Am J Epidemiol 2000; 152(8):716–26.

15. Uknowledge U, Coker AL, Hopenhayn C, et al. Violence against women raises risk of cervical cancer. Part of the Obstetrics and Gynecology Commons. J Womens Health (Larchmt) 2009. https://doi.org/10.1089/jwh.2008.1048.

16. Saraiya M, Unger ER, Thompson TD, et al. US Assessment of HPV types in cancers: implications for current and 9-valent HPV vaccines. JNCI Journal of the National Cancer Institute 2015;107(6):86.

17. Asiaf A, Ahmad ST, Mohammad SO, et al. Review of the current knowledge on the epidemiology, pathogenesis, and prevention of human papillomavirus infection. Eur J Cancer Prev 2014;23(3):206–24.

18. Alfonsi GA, Deblina Datta S, Mickiewicz T, et al. Prevalence of high-risk HPV types and abnormal cervical cytology in american indian/alaska native women, 2003–2005. Publ Health Rep 2011;126(3):330.

19. Products - Data Briefs - Number 280 - April 2017. Accessed July 19, 2023. https://www.cdc.gov/nchs/products/databriefs/db280.htm.

20. Davidson M, Schnitzer PG, Bulkow LR, et al. The prevalence of cervical infection with human papillomaviruses and cervical dysplasia in Alaska Native women. J Infect Dis 1994;169(4):792–800.

21. Lee NR, Winer RL, Cherne S, et al. Human Papillomavirus Prevalence Among American Indian Women of the Great Plains. J Infect Dis 2019;219(6):908–15.
22. Wheeler CM, Hunt WC, Cuzick J, et al. A Population-based Study of HPV Genotype Prevalence in the United States: Baseline Measures Prior to Mass HPV Vaccination. International Journal of Cancer Journal International du Cancer 2013;132(1):198–207.
23. Serrano B, Alemany L, Tous S, et al. Potential impact of a nine-valent vaccine in human papillomavirus related cervical disease. Infect Agent Cancer 2012;7(1). https://doi.org/10.1186/1750-9378-7-38.
24. Schmidt-Grimminger DC, Bell MC, Muller CJ, et al. HPV infection among rural American Indian women and urban white women in South Dakota: An HPV prevalence study. BMC Infect Dis 2011;11(1):1–8.
25. Melkonian SC, Henley SJ, Senkomago V, et al. Cancers Associated with Human Papillomavirus in American Indian and Alaska Native Populations — United States, 2013–2017. MMWR Morb Mortal Wkly Rep 2020;69(37):1283–7.
26. Kelly JJ, Unger ER, Dunne EF, et al. HPV genotypes detected in cervical cancers from Alaska Native women, 1980–2007. Int J Circumpolar Health 2013; 72(SUPPL.1). https://doi.org/10.3402/IJCH.V72I0.21115.
27. Schmidt-Grimminger D, Frerichs L, Black Bird AE, et al. HPV knowledge, attitudes, and beliefs among Northern Plains American Indian adolescents, parents, young adults, and health professionals. J Cancer Educ 2013;28(2): 357–66.
28. Estimated Adolescents Vaccination Coverage with Selected Vaccines, United States, 2020 | CDC. Accessed July 16, 2023. https://www.cdc.gov/vaccines/imz-managers/coverage/teenvaxview/pubs-presentations/NIS-teen-vac-coverage-estimates-2020-tables.html#table-01.
29. Bruegl AS, Emerson J, Tirumala K. Persistent disparities of cervical cancer among American Indians/Alaska natives: Are we maximizing prevention tools? Gynecol Oncol 2023;168:56–61.
30. Jacobs-Wingo JL, Jim CC, Groom AV. Human Papillomavirus Vaccine Uptake: Increase for American Indian Adolescents, 2013-2015. Am J Prev Med 2017; 53(2):162–8.
31. Increase the proportion of adolescents who get recommended doses of the HPV vaccine — IID-08 - Healthy People 2030 | health.gov. Accessed July 17, 2023. https://health.gov/healthypeople/objectives-and-data/browse-objectives/vaccination/increase-proportion-adolescents-who-get-recommended-doses-hpv-vaccine-iid-08.
32. Buchwald D, Muller C, Bell M, et al. Attitudes toward HPV vaccination among rural American Indian women and urban White women in the northern plains. Health Educ Behav 2013;40(6):704–11.
33. Toffolon-Weiss M, Hagan K, Leston J, et al. Alaska Native parental attitudes on cervical cancer, HPV and the HPV vaccine. Int J Circumpolar Health 2008;67(4): 363–73.
34. Gopalani SV, Janitz AE, Burkhart M, et al. HPV vaccination coverage and factors among American Indians in Cherokee Nation. Cancer Causes Control 2023; 34(3):267–75.
35. Jim CC, Wai-Yin Lee J, Groom AV, et al. Human papillomavirus vaccination practices among providers in Indian health service, tribal and urban Indian healthcare facilities. J Womens Health (Larchmt). 2012;21(4):372–8.
36. Winer RL, Gonzales AA, Noonan CJ, et al. A Cluster-Randomized Trial to Evaluate a Mother-Daughter Dyadic Educational Intervention for Increasing HPV

Vaccination Coverage in American Indian Girls. J Community Health 2016;41(2): 274–81.

37. Yzer M, Rhodes K, McCann M, et al. Effects of cultural cues on perceptions of HPV vaccination messages among parents and guardians of American Indian youth. Prev Med 2018;115:104–9.

38. Espey D, Castro G, Flagg T, et al. Strengthening breast and cervical cancer control through partnerships: American Indian and Alaska Native Women and the National Breast and Cervical Cancer Early Detection Program. Cancer 2014; 120(S16):2557–65.

39. Benard VB, Lee NC, Piper M, et al. Race-specific results of Papanicolaou testing and the rate of cervical neoplasia in the National Breast and Cervical Cancer Early Detection Program, 1991-1998 (United States). Cancer Causes Control 2001;12(1):61–8.

40. Coughlin SS, Uhler RJ, Blackman DK. Breast and cervical cancer screening practices among American Indian and Alaska Native women in the United States, 1992-1997. Prev Med 1999;29(4):287–95.

41. Health Service I. FY 2021 IHS National and Area GPRA Results. Published online 2021.

42. Increase the proportion of females who get screened for cervical cancer — C-09 - Healthy People 2030 | health.gov. Accessed July 17, 2023. https://health.gov/ healthypeople/objectives-and-data/browse-objectives/cancer/increase-proportion-females-who-get-screened-cervical-cancer-c-09#cit1.

43. Waxman AG, Haffner WHJ, Howe J, et al. A 50-year commitment to american indian and alaska native women. Obstet Gynecol 2020;136(4):739–44.

44. 2023 Indian Health Basic and Refresher Colposcopy Course | School of Medicine. Accessed July 13, 2023. https://hsc.unm.edu/medicine/education/cpl/ learn/cme-conferences/colpo2023.html.

45. Cervical Cancer Awareness and Prevention | January 2018 Blogs. Accessed July 13, 2023. https://www.ihs.gov/newsroom/ihs-blog/january2018/cervical-cancer-awareness-and-prevention/.

46. Gilbert T, Sugarman J, Cobb N. Abnormal papanicolaou smears and colposcopic follow-up among american indian and alaska native women in the Pacific Northwest. J Am Board Fam Pract 1995;8(3):183–8. Available at: https://oce-ovid-com. revproxy.brown.edu/article/00000101-199505000-00002/HTML. Accessed July 17, 2023.

47. Cervical Cancer Statistics | Key Facts About Cervical Cancer | American Cancer Society. Accessed November 1, 2023. https://www.cancer.org/cancer/types/ cervical-cancer/about/key-statistics.html.

48. Siegel RL, Miller KD, Wagle NS, et al. Cancer statistics, 2023. CA Cancer J Clin 2023;73(1):17–48.

49. Cervical Cancer — Cancer Stat Facts. Accessed November 1, 2023. https:// seer.cancer.gov/statfacts/html/cervix.html.

50. Kratzer TB, Jemal A, Miller KD, et al. Cancer statistics for A merican I ndian and A laska N ative individuals, 2022: Including increasing disparities in early onset colorectal cancer. CA Cancer J Clin 2023;73(2):120–46.

51. Becker TM, Bettles J, Lapidus J, et al. Improving Cancer Incidence Estimates for American Indians and Alaska Natives in the Pacific Northwest. Am J Public Health 2002;92(9):1469.

52. Frost F, Taylor V, Fries E. Racial misclassification of Native Americans in a surveillance, epidemiology, and end results cancer registry. J Natl Cancer Inst 1992;84(12):957–62.

53. White MC, Espey DK, Swan J, et al. Disparities in cancer mortality and incidence among American Indians and Alaska Natives in the United States. Am J Public Health 2014;104(Suppl 3). https://doi.org/10.2105/AJPH.2013.301673.
54. Becker TM, Espey DK, Lawson HW, et al. Regional differences in cervical cancer incidence among American Indians and Alaska Natives, 1999–2004. Cancer 2008;113(S5):1234–43.
55. Shaili Aggarwal N, McMillian N, David Gaffney MK, et al. NCCN Guidelines Cervical Cancer Version 1.2024. Published online 2023. Accessed November 1, 2023. https://www.nccn.org/home/member-.
56. Adegoke O, Kulasingam S, Virnig B. Cervical cancer trends in the united states: a 35-year population-based analysis. J Womens Health 2012;21(10):1031.
57. Javid SH, Varghese TK, Morris AM, et al. Guideline-concordant cancer care and survival among American Indian/Alaskan Native patients. Cancer 2014;120(14): 2183–90.
58. Markin A, Habermann EB, Zhu Y, et al. Cancer surgery among american indians. JAMA Surg 2013;148(3):277–84.
59. Amiri S, Greer MD, Muller CJ, et al. Disparities in access to radiation therapy by race and ethnicity in the united states with focus on american indian/alaska native people. Value Health 2022;25(12):1929–38.
60. Onega T, Duell EJ, Shi X, et al. Geographic access to cancer care in the U.S. Cancer 2008;112(4):909–18.
61. Dockery LE, Motwani A, Ding K, et al. Improving cancer care for American Indians with cervical cancer in the Indian Health Service (IHS) system - Navigation may not be enough. Gynecol Oncol 2018;149(1):89–92.
62. Fitch KC, Nguyen CGT, Vasquez Guzman CE, et al. Persistent cervical cancer disparities among American Indian/Alaska Native women: a systematic scoping review exploring the state of the science in this population. Cancer Causes Control 2023. https://doi.org/10.1007/S10552-023-01799-4.
63. Cervical Cancer: Statistics | Cancer.Net. Accessed November 5, 2023. https://www.cancer.net/cancer-types/cervical-cancer/statistics.
64. Jemal A, Ward EM, Johnson CJ, et al. Annual Report to the Nation on the Status of Cancer, 1975–2014, Featuring Survival. JNCI Journal of the National Cancer Institute 2017;109(9). https://doi.org/10.1093/JNCI/DJX030.
65. Bhatia S, Landier W, Paskett ED, et al. Rural-Urban Disparities in Cancer Outcomes: Opportunities for Future Research. J Natl Cancer Inst 2022;114(7): 940–52.
66. Warne D, Frizzell LB. American Indian Health Policy: Historical Trends and Contemporary Issues. Am J Public Health 2014;104(Suppl 3):S263.
67. O'Connell J, Yi R, Wilson C, et al. Racial disparities in health status: a comparison of the morbidity among American Indian and U.S. adults with diabetes. Diabetes Care 2010;33(7):1463–70.
68. Heck JL, Jones EJ, Bohn D, et al. Maternal Mortality Among American Indian/ Alaska Native Women: A Scoping Review. J Womens Health (Larchmt). 2021; 30(2):220–9.
69. Hutchinson RN, Shin S. Systematic review of health disparities for cardiovascular diseases and associated factors among American Indian and Alaska Native populations. PLoS One 2014;9(1). https://doi.org/10.1371/JOURNAL.PONE.0080973.
70. Ristevski E, Thompson S, Kingaby S, et al. Understanding Aboriginal Peoples' Cultural and Family Connections Can Help Inform the Development of Culturally

Appropriate Cancer Survivorship Models of Care. JCO Glob Oncol 2020;6(6): 124–32.

71. Takeshita J, Wang S, Loren AW, et al. Association of Racial/Ethnic and Gender Concordance Between Patients and Physicians With Patient Experience Ratings. JAMA Netw Open 2020;3(11):e2024583.

72. Cooper-Patrick L, Gallo JJ, Gonzales JJ, et al. Race, Gender, and Partnership in the Patient-Physician Relationship. JAMA 1999;282(6):583–9.

73. Cooper LA, Roter DL, Johnson RL, et al. Patient-centered communication, ratings of care, and concordance of patient and physician race. Ann Intern Med 2003;139(11). https://doi.org/10.7326/0003-4819-139-11-200312020-00009.

74. AAMC. Active physicians who identified as American Indian or Alaska Native. Published 2021. Accessed November 13, 2023. Available at: https://www.aamc.org/data-reports/workforce/data/active-physicians-american-indian-alaska-native-2021.

75. US Census Bureau. Facts for Features: American Indian and Alaska Native Heritage Month. Published 2022. Accessed November 13, 2023. Available at: https://www.census.gov/newsroom/facts-for-features/2022/aian-month.html.

76. Stubbe DE. Practicing Cultural Competence and Cultural Humility in the Care of Diverse Patients. Focus: Journal of Life Long Learning in Psychiatry 2020; 18(1):49.

77. Association of American Indian Physicians, Association of American Medical Colleges. Reshaping the Journey: American Indians and Alaska Natives in Medicine.; 2018. Accessed October 10, 2023. https://store.aamc.org/downloadable/download/sample/sample_id/243/.

78. Brodt E, Empey A, Mayinger P, et al. Shifting the Tide: Innovative Strategies to Develop an American Indian/Alaska Native Physician Workforce. Hawaii J Health Soc Welf 2019;78(12 Suppl 3):21.

79. Geana MV, Greiner KA, Cully A, et al. Improving Health Promotion to American Indians in the Midwest United States: Preferred Sources of Health Information and Its Use for the Medical Encounter. J Community Health 2012;37(6):1253.

80. Dick A, Holyk T, Taylor D, et al. Highlighting strengths and resources that increase ownership of cervical cancer screening for Indigenous communities in Northern British Columbia: Community-driven approaches. Int J Gynecol Obstet 2021;155(2):211–9.

81. Lin Y, Gong X, Mousseau R. Barriers of Female Breast, Colorectal, and Cervical Cancer Screening Among American Indians—Where to Intervene? AIMS Public Health 2016;3(4):891.

82. Caring for Patients Who Have Experienced Trauma | ACOG. Accessed October 10, 2023. https://www.acog.org/clinical/clinical-guidance/committee-opinion/articles/2021/04/caring-for-patients-who-have-experienced-trauma.

83. History of IHS | Gibagadinamaagoom. Accessed July 13, 2023. https://ojibwearchive.sas.upenn.edu/content/history-ihs.

84. Kunitz SJ. The history and politics of US health care policy for American Indians and Alaskan Natives. Am J Public Health 1996;86(10):1464.

85. Bergman AB, Grossman DC, Erdrich AM, et al. A Political History of the Indian Health Service. Milbank Q 1999;77(4):571.

86. Marcus JZ, Cason P, Downs LS, et al. The ASCCP Cervical Cancer Screening Task Force Endorsement and Opinion on the American Cancer Society Updated Cervical Cancer Screening Guidelines. J Low Genit Tract Dis 2021;25(3): 187–91.

87. HPV Vaccination Recommendations | CDC. Accessed July 25, 2023. https://www.cdc.gov/vaccines/vpd/hpv/hcp/recommendations.html.

88. S1701: POVERTY STATUS IN THE PAST - Census Bureau Table. Accessed July 15, 2023. https://data.census.gov/table?q=Income+and+Poverty&tid=ACSST 1Y2021.S1701.

89. Cornelius ME, Loretan CG, Wang TW, et al. Tobacco product use among adults-United States, 2020. MMWR Morb Mortal Wkly Rep 2022;. www.cdc.gov/nchs/washington_group/index.htm. Accessed July 15, 2023.

90. de Ravello L, Everett Jones S, Tulloch S, et al. Substance use and sexual risk behaviors among american Indian and alaska native high school students. J Sch Health 2014;84(1):25–32.

91. CDC. Youth Risk Behavior Survey Data Summary & Trends Report: 2011-2021.; 2021. Accessed July 15, 2023. https://www.cdc.gov/healthyyouth/data/yrbs/yrbs_data_summary_and_trends.htm.

92. Crossland C, Palmer J, Brooks A. NIJ's program of research on violence against american indian and alaska native women. Violence Against Women 2013;19(6): 771–90.

93. Hodge FS, Fredericks LO, Rodriguez B. American indian women's talking circle a cervical cancer screening and prevention project. Cancer 1996;78(7 Suppl): 1592–7.

94. Maar M, Burchell A, Little J, et al. A qualitative study of provider perspectives of structural barriers to cervical cancer screening among first nations women. Wom Health Issues 2013;23(5):e319.

95. Cervical Cancer Infographic - American Indian Cancer Foundation. Accessed October 10, 2023. https://americanindiancancer.org/acif-resource/cervical-cancer-infographic/.

96. Tailored Communication for Cervical Cancer Risk | Evidence-Based Cancer Control Programs (EBCCP). Accessed October 10, 2023. https://ebccp.cancercontrol.cancer.gov/programDetails.do?programId=26767713#.

97. HPV - American Indian Cancer Foundation. Accessed October 10, 2023. https://americanindiancancer.org/acif-resource/hpv/.

98. Training Resources | Division of Epidemiology and Disease Prevention. Accessed October 10, 2023. https://www.ihs.gov/epi/training-resources/.

99. Indian Health Service: Spending Levels and Characteristics of IHS and Three Other Federal Health Care Programs | U.S. GAO. Accessed October 10, 2023. https://www.gao.gov/products/gao-19-74r.

100. IHS Awards $1.2 Million in Tribal Management Grants to Support Tribal Self-Determination | 2023 Press Releases. Accessed October 10, 2023. https://www.ihs.gov/newsroom/pressreleases/2023-press-releases/ihs-awards-1-2-million-in-tribal-management-grants-to-support-tribal-self-determination/.

101. Native American Research Centers for Health (NARCH). Accessed October 10, 2023. https://www.nigms.nih.gov/capacity-building/division-for-research-capacity-building/native-american-research-centers-for-health-(narch).

Delivering Diversity and Inducing Inclusion
Evidence-Based Perspectives on Charting a Future of Equity in Obstetrics and Gynecology Residency Programs

Jasmin A. Eatman, MS[a,b,*], Cherie C. Hill, MD[c],
Agena R. Davenport-Nicholson, MD[c]

KEYWORDS

• Diversity • Equity • Inclusion • Residency • Advocacy

KEY POINTS

- Diversity, equity, and inclusion are principles that require active implementation.
- Residency programs must train technically excellent physicians who practice through self-interrogation of unconscious bias.
- The future of Obstetrics and Gynecology depends on the state of equity and justice in society and within the specialty.

INTRODUCTION

What is meant by the term "DEI," and why is it important? One of the most popular acronyms in modern-day society carries with it not only meaning but also charge to action. Diversity, equity, and inclusion (DEI) are most commonly represented as an acronym, but it is much more than three letters or words. It seeks to represent the importance of ensuring that groups of people working toward a common goal are diverse in identity, thought, and experience. Beyond identity, however, operationalizing principles of DEI requires a commitment to justice, safety, and accountability (**Fig. 1**). Whether the group's goal is commercial, political, creative, or educational in nature, the valuation of DEI determines how successful the group will be and the

[a] Emory University School of Medicine, Emory University, Atlanta, GA, USA; [b] Rollins School of Public Health, Emory University, Atlanta, GA, USA; [c] Department of Gynecology and Obstetrics, Emory University School of Medicine, Emory Women's Care, 550 Peachtree St NE, Atlanta, GA 30308, USA
* Corresponding author. Emory University School of Medicine, 100 Woodruff Circle, Atlanta, GA 30322.
E-mail address: jasmin.eatman@emory.edu

Obstet Gynecol Clin N Am 51 (2024) 143–155
https://doi.org/10.1016/j.ogc.2023.11.008
0889-8545/24/© 2023 Elsevier Inc. All rights reserved.

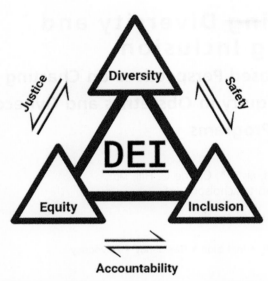

Accountability

Fig. 1. The interdependent triad of diversity, equity, and inclusion (DEI). Each term comprising the acronym, DEI is interdependent. Diversity in any group dynamic is important but suffers without inclusion. Equity allows diversity to thrive by actualizing inclusion.

impact that it will have. Throughout history, particularly in obstetrics and gynecology (OB/GYN), the perpetuation of homogeneity in legacy and leadership has been damaging and perilous.

The so-called father of gynecology, J Marion Sims, was once heralded as a hero in OB/GYN for performing experimental surgeries in pursuit of a repair for postpartum vesicovaginal fistulas.[1] In fact, he was known as a "plantation physician" by enslavers in Alabama seeking someone who would perform surgeries without patient consent and without the use of anesthesia.[1] The objective for the enslavers was to ensure that the individuals they considered property would be able to perform physical labor and that enslaved Black women would be able to work and reproduce. Despite decades of Sims' abhorrent experimentation, there are many physicians who continue to hold his legacy in high esteem. For example, a 2012 article published in the Annals of Surgery describes the core competencies in graduate medical education through a description of Sims' career as "exemplary."[2] Through the lens of heteronormative White patriarchy, one might believe that this physician—who was once the president of the American Medical Association—might be an exemplar in medicine. Figures that society chooses to uphold in history must also reflect ideals of the future. It was in this spirit that the statue of Sims was removed from Central Park on April 17, 2018, after citizen advocates successfully rallied to erase this relic of a painful past. However, to this day, over a thousand miles south, Sims statue remains in front of the Alabama state capital. In contrast, in 2022, The Mothers of Gynecology monument was erected in Montgomery, AL to honor the enslaved Black women who were the subjects of Sims' medical experiments.[3] Even in our modern society, the legacy of OB/GYN remains divided.

Forward movement in medicine must occur simultaneously with honest reckoning with the past. The word *Sankofa*, from the Akan tribe of Ghana, loosely translates to the phrase "go back for what you forgot, or left behind." Throughout history, OB/GYN has left behind the tenets of DEI. Although Sims' statue has fallen in some states and still stands in others, each OB/GYN provider has the opportunity to represent a more ethical and inclusive future. Through each patient care experience, teaching moment, and advocacy opportunity, OB/GYN providers can enact the principles of DEI to ensure that the legacy of divisiveness and bigotry in the medical field has more days behind it than ahead. The three tenets grounding this article—DEI—represent a steadfast commitment to *Sankofa*: reaching back for lessons from the past while moving forward on our journey to justice.

DISCUSSION
Recruitment

Diversity in residency cannot be fully evaluated without first taking a closer look at diversity within medical schools. With regard to diversity in medical schools, a 2022 press release from the Association of American Medical Colleges (AAMC) demonstrated an increasing number of applicants who identify as women in the 2022 to 2023 admissions cycle.[4] Unfortunately, this report also includes information on diversity of medical school applicants that is disappointing. With regard to race, numbers of Black and Latine applicants have both decreased by 19.2% and 14.2%, respectively, compared with the number of Black and Latine applicants in the previous year.[4] Numbers of Black and Latine matriculants also decreased by 9.9% and 3.0%, respectively, compared with the previous year.[4] In the same time frame, the number of American Indian or Alaska Native (AI/AN) applicants declined by 9%, and AI/AN medical students only compromise 1% of matriculants, currently. The tenet of equity is embedded within the term "DEI," and equity in all racial groups' ability to matriculate into medical school is crucial to diversifying the next generation of physicians.

With respect to residency applications, the Electronic Residency Application Service (ERAS) releases an annual report on number of applicants by specialty.[5] For OB/GYN, the 2022 to 2023 ERAS season saw 310 Black applicants, compared with 1494 White applicants.[5] Although the number of Black applicants decreased from 2021, numbers of White applicants increased. Furthermore, this report reveals that Black applicants are submitting, on average, fewer applications compared with White applicants (61.5 compared with 69.8 total applications, respectively). Considering the tremendous expense associated with applying to residency, where each application costs as much as $99 (depending on the number of applications) atop a $80 United States Medical Licensing Examination (USMLE) transcript fee, taxes, and additional fees, disparities in number of applications submitted by race may point to underlying issues in resource equity. In 2023, the American College of Obstetricians and Gynecologists (ACOG) released a specialty-wide initiative to implement a unique OB/GYN residency application.[6] This platform will officially open for the 2024 to 2025 residency application cycle and will be used in place of ERAS. The stated purpose of this transformed residency application platform is to "evaluate candidates holistically and better ensure that our OB/GYN trainees are able to meet the needs of the communities for whom we provide care."[6] The ACOG, in partnership with the Council on Resident Education in Obstetrics and Gynecology and the Association of Professors of Gynecology and Obstetrics, also highlights that this new application will be more efficient and less expensive for applicants. Initiatives to make applying to residency more inclusive and more accessible are a critical step in advancing DEI. OB/GYN, with the advent of this improved platform, is taking a step in a positive direction toward inclusion in residency education, starting at the application phase.

The current landscape of diversity in United States (US) OB/GYN residency programs exemplifies the best of all progress that has been made for DEI in medicine over the last century. The population of trainees in these programs is most closely representative of the racial diversity of the US population compared with other surgical residency training programs.[7] Although these metrics convey hope, the diversity of OB/GYN resident physicians still continues to lag behind evolving US demographics. A recent study through the University of California, Davis, which sought to measure racial and ethnic diversity among OB/GYN residents in the United States from 2014 to 2019, found that the number of Black OB/GYN residents has decreased, whereas the number of Latine[a] OB/GYN trainees has remained the same.[8] According to the AAMC 2022 Report on Residents, there are 4,804 resident trainees in OB/GYN nationwide who are graduates of MD-granting medical schools.[9] Of this total, 2,960 (61.6%) self-identify as White, 483 (10.1%) self-identify as Black or African American, and 471 (9.8%) self-identify as Latine.[9] Of all active MD residents in 2022, 48.8% reported White, 8.1% reported Latine, and 6.1% reported Black or African American race.[9]

It is imperative that OB/GYN residency programs operationalize strategies to promote and encourage recruiting diverse trainees. This is not just for the sake of meeting Accreditation Council for Graduate Medical Education (ACGME) metrics, but diversifying the physician workforce has been shown to improve patient outcomes.[10] Diversity in academic medical leadership is important to ensuring that policies and procedures exist for the recruitment of diverse trainees. A 2023 cross-sectional survey study on diversity in academic medical leadership revealed that OB/GYN saw a 53.2% increase in female representation in departmental chairperson leadership (although the term "female" is used here, the authors recognize that this term does not encompass all gender diverse communities and is used to cite prior data using this terminology).[11] However, this study also revealed dismal statistics capturing representation of Black individuals in academic medical leadership. Only 9.1% of OB/GYN residency program directors are Black, whereas only 3.5% of all residency program directors across all specialties are Black (the lowest percentage of all racial groups).[11] Increasing diversity of leadership will be important to improving diversity of the medical field. However, as sociopolitical landscapes continue to shift, diverse leadership alone cannot guarantee improvement in diversity of trainees.

The proverbial mammoth in the room with regard to diversity recruitment is the 2023 Supreme Court ruling on race conscious admissions. In their dissents, Justices Ketanji Brown Jackson, Sonya Sotomayor, and Elena Kagan posit that the implications of this decision are far-reaching and position our society at a point of criticality in terms of advancing racial equity. Justice Sotomayor urges readers of her dissent that "equal educational opportunity is a prerequisite to achieving racial equality in our Nation."[12] Affirmative action (AA) is a race-conscious recruitment policy designed to equalize access to jobs and professions, such as medicine, and is based on the premise that combatting illegal overt racial discrimination is not sufficient to equalize opportunity for minoritized groups.[13] Throughout the years, there has been staunch criticism of AA, particularly in admissions protocols for institutions of higher education including medical schools and residency training programs. However, racial diversity among medical trainees has demonstrated incredible benefit and a greater understanding of patient populations through racial concordance. In fact, peer-reviewed literature has demonstrated that health outcomes among patients belonging to minoritized racial groups are improved when racial identity is shared between patient and provider.[10,14–16] Following the Supreme Court ruling on AA, ACOG released a statement condemning the decision, urging medical schools to "take into account race, ethnicity,

---

[a] Latine is a gender-neutral term for individuals of Latin ancestry and/or Hispanic ethnicity.

and the lived experience that each candidate could bring to their career as a physician because of their background."[17] Further, ACOG's statement drew a strong, direct correlation between diversity in health care and the provision of high-quality care.[17] In a similar spirit, the American Medical Association recently passed policy through its House of Delegates, declaring that banning AA is a critical threat to health equity and that the recent decision by the Supreme Court will curtail racial diversity in medical schools.[18] Passed before the Supreme Court ruling, this policy urged medical training programs to proactively implement policies and procedures that support race-conscious admissions practices. Now that the landscape has changed, active measures must be taken to ensure progress toward racial equity through admissions in medical education.

In 2022, the Council of Residency Directors in Emergency Medicine published an article on the implementation of strategies in residency recruitment for DEI.[19] Although the nation's legal statutes have changed since its publication, this article provides concrete guidance for residency programs on recruitment of diverse residency applicants through holistic review. A holistic review, as it is described, includes assessing program readiness for recruits from groups who are underrepresented in medicine, engaging applicants through structured interviews, and programmatic consideration of potential bias in commonly used admissions metrics, such as clerkship grades, honor society membership, and standardized examinations.[19] Importantly, a recent study of the 20 largest ACGME resident specialties demonstrated that no residency program represented Black or Latine populations at rates that are comparable to the overall US population. The recruitment of trainees from diverse backgrounds is a critical issue that must be faced head-on. Admissions protocols should be anti-racist in their recruitment strategies, recognizing that ethnic and racial diversity are critical to their success. OB/GYN, representing the specialty with the highest mean percentage of applicants and matriculants who are underrepresented in medicine among surgical specialties at present, has an opportunity to lead the charge for equity in recruitment while navigating the complexities of the current political landscape.

Education and Engagement

Increasing representation of OB/GYN residents who are members of groups that are underrepresented in medicine is critically important to medicine and to the communities that they represent. Education of a diverse group of trainees in OB/GYN is enriched by partnership with the community throughout the curriculum. A 2022 study completed through a partnership between perinatal health care providers and a Nehiyawak (Plain Cree) community of Maskwacîs, Central Alberta (Canada) sought to measure interventions to improve cultural intelligence and sensitivity in health care through experiential learning opportunities encompassing anti-racism and cultural safety.[20] This study not only spoke to root causes of maternal health disparities disproportionately impacting Indigenous Peoples in Canada, but championed community-led strategies to improving health care delivery in this population. The title of this study, *Mâmawihitowin*, translates to "bringing the camps together for a common goal." Similarly, through incorporating principles of cultural safety and anti-racism while shining a light on implicit bias in health care delivery, researchers operationalized an explanatory sequential mixed method design to implement interventions that included cultural training for perinatal health care providers.

The effectiveness of this intentional approach was evidenced by the study's statistically significant results, which showed that providers' cultural intelligence scale scores and engagement with the community increased markedly post-intervention.[20] In addition, qualitative data evaluation demonstrated that interventions promoted awareness and acknowledgment of positive strengths within the community, contrasting negative, and pervasive stereotypes about Indigenous populations. Participants gained an immersive educational experience, noting an increased desire to meaningfully engage with patients on a personal level and to build empathy through cultural and social awareness. This consequentially allowed participants to feel better understood by their health care providers, as they were able to directly express a need for more empathy and compassion around common issues such as socioeconomic challenges, transportation barriers, and missed appointments. Mistrust between communities of color and OB/GYN has been thoroughly researched, evidenced, and documented. Increasing opportunities for partnership between the medical community and the populations we serve is an important but often forgotten opportunity to advance health equity. This is a ripe area in which OB/GYN residency programs can enhance DEI efforts in clinical care and integrate culturally compassionate care into their training.

Owing to resource limitations, purview, or other factors, some programs may navigate prohibitive challenges in interfacing directly with the community. There are, however, internal approaches to ensuring that the tenets of equity and inclusivity are thoroughly engaged, in these cases. In late 2022, The Journal of the American Medical Association released an article describing the benefits and drawbacks of mandated implicit bias training for health professionals.[21] This published issue describes more than 20 years of evidence that clinicians' implicit biases impact their clinical practice, and standardizing implicit bias training is beneficial on many fronts. First, requiring this type of training sends a powerful message about the importance of combatting conscious and subconscious bias among the health care workforce. In addition, focusing on specific clinical issues through implicit bias training can reveal areas in which inequities are particularly concerning or where bias is most deeply rooted. It is important to note that stark racial disparities in maternal morbidity and mortality helped to propel current laws mandating implicit bias training. In fact, perinatal care is the most consistent implicit bias training focus across the nation.[21] California, Maryland, Michigan, Minnesota, and Washington are currently the only states where implicit bias training for select categories of health professionals is required.[21] Outcomes related to maternal morbidity and mortality in states that have implemented mandatory implicit bias training have been mixed, but mandates without structural changes to address discrimination are futile at best. Training in the awareness of subconscious bias must be coupled with tools to intervene in situations where overt bias is present, along with pairing these actionable steps with practical tools for delivering health care through a culturally conscious lens.

Culturally Sensitive Training and Practice

In January 2018, ACOG released a committee opinion on the importance of social determinants of health and cultural awareness in the delivery of reproductive health care.[22] This opinion was reaffirmed in 2021. Important to highlight is the establishment of this opinion before the COVID-19 pandemic and resurgence of public awareness and outcry around issues of racial injustice. In addition to describing the importance of social determinants of health to patient outcomes, ACOG provides recommendations for OB/GYNs in practice who want to improve patient-centered care and decrease reproductive health care inequities. Among them is a recommendation that practicing OB/GYNs acknowledge that structural and institutionalized racism is a social determinant of health.

The committee opinion goes on to address the role of cultural awareness, humility, and sensitivity in addressing social determinants of health which impact patient outcomes. The use of the term "cultural sensitivity" or "cultural humility" intentionally contrasts the once widely used term "cultural competency." One cannot be competent in another person's culture, as there is no reality in which a person can be sufficiently versed or proficient in knowledge of another culture. In the context of patient care, it is important for health care providers to acknowledge that culture is a central identity for patients to whom they provide care, and it is important to approach this subject with humility in order to bring about awareness that can be applied to building trust and rapport.

Residency programs can aim to instill a sense of cultural humility and awareness among trainees through various approaches. One recommendation from the aforementioned ACOG committee opinion includes screening for social determinants of health, ensuring that resident trainees have reliable access to interpreter services (specifically in-person interpreters) and establishing medical–legal partnerships between the academic health care network and local legal practices. Medical–legal partnerships allow resident trainees and practicing physicians to provide patients with tangible assistance through legal services in the same site as the clinic. In this way, patients are able to receive medical care while simultaneously addressing aspects of health and well-being in their everyday lives, such as toxic environmental exposures, access to housing, and legal support with immigration challenges. Institutional support for resident training in addressing issues related to social determinants of health can directly improve residents' cultural awareness and humility, initiating momentum for lifelong medical practice that centers these tenets.

Throughout residency training, culturally sensitive care manifests through innovative approaches to operationalizing principles encompassed by DEI. At Emory University, in Atlanta, Georgia, the Department of Gynecology and Obstetrics implemented a Disparity Morbidity and Mortality (M&M) conference in response to the nationwide protests against racial injustice in the summer of 2020. The goal of Disparity M&Ms in this training program is to curate a more robust discussion of the social determinants of health, including racial and systemic barriers, that may have contributed to the outcomes seen among patients. Through this approach, residents are challenged to recognize how these factors are often interwoven. Residents also explore the implicit or explicit bias against patients that may impact medical decision-making in a case where an adverse outcome has been identified. In 2021, Emory went a step further to implement a monthly Justice Journal Club. These journal clubs are opportunities for both resident trainees, fellows, and faculty to explore topics such as "Mass Incarceration as a Driver of Reproductive Oppression" and "Associations Between Historically Redlined Districts and Racial Disparities in Current Obstetric Outcomes" (**Table 1**).

The Justice Journal Club series was developed with guidance from the Centers for Disease Control Health Equity Style Guide and a list of articles on anti-racist praxis in health care delivery. Data suggest a greater interest and higher attendance in these journal clubs than others hosted previously, which is supported by an increase in the average number of people who attend the Justice Journal Club compared with attendance at traditional journal clubs (**Table 2**). These spaces have created an increased appetite for these necessary and impactful conversations while cultivating community by drawing in various stakeholders from across the department including clinical faculty, research faculty, nonclinical staff, and community partners. Creative approaches to incorporating DEI into resident education, such as the Justice Journal Club, open the conversation to invite new perspectives. One of the great benefits of DEI programmatic engagement in residency is the opportunity to engage in self-reflection. The positive impact of programmatic engagement around principles of

Table 1
Emory University Department of Gynecology and Obstetrics, *Social Justice Journal Club*, presenter list and topics

Date	Presenters and Topics
1/26/21	Dr Joey Bahng and Dr Leah Rondon, "On Racism: A New Standard for Publishing on Racial Health Inequities" from the Health Affairs blog July, 2020
3/30/21	Dr Alex Forrest and Dr Jenn Reeves, "Reproductive Justice Disrupted: Mass Incarceration as a Driver of Reproductive Oppression"
5/25/21	Dr Nicole St Omer Roy and Dr Sharon Owusu-Darko, "Sterilization in US Immigration and Customs Enforcement's (ICEs) Detention: Ethical Failures and Systemic Injustice"
7/21/21	Dr Ashley Williams and Dr Chanhee Han, "Racial-Ethnic and Socioeconomic Disparities in Guideline-Adherent Treatment for Endometrial Cancer"
9/29/21	Dr Denise Jamieson and Dr Natalie Levey, "Race, Gender, and Generation: Reflections by Three Physicians in Three Parts" by Drs Kalinda Woods, Michael Lindsay and Kesley Robertson (all special guests) and StoryCorps interview with Dr Denise Raynor (also present as a special guest)
11/29/21	Dr Daniella Spielman and Dr Susan Davis, "Women or LARC First? Reproductive Autonomy and the Promotion of Long-Acting Reversible Contraceptive Methods"
2/9/22	Dr Caroline Wentworth and Dr Marisa Young, "Associations Between Historically Redlined Districts and Racial Disparities in Current Obstetric Outcomes" with special guest Professor LaDale Winling of the History Department at Virginia Tech
4/11/22	Dr Gia Garrett and Dr Austin Schirmer, "The pipeline problem: barriers to access of Black patients and providers in reproductive medicine" and "Health disparities of African Americans in reproductive medicine"
7/6/22	Dr Lisette Tanner and Dr Cynthia Abam, "Addressing systemic racism in birth doula services to reduce health inequities in the United States" with special guest Bradi Bishop-Stacker
9/27/22	Dr Damilola Olatunji and Dr Sana Ansari, "An American Crisis – The Lack of Black Men in Medicine" with special guests Dr. Kesley Robertson and Dr. Shenelle Wilson
1/23/23	Dr Raina Advani and Dr Nisha Verma, "Pathology of Racism — A Call to Desegregate Teaching Hospitals"
2/21/23	Dr Haben Debessai, Dr Lisa Flowers, and Dr Kelsey Schmidt, "Criminal Justice Involvement and Abnormal Cervical Cancer Screening Results Among Women in an Urban Safety Net Hospital"
3/29/23	Dr Alisha Kramer and Dr Agena Davenport "Toward the elimination of race-based medicine: replace race with racism as preeclampsia risk factor" with special guest Jasmin Eatman, Emory MD/PhD Candidate
5/31/23	Dr Stephanie Figueira and Dr Rafael Campos, "Racial and ethnic disparities in perinatal insurance coverage"

DEI is evidenced by Emory OB/GYN residents' positive ACGME survey responses to questions about resident preparation for interaction with diverse individuals, inclusivity in the work environment, and engagement in DEI recruitment and retention efforts. Across the program, residents' responses to these questions exceeded national percentages for compliance, with notable improvement from previous years. DEI is essential to holistic resident education and training. It equips the next generation of

Table 2 Participation in Justice Journal Clubs compared with Traditional Journal Clubs, Emory University Department of Gynecology and Obstetrics, December 2020 to Present ($N = 26$ sessions)		
	Mean Number of Participants per Session	Median Number of Participants per Session
Justice Journal Club	34	30
Traditional Journal Club	24	26

health care providers to be introspective in their interactions with patients and colleagues of all races, genders, sexual orientations, religions, ages, and abilities.

Retention

OB/GYN is a specialty that serves patients in some of the most vulnerable points in their lives. Just as patients served by this specialty are empowered to engage in wellness and self-expression, resident trainees must also be supported in this endeavor. Within institutional walls of academic hospitals nationwide, resident trainees battle emotionally and physically deleterious working conditions. In a study on resident burnout and coping mechanisms early in the COVID-19 pandemic, outcomes revealed that over half of all participants reported feeling burned out, with 69.9% reporting distress and emotional concerns regarding the pandemic.[23] Among the specialties with the highest number of respondents was OB/GYN and the majority of respondents self-reported being assigned female at birth. Of the specified support programs offered by residency programs, participants reported that meal support, structured mentorship, and mental health counseling services were the most helpful. Although some might argue that the COVID-19 pandemic is over, many current residents in OB/GYN programs started residency at the height of the pandemic and the lasting impacts of living and working through this international crisis are lasting.

Residents belonging to minoritized groups by race, ethnicity, and gender experience micro- and macroaggressions from patients and colleagues, compounded by exceedingly demanding working conditions of residency training. Alarmingly, Black trainees comprised approximately 20% of those dismissed from OB/GYN training programs.[24] In a 2020 study on physicians' experiences with mistreatment and discrimination, one in five physicians had experienced a patient or a member of the patient's family refusing to allow them to provide care because of the physician's personal physical attributes at least once in the previous year.[25] Further, outcomes revealed that Black physicians and physicians identifying as female were more likely to report discrimination in the past year. As might be expected, experiencing discrimination was independently associated with a higher likelihood of reporting burnout.[25] Black residents in particular demonstrate some of the lowest rates of matriculation throughout residency and experience over policing in their academic careers.[26] Peer-reviewed research into the impact of racism and gender discrimination in medical education has advocated for an inclusive educational environment that centers these experiences, termed trauma-informed medical education.[27] Data on weathering, burnout, and allostatic load on residents belonging to marginalized groups support the need for medical education that recognizes the impact of discrimination on trainee well-being and provides an opportunity for trauma-informed education.[28]

Stereotypes and prejudices against individuals of all minoritized identities are magnified in the context of medical and residency training, and these experiences are gravely consequential. An October 2021 study on experiences of LGBTQ+ residents in US general surgery training programs demonstrates that mistreatment is an experience that is pervasive among residents who are LGBTQ+. In this report, despite reporting similar career satisfaction, residents who are LGBTQ+ were twice as likely to consider leaving their training programs and significantly more likely to have thoughts of suicide.[29] In a recent study on OB/GYN resident experiences with training in provision of LGBTQ+ health care in Illinois, alarming outcomes demonstrated that 50% of OB/GYN residents felt unprepared to care for lesbian or bisexual patients and a staggering 76% did not feel prepared to care for transgender patients.[30] The current national landscape is one that would seek to marginalize and silence individuals who are minoritized in terms of their sexual orientation and gender identity. It is important that OB/GYN is a specialty composed of physicians who are equipped to serve patients who may face such daily discrimination and overt violence daily. Increasing the percentage of LGBTQ+ residents is an important aspect of this vision, and making sure that residency programs foster spaces that are inclusive and safe is equally critical.

Safety is a critical and necessary link between diversity and inclusion (see **Fig. 1**). Fostering wellness is as a critical component of cultivating a culture of safety. Programmatic development of a wellness curriculum, therefore, is an important step toward advancing DEI in OB/GYN training programs. A large and growing body of evidence demonstrates that residents benefit from programmatic commitment to incorporating wellness into the resident curriculum. At Emory University's OB/GYN residency program, wellness programming has been reimagined to include community engagement. For example, residents can choose to engage in events with community partners such as midwives and doulas to discuss opportunities for partnership. Importantly, these efforts also include investing in mental health resources for residents through partnership with psychologists in the department of Graduate Medical Education. Further examples of incorporating wellness in residency training programs include social gatherings, weekly protected administrative time, and offering mental health counseling resources including time to attend appointments. Engaging creative approaches to wellness and investment in these activities is critically important to resident success and relevant to fostering a DEI culture of safety.

Wellness, however, is not entirely a matter of the mind. In a cross-sectional study of more than 400,000 surgical residency programs, trainees from underrepresented racial or ethnic backgrounds were observed to be at significantly higher risk for attrition compared with White trainees. Professional safety and success is also critically important to promoting wellness, particularly among residents from backgrounds underrepresented in medicine. In a 2023 study on racial disparities in attrition rates, OB/GYN had the highest percentage of residents identifying as Black or African American (10.9%).[31] However, the representation of residents identifying as female and racially underrepresented in medicine increased over the study period for all specialties expect for OB/GYN.[7,31] As we advance DEI in medicine and, specifically, in the specialty of OB/GYN, it is important that our efforts are not temporally aligned with trends in matriculation. The recruitment of underrepresented students into residency programs is equally as important as ensuring that they are supported through graduation. In a 2023 publication of the American Journal of Surgery, a large team of residents and faculty representing medical training institutions across the United States developed an evidence-based framework to improve retention of Black surgical trainees.[32] Root causes of inequities in completion of surgical training included interpersonal discrimination and bias, social isolation, and increased socioeconomic and sociopolitical burden. Recommendations for increasing successful matriculation rates for residents of color were categorized by stakeholder type, including the ACGME, institution, program leadership, faculty and house staff, trainee, and professional societies. On part of the institution and program leadership, residency programs can support the successful matriculation of residents of color through interventions such as setting clear anti-discrimination policies, providing awareness for discrimination reporting avenues and transparency regarding the process of investigating these reports, recruiting and retaining diverse faculty and trainees, and ensuring diverse representation in performance review meetings.

Institutional accountability is an invaluable component of DEI work. Support for resident trainees who are doing the work of implementing DEI in residency training programs is nonnegotiable. A central component of infusing DEI into programmatic values is achieved through challenging institutions to move beyond the goal of simply satisfying DEI requirements. Fostering social justice through residency training requires commitment to DEI principles. Excellence in this arena is achieved through setting metrics for success, accountability through programmatic self-evaluation, and fostering a culture of both clinical and personal safety.

Allyship is also a critical component to fostering DEI in residency training programs. The term "minority tax" refers to the work that falls on individuals belonging to minoritized groups to represent and advocate for their communities. This burden of time, resources, emotional labor, and intellectual energy is compounded by the demands of job-related work. Inclusivity and diversity are linked by a sense of both personal and professional safety for trainees of all backgrounds and identities.

SUMMARY

In the spirit of the principle *Sankofa*, pressing forward while reaching back, OB/GYN will create powerful, multigenerational momentum that champions DEI through residency training and clinical practice. Actionable and evidence-based approaches to infusing DEI across the curricula in residency training programs will be critical to achieving outcomes that evidence progress. Although current literature and the present political landscape would suggest that achieving successful operationalization of DEI in medical training is out of reach, a more nuanced perspective reveals longitudinal success in the pursuit of equity and inclusion for our increasingly diverse trainee communities. OB/GYN is a specialty that has a higher percentage of underrepresented trainees than any other surgical specialty and with this diversity comes the power of perspective. The richness of experience must be leveraged through creative approaches to recruitment, education, community engagement, and retention. DEI is much more than an acronym, but a necessity for engaging a diverse community of OB/GYN providers for generations to come.

CLINICS CARE POINTS

- Diversity, equity, and inclusion (DEI) are three terms that represent actionable steps toward justice through acceptance and valuation of all people.
- Multidimensional approaches to actualizing DEI principles through obstetrics and gynecology (OB/GYN) residency training programs are essential to preparing the next generation of OB/GYN physicians.

> • The work of DEI requires collective action at both individual and institutional levels, which will create a more equitable tomorrow for patients and trainees alike.

ACKNOWLEDGMENTS

Dr Marisa Young, MD/PhD, Assistant Professor, Emory University Department of Gynecology and Obstetrics. Dr Haben Debessai, MD, Gilstrap Fellow, Centers for Disease Control and Prevention.

DISCLOSURE

The authors declare that they have nothing to disclose.

REFERENCES

1. Hallman JC. *Say Anarcha: A Young Woman, a Devious Surgeon, and the Harrowing Birth of Modern Women's Health*. First edition. New York: Henry Holt and Company; 2023.
2. Straughn JM Jr, Gandy RE, Rodning CB. The core competencies of James Marion Sims, MD. Ann Surg 2012;256(1):193–202.
3. Browder M. The More Up Campus. 2023. anarchalucybetsey.org.
4. AAMC. 2022 Fall Applicant, Matriculant, and Enrollment Data Tables 2022. 10/31/2022. Available at: chrome-extension://efaidnbmnnnibpcajpcglclefindmkaj/https://www.aamc.org/media/64176/download?attachment. Accessed July 10, 2023.
5. Colleges AoAM. ERAS® Statistics. 2022. Historical Specialty Specific Data (Obstetrics and Gynecology). https://www.aamc.org/media/39861/download.
6. Obstetrics AoPoGa. New Residency Application Platform for Obstetrics and Gynecology 2023. https://apgo.org/page/rrrapplicationplatform.
7. Nieblas-Bedolla E, Williams JR, Christophers B, et al. Trends in race/ethnicity among applicants and matriculants to US Surgical Specialties, 2010-2018. JAMA Netw Open 2020;3(11):e2023509.
8. López CL, Wilson MD, Hou MY, et al. Racial and ethnic diversity among obstetrics and gynecology, surgical, and nonsurgical residents in the US From 2014 to 2019. JAMA Netw Open 2021;4(5):e219219.
9. (AAMC) AAoMC. Report on Residents. https://www.aamc.org/data-reports/students-residents/data/report-residents/2022/table-b5-md-residents-race-ethnicity-and-specialty.
10. Jetty A, Jabbarpour Y, Pollack J, et al. Patient-physician racial concordance associated with improved healthcare use and lower healthcare expenditures in minority populations. J Racial Ethn Health Disparities 2022;9(1):68–81.
11. Meadows AM, Skinner MM, Hazime AA, et al. Racial, ethnic, and sex diversity in academic medical leadership. JAMA Netw Open 2023;6(9):e2335529.
12. Students for fair admissions, inc. v. president and fellows of harvard college; students for fair admissions, inc. v. University of North Carolina, et al., (Supreme Court of the United States of America 2023). https://www.supremecourt.gov/opinions/22pdf/20-1199_hgdj.pdf.
13. Curtis JL. Affirmative Action in Medicine: Improving Health Care for Everyone. Ann Arbor: University of Michigan Press; 2003.
14. Lakhan SE. Diversification of U.S. medical schools via affirmative action implementation. BMC Med Educ 2003;3(1):6.

15. Saha S, Guiton G, Wimmers PF, et al. Student body racial and ethnic composition and diversity-related outcomes in US medical schools. JAMA 2008;300(10): 1135–45.
16. Takeshita J, Wang S, Loren AW, et al. Association of racial/ethnic and gender concordance between patients and physicians with patient experience ratings. JAMA Netw Open 2020;3(11):e2024583.
17. ACOG Statement on Supreme Court Affirmative Action Ruling. ACOG; June 29, 2023, 2023. https://www.acog.org/news/news-releases/2023/06/acog-statement-on-supreme-court-affirmative-action-ruling.
18. AMA adopts policy for race-conscious admissions in higher education. AMA; June 13, 2023, 2023. https://www.ama-assn.org/press-center/press-releases/ama-adopts-policy-race-conscious-admissions-higher-education.
19. Gallegos M, Landry A, Alvarez A, et al. Holistic review, mitigating bias, and other strategies in residency recruitment for diversity, equity, and inclusion: an evidence-based guide to best practices from the council of residency directors in emergency medicine. West J Emerg Med 2022;23(3):345–52.
20. Bruno G, Bell RC, Parlee B, et al. Mâmawihitowin (bringing the camps together): Perinatal healthcare provider and staff participation in an Indigenous-led experiential intervention for enhancing culturally informed care-a mixed methods study. Int J Equity Health 2022;21(1):164.
21. Cooper LA, Saha S, van Ryn M. Mandated implicit bias training for health professionals—a step toward equity in health care. JAMA Health Forum 2022;3(8): e223250.
22. ACOG Committee Opinion No. 729. Importance of social determinants of health and cultural awareness in the delivery of reproductive health care. Obstet Gynecol 2018;131(1):e43–8.
23. Zoorob D, Shah S, La Saevig D, et al. Insight into resident burnout, mental wellness, and coping mechanisms early in the COVID-19 pandemic. PLoS One 2021; 16(4):e0250104.
24. McDade W. Diversity and inclusion in graduate medical education. Chicago: Accreditation Council for Graduate Medical Education presentation; 2019.
25. Dyrbye LN, West CP, Sinsky CA, et al. Physicians' experiences with mistreatment and discrimination by patients, families, and visitors and association with burnout. JAMA Netw Open 2022;5(5):e2213080.
26. Ellis J, Otugo O, Landry A, et al. Dismantling the overpolicing of black residents. N Engl J Med 2023;389(14):1258–61.
27. McClinton A, Laurencin CT. Just in time: trauma-informed medical education. Journal of Racial and Ethnic Health Disparities 2020;7(6):1046–52.
28. Miller HN, LaFave S, Marineau L, et al. The impact of discrimination on allostatic load in adults: An integrative review of literature. J Psychosom Res 2021;146: 110434.
29. Heiderscheit EA, Schlick CJR, Ellis RJ, et al. Experiences of LGBTQ+ residents in us general surgery training programs. JAMA Surgery 2022;157(1):23–32.
30. Guerrero-Hall KD, Muscanell R, Garg N, et al. Obstetrics and gynecology resident physician experiences with lesbian, gay, bisexual, transgender and queer healthcare training. Med Sci Educ 2021;31(2):599–606.
31. Haruno LS, Chen X, Metzger M, et al. Racial and sex disparities in resident attrition among surgical subspecialties. JAMA Surgery 2023;158(4):368–76.
32. Suraju MO, McElroy L, Moten A, et al. A framework to improve retention of Black surgical trainees: A Society of Black Academic Surgeons white paper. Am J Surg 2023;226(4):438–46.

Pelvic Floor Disorders in Black Women
Prevalence, Clinical Care, and a Strategic Agenda to Prioritize Care

Charelle M. Carter-Brooks, MD, MSc[a],*,
Oluwateniola E. Brown, MD[b], Mary F. Ackenbom, MD, MSc[c]

KEYWORDS

- Black women • Health disparities • Health equity • Pelvic floor disorders
- Pelvic organ prolapse • Urinary incontinence • Women of color

KEY POINTS

- Urinary incontinence (UI) and pelvic organ prolapse (POP) are common among Black women, with the prevalence of these disorders ranging from 3.3% to 45.9% for UI and 1% to 7.6% for POP.
- Studies show underutilization of evidence-based treatments for pelvic floor disorders (PFDs) among Black women. There are limited data on barriers to PFD care for this population.
- Large database studies consistently demonstrate that Black women experience poor outcomes after surgeries for UI and POP.
- Studies moving beyond identifying disparities in treatment are limited, yet necessary to improve outcomes.
- A strategic agenda to prioritize the care of Black women with PFDs should aim to address multiple influences on PFD care by increasing awareness of PFDs and treatments, optimizing clinical care, expanding representation of Black women in PFD research, and dismantling structural racism to achieve health equity.

INTRODUCTION

Pelvic floor disorders (PFDs) are a group of chronic conditions that include pelvic organ prolapse (POP) and urinary incontinence (UI). PFDs are prevalent, with 25% of

[a] The George Washington School of Medicine and Health Sciences, 2150 Pennsylvania Avenue NW, Suite 6A- 416, Washington, DC 20037, USA; [b] Northwestern University Feinberg School of Medicine, 250 East Superior Avenue Suite 05-2113, Chicago, IL 60601, USA; [c] Magee-Womens Research Institute, University of Pittsburgh, 3240 Craft Place, Suite 226, Pittsburgh, PA 15213, USA
* Corresponding author.
E-mail address: chbrooks@mfa.gwu.edu

Obstet Gynecol Clin N Am 51 (2024) 157–179
https://doi.org/10.1016/j.ogc.2023.11.002
0889-8545/24/© 2023 Elsevier Inc. All rights reserved.

obgyn.theclinics.com

women in the United States experiencing at least one PFD in their lifetime.[1,2] Although PFD conditions are benign, they can negatively impact quality of life (QoL).[3] In addition, PFDs are often underreported and subsequently undertreated in women due to embarrassment, normalization, and downplaying of symptoms by patients and health care professionals.[4–6]

Women from racial backgrounds that have been historically marginalized in the United States experience differences in PFD treatment and outcomes. In some instances, these differences constitute health care inequities.[7–9] Studies focusing on these differences often compare outcomes of Black and Hispanic women against the outcomes of White women. Research solely approached in this manner can be problematic as White women are made the reference group or "gold standard" for comparison. Women from historically marginalized groups require research performed through their own lens to increase understanding of their experiences with care and disease states and improve their outcomes.

This article focuses on PFDs, specifically POP and UI, in Black women in the United States. The authors explore what is known about PFDs in Black women, the clinical care they receive, and the associated outcomes and barriers they face to equitable care. Finally, the authors present action items to prioritize the care of Black women with PFDs in the United States.

PREVALENCE OF PELVIC FLOOR DISORDERS IN BLACK WOMEN

UI and POP are the most common PFDs in women, and their prevalence increases with age.[1,2] There are various subtypes of UI. Urgency urinary continence (UUI) is characterized by a sudden compelling desire to pass urine that is difficult to defer.[10] Overactive bladder is defined as urinary urgency, with or without UUI, usually with frequency and nocturia. In contrast, stress UI (SUI) refers to involuntary loss of urine with increases in intra-abdominal pressure such as exercise or coughing. POP is the descent of one or more of the anterior vaginal wall, posterior vaginal wall, the uterus (cervix) or the apex of the vagina through the pelvic floor to the level of the hymen or beyond.[11]

The prevalence and subtype of UI in Black women may vary based on the severity of leakage and screening methodology. Several studies report varied prevalence rates of UI among Black women with rates ranging from 3.3% to 45.9% (**Tables 1** and **2**). A study of women aged 35 to 64 years in Michigan from 2002 to 2004 found that the prevalence of UI was 14.6% for Black women. Of women with UI, Black women reported high frequency of urge symptoms (23.8%).[12] Another study of women aged 40 to 69 years found that the prevalence of UI was 64.8% in Black women. In a cross-sectional, population Internet-based survey, the prevalence of UUI among Black women was 14.2%. In another study of women aged 66 years and older, overactive bladder was diagnosed in 5.5% of Black women. Overall rates of SUI in Black women range from 3% to 25% compared with 6% to 40% in White women in cross-sectional studies based on patient-reported symptoms.[12–18] Of note, these studies overwhelmingly show that Black women have similar rates of UI as White women yet Black women are more likely to report urge symptoms than SUI.

POP is also prevalent among Black women. Population-based studies found that the prevalence in Black women ranged from 1% to 7.6%. In a systematic review, the pooled prevalence rates of symptomatic POP were 3.8% (95% CI, 3.22%–4.38%) for Black women.[19]

PFD prevalence studies also suggest racial differences in PFD prevalence. In particular, studies suggest lower overall UI prevalence, higher UUI prevalence, and

Table 1
Prevalence of overactive bladder/urgency urinary incontinence by patient-reported symptoms in validated questionnaires

Author	Year	Type of Study	Age (years)	N Total Study	N = Black Women	N = White Women	Overall OAB/ UUI Prevalence	OAB/UUI in Black Women	OAB/UUI in White Women*
Fenner	2008	Phone questionnaire	35–64	2814	892	1922	26.5%	23.8%	11%
Jackson	2004	Interview	70–79	1558	717	841	11.6%	7%	11%
Thom	2006	Interview	Middle-aged	2109	383	1003	–	13.6%	8.8%
Coyne	2013	Internet questionnaire	18–70	5023	1026	3032	20.0%	19.0%	19%
Coyne	2012	Internet questionnaire	18–70	4482	514	3499	–	45.9%	43.4%
Townsend	2010	Mailed questionnaires	37–79	76,724	1138	74,734	–	0.5	0.4
Tennstedt	2008	In-person interview/ questionnaire	37–79	3205	1070	1024	10.4%	3.3%	13.4%
Akbar	2021	Questionnaire	Mean 70	1749	443	641	–	10.2%	7.6%

Abbreviations: OAB, overactive bladder; UUI, urgency urinary incontinence.

Table 2
Prevalence of stress urinary incontinence by patient-reported symptoms in validated questionnaires

Author	Year	Type of Study	Age (years)	Total N in Study	N = Black Women*	N = White Women*	Overall SUI Prevalence	SUI in Black Women*	SUI in White Women*
Fenner	2008	Phone questionnaire	35–64	2814	892	1922	26.50%	25%	39.2%
Jackson	2004	Interview	70–79	1558	717	841	12%	5%	12%
Thom	2006	Interview	Middle-aged	2109	383	1003	–	7.5%	15.1%
Coyne	2013	Internet questionnaire	18–70	5023	1026	3032	–	24.8%	40.15%
Townsend	2010	Mailed questionnaires	37–79	76,724	1138	74,734	–	0.1	0.8
Tennstedt	2008	In-person interview/questionnaire	37–79	3205	1070	1024	26.4%	9.4%	35.4%
Akbar	2021	Questionnaire	Mean 70	1749	443	641	–	3.1%	6.2%

Abbreviation: SUI, stress urinary incontinence.

lower POP prevalence for Black women compared with White women.[2,12–24] It is noteworthy that there have been studies aimed at understanding differences in the prevalence of PFD in Black women compared with White women by examining biological and anatomic differences including differences in genetic loci, pelvic floor musculature, and urodynamic parameters.[25,26] Giri and colleagues evaluated the association of specific genetic loci and POP across races. This study demonstrated that being of European ancestry did not increase the risk of POP.[25] Derpapas and colleagues assessing pelvic floor musculature using translabial sonography found that nulliparous Black women had larger rhabdosphincters than White women (8.88 cm^3 ± 1.65 vs 5.97 cm^3 ± 1.82, P=.001). Black women also had a significantly wider transverse diameter at rest (levator hiatal dimension) than White women.[26] However, the reported findings from these studies did not examine how these differences relate to associated PFDs. The caution and critique of genetic and anatomic studies is that the data can be misinterpreted to infer that Black women have protective factors against certain PFDs. Yet, it is well established that race does not denote genetics or biology. Race is a social political construct that has biological consequences but indicates inherent biological differences.[27] Hence, the focus on biological differences to explain racial differences in prevalence is flawed and detracts from social and structural determinants of health that may impact a population's manifestation of symptoms and attitudes toward reporting of PFD symptoms. Furthermore, an assumption of inherent biological differences by race that explain the discrepancies in PFD prevalence could place Black women at risk for inequities in care such as not being asked about PFD symptoms by providers, leading to subsequent underdiagnosis and undertreatment.

The prevalence data for PFD in Black women obtained from questionnaires should also be interpreted with caution as there is a possibility for underreporting. A mixed methods study involved surveying participants on knowledge and experience of PFDs, followed by a focus group. The investigators found that Black women were less likely to report having PFD in the initial questionnaire; however, in the follow-up focus group discussion, many women reported the incidence of UI and indecision whether to classify UI as a health problem.[28]

CLINICS CARE POINTS

- prevalence of UI in Black women ranges from 3.3% to 45.9%.
- prevalence of POP in Black women ranges from 1% to 7.6%.
- There is little evidence to attribute biologic, anatomic, or genetic variation to account for differences in the prevalence of POP by race.
- Underreporting of PFD symptoms may occur among Black women.

KNOWLEDGE AND EXPERIENCE OF PELVIC FLOOR DISORDERS AMONG BLACK WOMEN

Overall, studies estimate that at least 50% of women do not seek care for UI.[29,30] In particular, the data on care-seeking for PFD treatment for Black women are sparse and conflicting. A study of Black and White community-dwelling women (not residing in nursing homes) in Michigan with UI previously identified that there were no differences in care-seeking for PFDs (53% Black vs 50.6% White, P=.64).[29] Another study assessing treatment-seeking behavior for POP found no difference between Black and White community-dwelling women.[21] However, in a large study from an integrated health care system in California, women with at least moderate bother from UI were less likely to discuss their incontinence with a health care provider. Race and income were influencing factors (Black race adjusted odds ratio (aOR) 0.45, 95%CI [0.25–0.81] compared with White race and income less than $30,000 per year aOR 0.37, 95% CI [0.17–0.81] compared with ≥ $120,000 per year).[31] A systematic review and meta-analysis of studies on care-seeking behavior found that Black race was predictive of decreased health care utilization for women with PFDs (OR 0.77; 95% CI [0.55–1.08]).[32] Other factors associated with decreased utilization were normalization of symptoms due to aging, fear, and misinformation. As race is an indicator of sociopolitical conditions and is not in of itself a risk factor, a critical step to understanding these data would be determining how social and structural determinants of health including systemic racism impact health care utilization and care-seeking for Black women with PFD. Of note, this dynamic is not well elaborated in prior PFD research.

Insufficient knowledge and misconceptions about PFD are often suggested as potential reasons for lower health care utilizations and care-seeking among populations. There are few studies that examine PFD knowledge among women from different racial groups. One study found no differences in knowledge of UI when controlling for relevant confounders between Black and White women.[33] Another analysis of community-dwelling women found differences in knowledge about modifiable risk factors and treatment options for UI and POP.[34] Black women in this study were less likely to recognize childbirth as a risk factor for UI, less likely to know that pelvic floor exercises could help control leakage, and less likely to recognize pessaries as a treatment for UI.[34] Although there may be opportunities to enhance knowledge about PFD among Black women, knowledge proficiency alone is insufficient to optimize care utilization for Black women with PFD.

Understanding barriers to care can provide insights to improving care-seeking and health care utilization. There are a paucity of data examining barriers to PFD care among Black women. One study by Willis-Gray and colleagues used a validated barrier assessment questionnaire, known as the Barriers to Incontinence Care-Seeking Questionnaire, to assess barriers to care for PFDs between Black, White, and Latina women. Barrier scores were higher in Black women compared with White women (2.9 vs 7.3, P < .0001).[35] However, when adjusting for demographics such as age, income, and education, there were no differences in barrier scores between Black and White women. Only one published study has examined barriers to PFD care specific to Black women and not in comparison to another racial group. The study found that insurance concerns were a significant barrier for Black community-dwelling women when adjusting for health status and embarrassment (aOR, 3.80; 95%CI [1.39–10.33]).[36]

A significant gap in the literature on knowledge and care seeking for PFDs is comprehensive data focused on the lived experiences of Black women with PFDs and their perceptions of treatment options (not in comparison to other racial groups). Such data would highlight opportunities for interventions in improving knowledge and care-seeking for Black women with PFD.

CLINICS CARE POINTS

- Data suggest that Black women with PFDs underuse PFD care.
- Our understanding of the drivers of lower PFD care utilization among Black women is limited.

- There is a paucity of literature aimed to increase our understanding of barriers to care of PFDs specifically in Black women.
- Data suggests that Black women with PFDs underutilize PFD care.

TREATMENT AND OUTCOMES IN BLACK WOMEN WITH PELVIC FLOOR DISORDERS

For both UI and POP, pelvic floor physical therapy (PFPT) is the cornerstone of conservative therapy and is a first-line treatment for UUI. Although PFPT can improve urinary symptoms by up to 50%, there are little data on PFPT utilization, responsiveness, and outcomes in Black women. Regarding referrals, utilization, and adherence, data are conflicting concerning race, with some showing lower rates[37] and others showing higher rates among Black women.[37–39] In all studies, except for one, Black women were largely underrepresented (2%, 10.3% vs 33.4%).[37,38,40]

Urinary Incontinence Treatment

Second-line therapies for UUI/overactive bladder (OAB) diverge from SUI treatment and include medical management of symptoms with anticholinergic and beta-3-agonist medications. Globally, medical management of UI/OAB is low, with some studies showing only 1.6% of Medicare visits being associated with OAB medication prescribing.[39] Data suggest that Black women receive anticholinergics at similar rates to White women; however, they are less likely to receive the newer beta-3-agonists.[9,39,41,42] Data regarding medication continuation are controversial as only two studies showed Black race was associated with decreased adherence compared with White race,[43,44] whereas another large cross-sectional study found overall drug use was low with no difference in adherence by race.[45]

Third-line therapies for UUI/OAB include percutaneous nerve stimulation (PTNS), chemodenervation of the bladder with onabotulinum, and sacral neuromodulation (SNM). Overall SNM and PTNS are used infrequently (<1%) but began increasing in the early 2000s.[46,47] However, in a recent study by Edge and colleagues using medical claims data from 2010 to 2020, SNM actually decreased from 2010 onward. Conversely, intradetrusor onabotulinum utilization increased, accounting for 50% of third-line therapies in women with OAB.[46,47] Laudano and colleagues found that racially minoritized Medicare patients were less likely to receive third-line treatments compared with White patients.[48] Similar findings were noted in a commercially insured population.[49] For SNM specifically, a study using California state ambulatory surgery data from 2005 to 2011 found that Black patients had similar SNM treatment success compared with White patients.[50] However, only 4.5% of total study participants were Black. There is a paucity of research specifically assessing drivers of advanced OAB/UUI treatment (PTNS, intradetrusor onabotulinum, SNM) utilization in Black women.

Patients who demonstrate SUI on examination in the office are candidates for surgical-based treatments. Of note, SUI procedures have decreased over time by at least 25%, with sling procedures (fascial and synthetic) decreasing by 50%.[51,52] Most studies using large hospital-based or insurance databases demonstrate that Black women undergo SUI or sling procedures less than White women, yet they experience higher rates of postoperative complications including unplanned readmissions, urinary obstruction, and new-onset POP.[51–55]

Overall, the data suggest that Black women are less likely to receive beta agonist medications, advanced UI therapies, and surgical management of UI. For SUI procedures, Black women experience worse outcomes than White women.

Pelvic Organ Prolapse Treatment

QoL is an important surgical outcome to evaluate the long-term impact of surgery. There are no specific data assessing QoL after POP or UI surgery using validated measures in Black women in the United States. A prospective observational study of Ugandan women showed a significant improvement in physical, social, sexual, emotional, and sleep QoL domains after surgical repair at 1 year.[56] In addition, we know that after surgery and incontinence procedures, most women across race and ethnicity have improvement in various areas including sexual function, bladder function, and prolapse symptoms.[57] However, QoL improvement among Black women after POP/UI procedures is an area that has not been largely or explicitly studied to date and represents a significant research gap.

There is emerging evidence that Black women are less likely to receive surgery for their POP. When they do receive surgery, the approach and procedures vary by race. A large cohort study using an administrative database found that Black women were less likely to have surgery for POP than White women (5.6 vs 14.8 per 10,000 women).[58] Black women in this study were more likely to be on public assistance (27% vs 5.9%) and have surgery at a government hospital (20.2% vs 11.9%) than White women[58] suggesting that socioeconomic status may influence the receipt of surgery for POP. A limitation of this study however is that the investigators could not evaluate other potential drivers of this observation such as clinicians' recommendations for surgery among all women presenting for prolapse management.

There are six studies using the National Surgical Quality Improvement Program (NSQIP) Database and two additional studies using the National Inpatient Sample database to assess surgical treatment of POP and associated outcomes in Black women.[7,8,59–64] Black women underwent disproportionately less surgery for POP than White women.[7,8,59–62] Although NSQIP studies demonstrate similar rates of vaginal apical suspensions and sacrocolpopexy between Black and White women,[60–62] Cardenas-Trowers and colleagues found that Black women were also more likely to have a hysterectomy without a concomitant prolapse procedure than White women.[61] This is an important finding, as current practice guidelines recommend apical procedures at the time of surgery for symptomatic prolapse. Hysterectomy alone or with anterior and posterior repairs alone is rarely the correct procedure for women with symptomatic POP. Not only are Black women receiving surgical treatment less often but they are also undergoing surgeries that may not appropriately treat their symptoms. These conflicting data need to be further explored to better understand why treatment disparities exist.

Finally, Black women were more likely to have obliterative procedures (ie, colpocleisis), which have the lowest rates of surgical failure but preclude women from being able to have penetrative intercourse postoperatively.[7,59,61] Although these surgeries are associated with low risk of regret, we must critically examine this finding to ensure that Black women's desires for future coital function is being supported.

Black women experience more morbidity after surgery for POP than White women. Using the same databases that determined differential surgical approaches, Shah and colleagues found that Black women had higher rates of postoperative complications compared with White women (34.1% vs 19.4%, respectively), even though they were less likely to have surgery for POP.[58] Numerous studies have found increased perioperative morbidity including increased surgical injury, blood transfusion, venous thromboembolic event, and longer operative times.[8,60–64]

It is difficult to extrapolate why Black women have worse outcomes than White women after surgery for POP. The data are limited to large national databases with limited meaningful variables and underrepresentation of Black women. In addition,

Black women in these databases have more medical comorbidities than White women which predisposes them to higher perioperative morbidity, a factor that may influence a surgeon to choose a different surgical/management approach.[7,8,59–62]

Much of the current disparities research has focused on patient factors associated with poor outcomes including obesity, large uteri, and markers of poor health. When the focus is on these types of patient factors, it implies that the population is in part responsible for their poor outcomes. This is problematic and inhibits our ability to understand other variables, such as the contribution of bias, racism, and discrimination. Future research is needed to evaluate these outcomes through a health equity lens, specifically understanding how racism impacts Black women in the health care system. **Tables 3** and **4** outline the key findings related to SUI and POP outcomes.

CLINICS CARE POINTS

- There are disparities in the receipt of evidence-based treatments for PFDs for Black women.
- Outcome data for urgency UI advanced treatments in Black women are limited.
- Black women experience poorer outcomes after surgeries for PFD and SUI.
- Studies moving beyond identifying disparities in treatment are limited, yet necessary to improve outcomes.

REPRESENTATION OF BLACK WOMEN IN BIOMEDICAL RESEARCH AND THE IMPACT OF EVIDENCE-BASED GUIDELINES
Research

There is a paucity of research on Black women with PFDs, their lived experiences, how they perceive their symptoms, at what threshold they would seek treatment, barriers to treatment, how they view conservative versus surgical treatment options, and perceptions of how racism directly impacts the care they receive. Not only are Black women underrepresented in the research but they are also underrepresented in the teams performing the research.

Recent research has focused on the lack of Black women in research studies used to create evidence-based guidelines. Brown and colleagues analyzed 387 studies referenced in the 2019 American Urologic Association and Society of Urodynamics and the Female Pelvic Medicine and Urogenital Reconstruction nonneurogenic OAB Diagnosis and Treatment Guidelines.[65] Of note, only 35% of all studies reported the patient's race. They found White and Asian patients were overrepresented (representation quotients 1.06, 1.62), whereas Black, Hispanic, and Native American/Alaska Native patients were underrepresented (representation quotients 0.85, 0.56, and 0.02, respectively). There was no change in representation over the study period of 1990 to 2019.[65] A similar study by Gonzalez and colleagues evaluated racial and ethnic representation in the evaluation and management of SUI. They found that less than half of studies were from populations within the United States (17/52 studies) and even fewer reported race of the study participants (9/52 studies). Of these 9 studies, 80% of participants were non-Hispanic White women.[66]

A similar study by Grimes and McKay reviewed racial representation in the PFD NIH-funded research network including the Pelvic Floor Disorders Network (PFDN) and Urinary Incontinence Treatment Network (UITN).[67,68] Data demonstrate that 90/111 studies reported race. Overall 9.9% of patients were Black compared with 79% White. Of note, racial and ethnic representation varied, with higher representation of non-White

Table 3
Summary of urinary incontinence treatment data

Author Journal Year	Database N(%) Black Women	Methods	Relevant Findings
Mckellar Neuro Uro 2019	Single Healthcare System 2013–2016 39,933 (33.4%)	Cohort study Prevalence and treatment SUI	• Pessary placement was the least used form of active treatment (2.31%) and was more likely in White women* (P=.03) • Black women were less likely to consult with a specialist and undergo active treatment (physical therapy, pessary placement, and sling surgery) compared with all other racial groups • Rates of sling surgery were similar between Black and White women (2.15 vs 2.04%)
Anger Urology 2007	Medicare Claims 1999–2001 1,789,155 (8.7%)	Cohort study Prevalence and surgical treatment SUI	• 7.1% of Black women underwent a sling compared with 13.1% of White women (P<.01) • Non-White women had more non-urologic complications (aOR 2.02 95%CI [1.22–3.34]), new-onset pelvic prolapse (aOR 2.04 95%CI [1.19–3.50]), and urinary obstruction (aOR 2.30 95%CI [1.07–4.91])
Waetjen Obstet Gyn 2003	National Hospital Discharge Survey 1998[a]	Cohort study Prevalence and surgical treatment SUI	• Black Women were less likely to have a surgery for SUI (2.6 per 10,000 vs 11.6 per 10,000). • Black Women had higher rate of complications (20.6% vs 9.7%)
Shah Int Urogyn 2008	National Hospital Discharge Survey 2003 4352 (3.4%)	Cohort study Prevalence and surgical treatment SUI	• 12 surgical procedures per 10,000 women were performed in the United States, for SUI, the majority were 10 per 10,000 in White women (66.7%) vs 3 per 10,000 women (3.4%) in Black women • Surgical complications were not different in Black vs White women • Women in the other group (26.8% of surgeries) had the highest rates of complications

Source	Database	Study Type	Findings
Dallas *Urology* 2017	California State Ambulatory Surgery Database 2005–2011 474 (1.7%)	Cohort study Surgical treatment SUI: Sling surgery	• Increased postoperative complications within 30 d in Black women • Black race increased the odds of unplanned hospital visits (OR 1.8) • Black women had more unplanned events (10.5%, $P < .01$), including higher surgical revision rates than all other groups (0.6%, $P < .05$) even in adjusted models
Luchristt *JAMA Open* 2023	Medical Expenditure Panel Survey 2019[a]	Cross-sectional Analysis Assessing OAB Prescriptions Filled	• Black women were 90% less likely to fill a β3-agonist prescription (adjusted OR, 0.10; 95%CI [0.04–0.27]) compared with White women
Ju *Int Urogyn* 2014	Ambulatory Medical Care Survey database (NAMCS) 2009[a]	Cross-sectional analysis assessing OAB prescriptions filled	• 1.6% of Medicare visits in women were associated with an anticholinergic (ACh) prescription • No differences between Black and White women in prescriptions for ACh
Mckellar *Urology* 2019	Single Healthcare System 2013–2016 41,710 (34.02%)	Retrospective cohort Prevalence and Treatment OAB	• No difference in treatment of OAB with medication prescriptions between Black and White women (21.5% vs 23.9%) • Black women were less likely to consult with a specialist
Benner *BJU Int* 2010	Survey of USA Households 2009 453 (8.4%)[b]	Cross-sectional study Discontinuation OAB meds	• Overall OAB drug use was low, 24.5% reported discontinuing prescription OAB medication within the last 12 mo • No difference in discontinuation by race
Shaya *Am J Manag* 2005	Medicaid Managed Care 2000–2003 737 (45%)[b]	Retrospective Cohort Study Continuation OAB meds	• Black women had decreased adherence compared with White race (continuation 15% of Black vs 27% White)
Rashid *J Mang Care Spec Pharm* 2017	Kaiser Permanente Southern California (KPSC) Electronic Medical Records (EMR) 977 (10.8%)[b]	Retrospective cohort study Prescribing new OAB med prescriptions	• Black women had increased odds of non-adherence after OAB medication was prescribed (aOR 1.56 95%CI [1.24–1.96])

(continued on next page)

Table 3
(continued)

Author Journal Year	Database N(%) Black Women	Methods	Relevant Findings
Lee *Urology* 2021	CDM (Optum de-identified Clinformatics Data Mart) for women 18–64 year old and the CMS (Centers for Medicare and Medicaid Services) Medicare 5% Sample 2004–2013[a]	Retrospective cohort study Surgical management of urinary incontinence	• Decline in the percent of women with UI who underwent surgical treatment according to the CMS from 4.7% in 2004–2.7% in 2013 and the CDM from 12.5% in 2004–9.1% in 2013 • Slings decreased by 50% over study period • Younger and older White women were more likely than Black women to have surgery for UI • Slings were also more common in white women • UI surgery prevalence of 1% or less among Black women
Laudano *J Uro* 2015	Medicare Claims Data 2001, 2004, 2007, 2010[a]	Retrospective cohort study Sacral neuromodulation (SNM) trends	• SNM implantation increased from 0.03% to 0.91% (P<.0001) for a total of 13,360 (0.58%) • Minority patients (OR 0.38, P<.0001) were less likely to receive SNM
Syan *Urology* 2020	Optum, a national claims database 2003–2017 368,568 (9%)[b]	Retrospective cohort study Treatment of OAB/UUI	• SNM was no different between Black and White patients • Onabotulinum was similar between races/ethnicities (P <.05) • Non-White race was associated with decreased odds of receiving advanced therapies for OAB/UUI (OR 0.89, 95% CI [0.87,0.91])
Dobberfuhl *FPMRS* 2018	California State Ambulatory Surgery Database 2005–2011 124 (4.5%)[b]	Retrospective cohort study Sacral neuromodulation (SNM) success rates	• Race was not associated with SNM treatment success

Abbreviations: OAB, overactive bladder; UI, urinary incontinence;UUI, urgency urinary incontinence; SNM, sacral neuromodulation; SUI, stress urinary incontinence.

[a] Race numerators not given.
[b] Includes population numbers where males are included.

Table 4
Summary pelvic organ prolapse treatment data

Author Journal Year	Database N(%) Black Women	Methods	Relevant Findings
Cardenas-Trowers *FPMRS* 2021	National Surgical Quality Improvement Project 2005–2015 2299 (4.7%)	Cohort study surgical treatment POP	• Minority women* were less likely to undergo an apical suspension than White women (aOR 0.78 95%CI [0.71–0.86]) • Obliterative procedures were more likely to be performed in Black women (aOR, 1.53 95%CI [1.20–1.92]) compared with White women • Black women experienced higher complication rates (10.7%) compared with White women (8.9%, $P < .01$) including higher rates of major complications, blood transfusion surgical site infection, sepsis, and readmission
Winkelman *FPMRS* 2021	National Surgical Quality Improvement Project 2010–2018 2353 (5%)	Cohort study Surgical treatment POP	• Black patients were more likely to undergo obliterative procedures compared with White patients (RR 1.2 95% CI [1.03–1.3]), which persisted in adjusted models • Black patients had increased risk of a postoperative complication (RR, 1.2 95% CI [1.1–1.4]); in the adjusted model, this difference was not statistically significant
Roberts *FPMRS* 2020	National Surgical Quality Improvement Project 2010–2015 738 (5.5%)	Cohort study Sacrocolpopexy for treatment POP	• Overall complications were higher in Black patients 15.0% vs 11.5% ($P=.006$), persisted on multivariable regression (aOR 1.29) • Most common complication for Black patients was postoperative transfusion
Yadav *FPMRS* 2022	National Inpatient Sample 2008–2018 3404 (4.8%)	Cohort study Surgical treatment POP	• Non-White (Black, Hispanic, and other races), Medicaid patients, and patients at urban teaching hospitals were less likely to receive reconstructive prolapse repairs compared with obliterative procedures in adjusted analyses • Non-White (Black, Hispanic, and "other" races), uninsured/Medicaid patients, and patients in the Midwest, South, and West were more likely to receive a native tissue repair compared with a sacrocolpopexy in adjusted analyses

(continued on next page)

Table 4
(continued)

Author Journal Year	Database N(%) Black Women	Methods	Relevant Findings
Rodriguez *Urology* 2023	National Surgical Quality Improvement Project 2012–2017 2776 (5.5%)	Cohort study Surgical treatment POP	• Black patients were more likely to undergo apical repair procedures (*P*<.001) and less likely to undergo combination POP procedures (*P*<.001) than White or other patients • Black were more likely to undergo POP repair with a concomitant hysterectomy as compared with White patients (*P*<.001) • Blood transfusion was more common in Blacks (2.4% vs 1.1%, *P*<.001) • Black patients were more often readmitted (3.2%; *P*=.014) • Operative time was longer for Black patients (146 min vs 132 min, *P*<.001)
Brown *Int Urogyn* 2022	National Surgical Quality Improvement Project 2012–2014 1460 (5.0%)	Cohort study Surgical treatment POP and cost analysis	• Postoperative complications were significantly higher among Black women (20%) compared with White women of other races (16%, *P* <.01) • Black race had an increased odds of complications compared with White women (aOR 1.21) controlling for confounders
Ringel *Urology* 2022	National Surgical Quality Improvement Project 2010–2018 3756 (5%)	Cohort study Surgical treatment POP	• Black women had the highest complication rates (11% vs 9% for both White women, p<0.01) • In adjusted models, Black women still experienced higher odds of any complication (aOR 1.15, 95% CI [1.03–1.29]) and vascular complication (aOR 2.50, 95% CI [2.05–3.04]) • Trends in vascular complications showed a decrease from 2010 to 2018 in non-Black women after prolapse repair, the same decrease was not seen in Black women

Shah *AJOG* 2007	National Hospital Discharge Survey and National Census 2003 7668 (3.8%)	Cohort study	Surgical treatment POP	• 5.5 per 10,000 Black women had surgery for POP in 20,023 compared with 14.1 per 10,000 White women • Of Black women, 27% were on public assistance, compared with 5.9% White women • Complications were higher in Black women (34.1% vs 19.4%) of White women
Boyd *AJOG* 2021	National Surgical Quality Improvement Project 2014–2017 1281 (6%)	Cohort study	Sacrocolpopexy and vaginal colpopexy for treatment POP	• No differences in sacrocolpopexy vs vaginal colpopexy performed between Black and White women in adjusted analyses • Black women were more likely to need a blood transfusion after vaginal colpopexy (OR 3.04; 95% CI [1.95–4.73], $P{\leq}.001$) and have a deep vein thrombosis or pulmonary embolus (OR 2.46; 95% CI [1.10–5.48], $P=.028$) than White women in multivariable regression models

Abbreviations: aOR, adjusted odds ratio; CI, confidence interval; OR, odds ratio; POP, pelvic organ prolapse; RR, relative risk.

participants in pregnancy-related and fecal incontinence studies.[67] McKay and colleagues found that White women composed 70% to 89% of total participants, whereas Black women represented 6% to 16% of participants in PFD trials. White women were overrepresented in 13 of 18 PFDN studies, whereas Black women were underrepresented or absent in 10 of 18 studies.[68]

Of note, in all NSQIP and large administrative database studies, Black women are underrepresented (3%–6% total cohort), and missing race data were common (up to 25%). Although this could be due to lower rates of bothersome or symptomatic POP among this population, there is also the possibility that these large databases are unable to capture disparities in the symptom reporting, diagnosis, and treatment of this particular patient population.

Despite numerous studies describing disparities for women from minoritized racial groups, our understanding of how to alleviate these disparities remains limited. This is further highlighted by the fact that women from minoritized racial groups remain underrepresented in PFD research.[63,67,68] Underrepresentation of Black communities in PFD research poses missed opportunities for a deeper understanding of how nonclinical factors (such as systemic racism) may impact clinical outcomes. There is an opportunity to reimagine how we approach and study PFDs for women from minoritized racial groups. Further, although it is important to identify disparities, the transformative work lies in designing care delivery that optimizes outcomes for historically marginalized populations.

Risk Calculators

Studies published from the PFDN and UITN were not only used to create guidelines for management of PFDs. Treatment recommendations are often created and supported based on these research findings, which would be more generalizable if all races/ethnicities were represented in these large trials.[69] Data from these large network trials are also used to create decisions calculators for risk stratification and treatment. Risk calculators have been used throughout medicine to stratify severity of an illness or risk associated with a treatment based on patient- and hospital-level factors.

Getaneh and colleagues called attention to a calculator created to predict success of treatment with intradetrusor onabotulinum, which uses race as a factor.[70] Black and other non-White women in this model have a decreased risk of treatment success. This model and the studies from which it is derived do not provide insight into why or how Black race—a social construct—could decrease treatment efficacy. Authors postulated that including race may be harmful for non-White patients by exacerbating treatment disparities that are already present. In addition, it perpetuates the ideology that Black race denotes genetic differences leading to treatment disparities, which is false. Similar editorials have been published in the obstetric and urology literature critiquing the vaginal birth after cesarean delivery calculator, the estimated glomerular filtration rate calculator, and STONE Score for uncomplicated ureteral stone for their inclusion of race as a mitigating factor.[71,72]

CLINICS CARE POINTS

- Black women are underrepresented in major clinical trials guiding treatment decisions and algorithms for UI and POP.
- Calculators driving treatment for PFDs may introduce bias when including race as variable.
- Black women are underrepresented in major clinical trials guiding treatment decisions and algorithms for UI and POP.

> - Calculators driving treatment for PFDs may introduce bias when including race as a variable.

STRATEGIC AGENDA TO PRIORITIZE THE CARE OF BLACK WOMEN WITH PELVIC FLOOR DISORDERS

There remains a gap in alleviating inequities in Black women's outcomes and experiences with care and treatment for PFDs. To address this gap, health care professionals and advocates alike must be intentional in our actions to improve PFD care for Black women. Impact plans to address health inequities should incorporate elements that both address individual and population level needs.[73] The following incorporates our proposed impact plan "Strategic Agenda to Prioritize the Care of Black Women with PFDs," which includes a multilevel approach to minimizing health inequity in Black women with PFDs (**Box 1**).

STRATEGY 1: ENHANCE KNOWLEDGE AND AWARENESS OF THE EXISTENCE AND IMPACT OF PELVIC FLOOR DISORDERS AMONG HEALTH CARE PROFESSIONALS, PATIENTS, AND THE COMMUNITY

One element that impedes the narrowing of health inequities for Black women with PFDs is variations in awareness of PFDs and PFD treatment not only among patients but also among health care practitioners. In order *to enhance knowledge and awareness of the existence and impact of PFDs among healthcare professionals, patients, and the community,* the authors proposed increasing efforts to help patients improve reporting of symptoms by increasing clinician screening and inquiry during health assessments in various health care settings.[74] Black women may under report their PFD symptoms due to personal and cultural beliefs. In addition, health care professionals may minimize or ignore their symptoms leading to underdiagnosis. Targeting these phenomena is key to eradicating these care disparities.

STRATEGY 2: OPTIMIZE THE QUALITY OF CLINICAL CARE FOR BLACK WOMEN WITH PELVIC FLOOR DISORDERS

Significant efforts must be made *to optimize the quality of clinical care for Black women with PFDs.* Perpetuation of public education and community awareness of

---

Box 1
Strategic agenda to prioritize the care of Black women with pelvic floor disorders

Strategy 1: Enhance knowledge and awareness of the existence and impact of PFDs in health care professionals, patients, and the community

Strategy 2: Optimize the quality of clinical care for Black women with PFDs
 i. Educating health care providers
 ii. Facilitation and promotion of connections between medical community and Black women by
  a. Supporting programs/patient navigators
  b. Improving access and insurance coverage
  c. Diversification of workforce
 iii. Advocacy
 iv. Policy changes

Strategy 3: Expand representation of Black women in biomedical research

Strategy 4: Dismantle structural racism in PFD care to achieve health equity

PFDs is an essential element of optimizing clinical care, but it is insufficient to eliminate racial health disparities. Facilitation and promotion of connections between the medical community and Black communities are critical to the achieving equitable PFD care for Black women. Authentic community partnerships ensure that the efforts of professionals that treat PFDs are aligned with the needs of the communities, for which there is a dearth of community-based partnerships and initiatives.

Efforts should also be made to identify and address structural barriers to health care professional PFD screening and referrals for Black women. At both the individual and institutional levels, equitable patient counseling on PFD management options must be prioritized. In addition, efforts should be made to mitigate the effects of differential care through insurance access and universal coverage for PFD treatment. Insurance status/coverage is a known barrier to PFD treatment for underrepresented racial and ethnic minority women and should be addressed.[75] The use of patient navigators can help address these barriers. There should be collective efforts to advocate for policy changes at state and federal levels with outputs that directly improve access to health care and health care quality.[76]

Diversification of the health care/medical workforce is also an actionable step that can directly improve the QoL for Black women.[74,76] There should be intentional efforts to increase racial and ethnic diversity at the trainee level by program leadership, specifically for obstetrics and gynecology residency and urogynecology and reconstructive surgery fellowship programs. In addition, once trainees are accepted into the program they should be supported with the knowledge that those underrepresented in medicine face unique challenges that may not be readily apparent. Mentorship programs that increase exposure to urogynecology as a subspecialty should also be considered.

STRATEGY 3: EXPAND REPRESENTATION OF BLACK WOMEN IN BIOMEDICAL RESEARCH

Approaches to clinical care are often developed through evidence-based medicine supported by research. Given that research findings greatly influence recommendations for clinical care as well as insurance coverage and policy guidelines, it is essential *to expand representation of Black women in biomedical research*. This strategy can be achieved through focus on community-based participatory research efforts, promotion of Black researchers to lead scientific efforts, and inclusion of appropriate honorariums for participation in research studies.[76] In addition, efforts should be made to report race and ethnicity in study populations, understanding the limitations of underrepresentation and required reporting of such limitations. Larger databases should reflect the diversity of our communities and report the demographic breakdown of the entire population to minimize bias in case selection.

STRATEGY 4: DISMANTLE STRUCTURAL RACISM IN PELVIC FLOOR DISORDER CARE TO ACHIEVE HEALTH EQUITY

Finally, efforts must be made *to dismantle structural racism in PFD care to achieve health equity*. We acknowledge that this is a grand task. However, we also appreciate the fact that structural racism is not well measured or appreciated in efforts to understand and reduce health disparities. Actions made toward dismantling structural racism directly influence all of the proposed strategies, which emphasize its importance in developing a plan to improve health equity for Black women. There is currently a dearth of research models that actually highlight the role of racism in sexual and reproductive health, with many studies focused on the reproductive (ie, perinatal) health of African American women.[73] The lived experiences of Black women should be acknowledged and measured through research to capture the impact of racism. In addition, other suggested efforts include professional development that addresses anti-Black racism in the medical profession as well as efforts to fight against anti-Black interpersonal racism.[77] All women, including Black women themselves, may benefit from opportunities that increase their own understanding of the historical impact of racism and its links to contemporary health outcomes. Subsequently, this interaction should promote further learning and support individual and community advocacy opportunities.[73]

In summary, White PFDs are prevalent in Black women, their experiences with those PFDs are lacking in the literature. Black women deserve dedicated efforts to optimize their PFD care and representation in PFD research.

CLINICS CARE POINTS

- The prevalence of UI in Black women ranges from 3.3% to 45.9%.
- The prevalence of POP in Black women ranges from 1% to 7.6%.
- There is little evidence to attribute biologic, anatomic, or genetic variation to account for differences in prevalence of POP by race.
- Data suggest that Black women with PFDs underuse PFD care; there is a paucity of literature to increase our understanding of barriers to care of PFDs specifically in Black communities.
- There are disparities in the receipt of evidence-based treatments for PFDs for Black women.
- Black women experience poorer outcomes after surgeries for PFD and SUI.
- Studies moving beyond identifying disparities in treatment are limited, yet necessary to improve outcomes.

ACKNOWLEDGMENTS

Although this work focuses on the published literature of pelvic floor disorder in women, the authors acknowledge that gender identity is diverse and the use of this term may not be fully representative of the people studied. Furthermore, terms such as "Latina" are used in this article to report study findings as researchers have reported them. The authors recognize that gender inclusive terminology is evolving.

DISCLOSURES

Dr M.F. Ackenbom received grant funding from the NIH National Institute on Aging (K23AG073517–01), the Pennsylvania Department of Health (4,100,088,553), and the Alzheimer's Association.

REFERENCES

1. Nygaard I, Barber MD, Burgio KL, et al. Prevalence of symptomatic pelvic floor disorders in US women. JAMA 2008;300(11):1311–6.
2. Wu JM, Vaughan CP, Goode PS, et al. Prevalence and trends of symptomatic pelvic floor disorders in U.S. women. Obstet Gynecol 2014;123(1):141–8.
3. Cox CK, Schimpf MO, Berger MB. Stigma associated with pelvic floor disorders. Female Pelvic Med Reconstr Surg 2021;27(2):e453–6.

4. Abrams P, Kelleher CJ, Kerr LA, et al. Overactive bladder significantly affects quality of life. Am J Manag Care 2000;6(11 Suppl):S580–90.
5. Ricci JA, Baggish JS, Hunt TL, et al. Coping strategies and health care-seeking behavior in a US national sample of adults with symptoms suggestive of overactive bladder. Clin Therapeut 2001;23(8):1245–59.
6. Minassian VA, Yan X, Lichtenfeld MJ, et al. Predictors of care seeking in women with urinary incontinence. Neurourol Urodyn 2012;31(4):470–4.
7. Yadav GS, Rutledge EC, Nisar T, et al. Health care disparities in surgical management of pelvic organ prolapse: A contemporary nationwide analysis. Female Pelvic Med Reconstr Surg 2022;28(4):207–12.
8. Boyd BAJ, Winkelman WD, Mishra K, et al. Racial and ethnic differences in reconstructive surgery for apical vaginal prolapse. Am J Obstet Gynecol 2021;225(4):405.e1–7.
9. Luchristt D, Bretschneider CE, Kenton K, et al. Inequities in filled overactive bladder medication prescriptions in the US. JAMA Netw Open 2023;6(5):e2315074.
10. Abrams P, Andersson KE, Birder L, et al. Fourth International Consultation on Incontinence Recommendations of the International Scientific Committee: Evaluation and treatment of urinary incontinence, pelvic organ prolapse, and fecal incontinence. Neurourol Urodyn 2010;29(1):213–40.
11. Haylen BT, Maher CF, Barber MD, et al. An International Urogynecological Association (IUGA)/International Continence Society (ICS) joint report on the terminology for female pelvic organ prolapse (POP). Int Urogynecol J 2016;27(2):165–94.
12. Fenner DE, Trowbridge ER, Patel DA, et al. Establishing the prevalence of incontinence study: racial differences in women's patterns of urinary incontinence. J Urol 2008;179(4):1455–60.
13. Jackson RA, Vittinghoff E, Kanaya AM, et al. Urinary incontinence in elderly women: findings from the Health, Aging, and Body Composition Study. Obstet Gynecol 2004;104(2):301–7.
14. Thom DH, van den Eeden SK, Ragins AI, et al. Differences in prevalence of urinary incontinence by race/ethnicity. J Urol 2006;175(1):259–64.
15. Akbar A, Liu K, Michos ED, et al. Racial differences in urinary incontinence prevalence and associated bother: the Multi-Ethnic Study of Atherosclerosis. Am J Obstet Gynecol 2021;224(1):80.e1–9.
16. Tennstedt SL, Link CL, Steers WD, et al. Prevalence of and risk factors for urine leakage in a racially and ethnically diverse population of adults: the Boston Area Community Health (BACH) Survey. Am J Epidemiol 2008;167(4):390–9.
17. Townsend MK, Curhan GC, Resnick NM, et al. The incidence of urinary incontinence across Asian, black, and white women in the United States. Am J Obstet Gynecol 2010;202(4):378.e1–7.
18. Coyne KS, Sexton CC, Bell JA, et al. The prevalence of lower urinary tract symptoms (LUTS) and overactive bladder (OAB) by racial/ethnic group and age: results from OAB-POLL. Neurourol Urodyn 2013;32(3):230–7.
19. Mou T, Warner K, Brown O, et al. Prevalence of pelvic organ prolapse among US racial populations: A systematic review and meta-analysis of population-based screening studies. Neurourol Urodyn 2021;40(5):1098–106.
20. Townsend MK, Curhan GC, Resnick NM, et al. Original research: rates of remission, improvement, and progression of urinary incontinence in Asian, Black, and White women. Am J Nurs 2011;111(4):26–33, quiz 34.
21. Brazell HD, O'Sullivan DM, Tulikangas PK. Socioeconomic status and race as predictors of treatment-seeking behavior for pelvic organ prolapse. Am J Obstet Gynecol 2013;209(5):476.e1–5.

22. Whitcomb EL, Rortveit G, Brown JS, et al. Racial differences in pelvic organ prolapse. Obstet Gynecol 2009;114(6):1271–7.

23. Kudish BI, Iglesia CB, Gutman RE, et al. Risk factors for prolapse development in white, black, and Hispanic women. Female Pelvic Med Reconstr Surg 2011; 17(2):80–90.

24. Rortveit G, Brown JS, Thom DH, et al. Symptomatic pelvic organ prolapse: prevalence and risk factors in a population-based, racially diverse cohort. Obstet Gynecol 2007;109(6):1396–403.

25. Giri A, Hartmann KE, Aldrich MC, et al. Admixture mapping of pelvic organ prolapse in African Americans from the Women's Health Initiative Hormone Therapy trial. PLoS One 2017;12(6):e0178839.

26. Derpapas A, Ahmed S, Vijaya G, et al. Racial differences in female urethral morphology and levator hiatal dimensions: an ultrasound study. Neurourol Urodyn 2012;31(4):502–7. https://doi.org/10.1002/nau.21181.

27. Roberts D. Fatal invention: how science, politics, and big business Re-create race in the twenty-first century. 50852nd ed. The New Press; 2012. p. 400.

28. Hatchett L, Hebert-Beirne J, Tenfelde S, et al. Knowledge and perceptions of pelvic floor disorders among african american and latina women. Female Pelvic Med Reconstr Surg 2011;17(4):190–4.

29. Berger MB, Patel DA, Miller JM, et al. Racial differences in self-reported healthcare seeking and treatment for urinary incontinence in community-dwelling women from the EPI Study. Neurourol Urodyn 2011;30(8):1442–7.

30. Morrill M, Lukacz ES, Lawrence JM, et al. Seeking healthcare for pelvic floor disorders: a population-based study. Am J Obstet Gynecol 2007;197(1):86.e1–6.

31. Duralde ER, Walter LC, Van Den Eeden SK, et al. Bridging the gap: determinants of undiagnosed or untreated urinary incontinence in women. Am J Obstet Gynecol 2016;214(2):266.e1–9.

32. Mou T, Gonzalez J, Gupta A, et al. Barriers and Promotors to Health Service Utilization for Pelvic Floor Disorders in the United States: Systematic Review and Meta-analysis of Qualitative and Quantitative Studies. Urogynecology (Phila). 2022;28(9):574–81.

33. Kubik K, Blackwell L, Heit M. Does socioeconomic status explain racial differences in urinary incontinence knowledge? Am J Obstet Gynecol 2004;191(1):188–93.

34. Mandimika CL, Murk W, Mcpencow AM, et al. Racial Disparities in Knowledge of Pelvic Floor Disorders Among Community-Dwelling Women. Female Pelvic Med Reconstr Surg 2015;21(5):287–92.

35. Willis-Gray MG, Sandoval JS, Maynor J, et al. Barriers to urinary incontinence care seeking in White, Black, and Latina women. Female Pelvic Med Reconstr Surg 2015;21(2):83–6.

36. Washington BB, Raker CA, Mishra K, et al. Variables impacting care-seeking for pelvic floor disorders among African American women. Female Pelvic Med Reconstr Surg 2013;19(2):98–102.

37. Mckellar K, Abraham N. Prevalence, risk factors, and treatment for women with stress urinary incontinence in a racially and ethnically diverse population. Neurourol Urodyn 2019;38(3):934–40.

38. Brown HW, Barnes HC, Lim A, et al. Better together: multidisciplinary approach improves adherence to pelvic floor physical therapy. Int Urogynecol J 2020; 31(5):887–93.

39. Ju R, Garrett J, Wu JM. Anticholinergic medication use for female overactive bladder in the ambulatory setting in the United States. Int Urogynecol J 2014; 25(4):479–84.

40. Washington BB, Raker CA, Sung VW. Barriers to pelvic floor physical therapy utilization for treatment of female urinary incontinence. Am J Obstet Gynecol 2011; 205(2):152.e1–9.

41. Mckellar K, Bellin E, Schoenbaum E, et al. Prevalence, risk factors, and treatment for overactive bladder in a racially diverse population. Urology 2019;126:70–5.

42. Hall SA, Link CL, Hu JC, et al. Drug treatment of urological symptoms: estimating the magnitude of unmet need in a community-based sample. BJU Int 2009; 104(11):1680–8.

43. Shaya FT, Blume S, Gu A, et al. Persistence with overactive bladder pharmacotherapy in a Medicaid population. Am J Manag Care 2005;11(4 Suppl):S121–9.

44. Rashid N, Vassilakis M, Lin KJ, et al. Primary nonadherence to overactive bladder medications in an integrated managed care health care system. J Manag Care Spec Pharm 2017;23(4):484–93.

45. Benner JS, Nichol MB, Rovner ES, et al. Patient-reported reasons for discontinuing overactive bladder medication. BJU Int 2010;105(9):1276–82.

46. Lee UJ, Ward JB, Feinstein L, et al. National Trends in Neuromodulation for Urinary Incontinence Among Insured Adult Women and Men, 2004-2013: The Urologic Diseases in America Project. Urology 2021;150:86–91.

47. Edge P, Scioscia NF, Yanek LR, et al. National Trends in Third-Line Treatment for Overactive Bladder Among Commercially Insured Women, 2010-2019. Urology 2023;175:56–61.

48. Laudano MA, Seklehner S, Sandhu J, et al. Disparities in the Use of Sacral Neuromodulation among Medicare Beneficiaries. J Urol 2015;194(2):449–53.

49. Syan R, Zhang CA, Enemchukwu EA. Racial and socioeconomic factors influence utilization of advanced therapies in commercially insured OAB patients: an analysis of over 800,000 OAB patients. Urology 2020;142:81–6.

50. Dobberfuhl AD, Mahal A, Dallas KB, et al. Statewide Success of Staged Sacral Neuromodulation for the Treatment of Urinary Complaints in California (2005-2011). Female Pelvic Med Reconstr Surg 2020;26(7):437–42.

51. Anger JT, Rodríguez LV, Wang Q, et al. Racial disparities in the surgical management of stress incontinence among female Medicare beneficiaries. J Urol 2007; 177(5):1846–50.

52. Lee JA, Johns TS, Melamed ML, et al. Associations between Socioeconomic Status and Urge Urinary Incontinence: An Analysis of NHANES 2005 to 2016. J Urol 2020;203(2):379–84.

53. Shah AD, Shott S, Kohli N, et al. Do racial differences in knowledge about urogynecologic issues exist? Int UrogynEcol J Pelvic Floor Dysfunct 2008;19(10): 1371–8.

54. Dallas KB, Sohlberg EM, Elliott CS, et al. Racial and Socioeconomic Disparities in Short-term Urethral Sling Surgical Outcomes. Urology 2017;110:70–5.

55. Waetjen LE, Subak LL, Shen H, et al. Stress urinary incontinence surgery in the United States. Obstet Gynecol 2003;101(4):671–6.

56. Kayondo M, Kaye DK, Migisha R, et al. Impact of surgery on quality of life of Ugandan women with symptomatic pelvic organ prolapse: a prospective cohort study. BMC Wom Health 2021;21(1):258.

57. Ghanbari Z, Ghaemi M, Shafiee A, et al. Quality of Life Following Pelvic Organ Prolapse Treatments in Women: A Systematic Review and Meta-Analysis. J Clin Med 2022;11(23).

58. Shah AD, Kohli N, Rajan SS, et al. Racial characteristics of women undergoing surgery for pelvic organ prolapse in the United States. Am J Obstet Gynecol 2007;197(1):70.e1–8.

59. Winkelman WD, Hacker MR, Anand M, et al. Racial and ethnic disparities in obliterative procedures for the treatment of vaginal prolapse. Female Pelvic Med Reconstr Surg 2021;27(12):e710–5.

60. Rodríguez D, Goueli R, Lemack G, et al. Carmel M. Racial and Ethnic Disparities in Pelvic Organ Prolapse Surgery in the United States: An Analysis of the ACS-NSQIP Clinical Registry. Urology 2023;174:70–8.

61. Cardenas-Trowers OO, Gaskins JT, Francis SL. Association of patient race with type of pelvic organ prolapse surgery performed and adverse events. Female Pelvic Med Reconstr Surg 2021;27(10):595–601.

62. Roberts K, Sheyn D, Emi Bretschneider C, et al. Perioperative complication rates after colpopexy in african american and hispanic women. Female Pelvic Med Reconstr Surg 2020;26(10):597–602.

63. Brown O, Mou T, Kenton K, et al. Racial disparities in complications and costs after surgery for pelvic organ prolapse. Int Urogynecol J 2022;33(2):385–95.

64. Ringel NE, Brown O, Moore KJ, et al. Disparities in Complications After Prolapse Repair and Sling Procedures: Trends From 2010-2018. Urology 2022;160:81–6.

65. Brown O, Siddique M, Mou T, et al. Disparity of racial/ethnic representation in publications contributing to overactive bladder diagnosis and treatment guidelines. Female Pelvic Med Reconstr Surg 2021;27(9):541–6.

66. Gonzalez DC, Khorsandi S, Mathew M, et al. A systematic review of racial/ethnic disparities in female pelvic floor disorders. Urology 2022;163:8–15.

67. Grimes CL, Clare CA, Meriwether KV, et al. Inadequacy and underreporting of study subjects' race and ethnicity in federally funded pelvic floor research. Am J Obstet Gynecol 2021;225(5):562.e1–6.

68. Mckay ER, Davila JL, Lee JA, et al. Representation of minority groups in key pelvic floor disorder trials. Female Pelvic Med Reconstr Surg 2021;27(10):602–8.

69. Northington GM, Minaglia S. Diversity in pelvic floor disorders research: A matter of equity and inclusion. Urogynecology (Phila). 2023;29(1):1–4.

70. Getaneh FW, Ackenbom MF, Carter-Brooks CM, et al. Race in clinical algorithms and calculators in urogynecology: what is glaring to us. Urogynecology (Phila). 2023;29(8):657–9.

71. Kessler L, Watts K, Abraham N. Should we correct the use of race in urological risk calculators? J Urol 2023;209(1):17–20.

72. Grobman WA, Sandoval G, Rice MM, et al. Prediction of vaginal birth after cesarean delivery in term gestations: a calculator without race and ethnicity. Am J Obstet Gynecol 2021;225(6):664.e1–7.

73. Prather C, Fuller TR, Marshall KJ, et al. The impact of racism on the sexual and reproductive health of african american women. J Womens Health (Larchmt) 2016;25(7):664–71.

74. Negbenebor NA, Garza EW. Black lives matter, but what about our health? J Natl Med Assoc 2018;110(1):16–7.

75. Ackenbom MF, Carter-Brooks CM, Soyemi SA, et al. Barriers to urogynecologic care for racial and ethnic minority women: A qualitative systematic review. Urogynecology (Phila). 2023;29(2):89–103.

76. Sanses TVD, Zillioux J, High RA, et al. Evidence-Informed, Interdisciplinary, Multidimensional Action Plan to Advance Overactive Bladder Research and Treatment Initiatives: Directives From State-of-the-Science Conference on Overactive Bladder and Cognitive Impairment. Urogynecology (Phila). 2023;29(1S Suppl 1):S20–39.

77. Leitch S, Corbin JH, Boston-Fisher N, et al. Black Lives Matter in health promotion: moving from unspoken to outspoken. Health Promot Int 2021;36(4):1160–9.

Diversity in Academic Obstetrics and Gynecology

William F. Rayburn, MD, MBA

KEYWORDS

- Academic • Diversity • Faculty • Female • Obstetrics and gynecology • Residents
- Underrepresented

KEY POINTS

- As medical school classes become more diverse, faculty who are more diversRevie offer advantages in services, teaching, mentoring, and scholarly works.
- Academic obstetrics and gynecology (OB/GYN) has had a surge of female representation and a slow increase in the representation of historically underrepresented physicians.
- Racial and ethnic diversity in OB/GYN is evenly distributed between residents and faculty and is among the highest of the major medical/surgical specialties.
- The percentage of male OB/GYN faculty will continue to decline, allowing more female faculty to advance in rank and leadership in higher positions.

INTRODUCTION

Diversity is defined as the spectrum of individual differences and the corresponding group memberships and identities that human beings have in society.[a] Enhancing diversity in the medical profession has continued to gain attention as a strategy to recruit practitioners who better represent patient populations.[1,2] Patients cared for by race-concordant or ethnicity-concordant physicians report greater satisfaction with their care, are more likely to adhere to care recommendations, and demonstrate improved health outcomes.[3] Despite more females entering the medical profession, the proportion of physicians who were historically excluded in medicine and science still lags behind corresponding US demographic changes.[4,5] For example, Black and Hispanic people in 2018 represented 30% collectively of the US population, yet accounted for only 13% of all medical students and 9% of all medical school faculty.[6]

Department of Obstetrics and Gynecology, Medical University of South Carolina, 171 Ashley Avenue, Charleston, SC 29425, USA
E-mail address: wrayburnmd@gmail.com

[a] Of note, we recognize that the terms "female" and "male" do not fully encompass the breadth of gender diversity. These terms are used throughout this article to best characterize the historical identification and categorization of those assigned female at birth and those assigned male at birth.

Obstet Gynecol Clin N Am 51 (2024) 181–191
https://doi.org/10.1016/j.ogc.2023.11.003
0889-8545/24/© 2023 Elsevier Inc. All rights reserved.

obgyn.theclinics.com

A diverse resident and faculty body plays a significant role in medical education settings where care needs, diagnostic accuracy, and treatment outcomes often vary by the patient's gender identity, race, ethnicity, and cultural status. Training by faculty who understand these differences may lead to more effective teaching and better patient care.[7–9] Such diversity among faculty also helps ensure a more comprehensive research agenda and drives institutional excellence.[10,11]

The continued change in resident and faculty composition and flexibility in career pathways prompts an examination of academic diversity in obstetrics and gynecology (OB/GYN).

EVOLUTION FROM A MALE TO FEMALE DOMINANT SPECIALTY

OB/GYN became a recognized specialty in 1927 when the American Board of Obstetrics and Gynecology (ABOG) was founded. Residency training programs began in 1930. For many years, more than 90% of all US medical school graduates and OB/GYN residents were males.[12] Gynecology was viewed by many as being a surgical specialty of the female reproductive tract, and obstetrics was associated with long hours of clinical responsibilities and frequent night calls.

In the 1960s and 1970s, 2 major events unfolded, which affected the diversity of persons entering the medical professions: affirmative action and expansion of US medical school enrollment. The Women's Movement in the 1960s and President Johnson's subsequent inclusion of women as part of the existing Affirmative Action policy in 1967 were examples of momentous actions. As ordered by President Johnson (Section 717 of Title VII of the Civil Rights Act of 1964), federal contractors used affirmative action to recruit and advance qualified minorities, women, persons with disabilities, and veterans. In its simplest terms, affirmative action continues to involve initiatives that compensate for societal barriers that hinder specific groups from being represented equally.

A wave of new medical schools in the United States in the 1960s and 1970s led to a previously unseen growth in the number and percentage of female medical students.[13] Another expansion in the 1990s to 2010s led to more growth of female and minoritized students. By 2017, more than half of all US medical school matriculants were female.[14] Male students began to feel more disadvantaged while female students may have considered their gender as advantageous in core rotations such as OB/GYN.[13,15] A lesser expansion of residency positions and lower proportion of male applicants led to an increasing number and proportion of OB/GYN first-year positions filled by females.[13,15–17]

The most recent 50 years demonstrated an increase in numbers of OB/GYN residents and faculty.[12,18] Faculty numbers increased 6.2-fold (from 1801 in 1972 to 6606 in 2021), whereas resident numbers increased 1.4-fold (from 4221 in 1980 to 5738 in 2021). By 2006, the number of faculty exceeded the number of residents. More female OB/GYN resident graduates contributed to more faculty being female. A notable difference was the 8-fold increase in percent of faculty being female (from 8.0% in 1972 to 67.3% in 2021), which was more than any other specialty.

A gender analysis of OB/GYN faculty, residents, and active physicians since 1972 was reported by Romero and colleagues using data from the Association of American Medical Colleges 9 (AAMC; Faculty Roster and GME Track) and the American Medical Association (Physician Characteristics and Distribution).[12] In 1972, 85% of OB/GYN faculty and 90% of OB/GYN residents were male. Because of rapidly shifting demographics, there has been a complete reversal of the gender make-up of OB/GYN

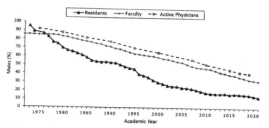

Fig. 1. Percentage decline of males who were OB/GYN residents, faculty, and physicians in practice from 1972 to 2021. (*From* abstract, Central Association of Obstetrics and Gynecology meeting, November 28, 2023, with permission.)

(Fig. 1).[12] During this 50-year period, males decreased by 63% for faculty, 85% for residents, and 63% for practicing OB/GYN physicians.

Between 2008 and 2019, the number of matriculating medical students increased 30% during another wave of medical school expansion, with nearly half (48%) being female.[13,14] Residency positions increased and filled, and the numbers and percentages by female students matching for first year OB/GYN positions were high.[15] As more were added, OB/GYN faculty began to be recognized as more racial and ethnically diverse, and largely female.[12,13]

Rotations for students and residents were more subspecialty-driven, and the evolution of subspecialties likely enhanced the appeal of OB/GYN being a more complete women's health-care specialty and a career pathway for future residents and faculty.[13,16] Gynecologic oncology, maternal–fetal medicine, and reproductive endocrinology and infertility became board-approved in 1972. Further subspecialization included female pelvic medicine and reproductive surgery in 2011 and complex family planning in 2018. The American Board of Medical Specialties approved ABOG to offer focused practice designation in pediatric and adolescent gynecology and minimally invasive gynecologic surgery in 2019. Although numbers are inexact, there has been diversity of OB/GYN residency graduates accepted into these fellowship programs and as eventual faculty.[13]

COMPARISON WITH OTHER CLINICAL DEPARTMENTS

Evidence exists of specialty-specific gender disparities in resident recruitment and selection. Bowe and colleagues examined applicant data between 2013 and 2018 from the Electronic Residency Application Service and resident data from the Accreditation Council for Graduate Medical Education (ACGME).[17] Eleven specialties represented the highest number of applications per applicant. OB/GYN demonstrated the lowest gender diversity (mostly female) of all the specialties in residency applicants and filled positions, whereas general surgery and neurologic surgery showed increased gender diversity over time (see **Fig. 1**).

In a retrospective, cross-sectional study, Xierali and colleagues used data from the AAMC Faculty Roster from 1979 to 2018 to identify diversity trends in all clinical department faculty by sex and underrepresented in medicine (URM) status.[18] As shown in **Fig. 2**, the substantial increase in diversity was mostly among females overall than male or female URM faculty separately. OB/GYN, dermatology, and psychiatry experienced the fastest increase in proportions of female faculty, whereas anesthesiology, physical rehabilitation, and orthopedic surgery experienced the slowest

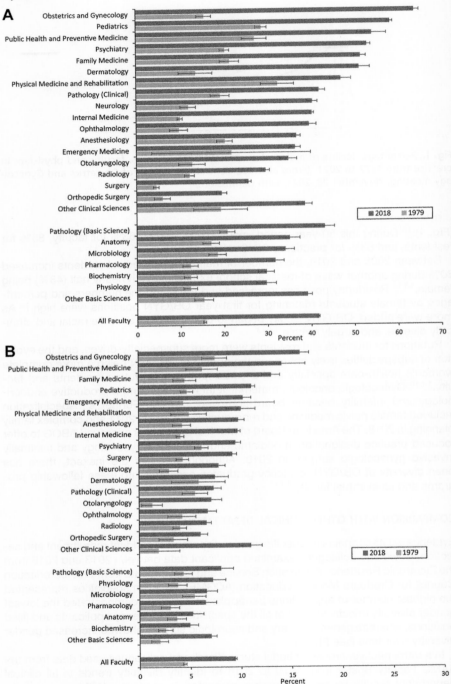

Fig. 2. Department-specific comparisons between proportions of full-time faculty at US medical schools who are female (*A*) and who are underrepresented minorities (*B*) in 1979 and 2018. (Xierali, Imam M. PhD; Nivet, Marc A. EdD, MBA; Rayburn, William F. MD, MBA. Full-Time Faculty in Clinical and Basic Science Departments by Sex and Underrepresented in Medicine Status: A 40-Year Review. Academic Medicine 96(4):p 568-575, April 2021. | DOI: 10.1097/ACM.0000000000003925).

increase. A 4-fold growth in the proportion of female faculty was noted in 4 departments: OB/GYN, pediatrics, ophthalmology, and internal medicine. More than half of the female faculty in 2018 represented just 6 departments: OB/GYN (63.8%), pediatrics (58.3%), public health and preventive medicine (54.1%), psychiatry (53%), family medicine (51.5%), and dermatology (51.2%).

Family medicine, public health and preventive medicine, and OB/GYN experienced the fastest annual rates of increases in proportions of URM faculty, whereas pathology, radiology, and dermatology experienced the slowest (see **Fig. 2**).[18] The highest proportions of all URM faculty in 2018 were found in 4 departments: OB/GYN (15.9%), public health and preventive medicine (14.1%), family medicine (13.1%), and pediatrics (11.1%). Even in those departments, the proportion of URM faculty was less than 16.0%

DIVERSITY BETWEEN OBSTETRICS AND GYNECOLOGY DEPARTMENTS AND UNITED STATES POPULATION

The US population is diversifying at a fast pace. Rayburn and colleagues used data from the 2021 AAMC Faculty Roster, ACGME Data Resource Book, and American Community Survey to compare the racial and ethnic diversity of OB/GYN faculty with the US adult female population.[19] The distribution of racial and ethnic groups was not different between OB/GYN residents and faculty who were Asian (11.9% vs 12.9%, respectively), Black (8.3% vs 8.5%, respectively), Hispanic (7.2% vs 7.3%, respectively), or Native American (0.4% vs 0.5%, respectively).

The racial and ethnic distribution of faculty was compared with the US population according to faculty rank (**Fig. 3**). Female and male faculty were subdivided into junior

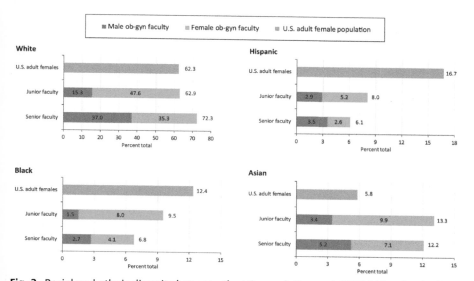

Fig. 3. Racial and ethnic diversity between the US population and OB/GYN faculty. (William F. Rayburn, Imam M. Xierali, William A. McDade, Racial-ethnic diversity of obstetrics and gynecology faculty at medical schools in the United States, American Journal of Obstetrics and Gynecology, 226 (6), 2022, 862-864, https://doi.org/10.1016/j.ajog.2022.02.007.)

(instructor or assistant professor) and senior (associate professor or professor) levels. Females constituted two-thirds of all faculty and were more likely to be junior than seniors (75.6% vs 50.5%). Junior faculty were less likely to be White and more likely to reflect the White US female population (62%–63%). Junior faculty were more likely to be Black or Hispanic than senior faculty, although these proportions were lower than the adult female population (Black: 8.5% vs 12.4%; Hispanic: 7.4% vs 16.7%). Asian faculty were more common than US adult females (12.9% vs 5.8%).

OTHER CONSIDERATIONS
A Departmental Approach to Diversity, Equity, and Inclusion

As at other academic institutions, an institutional mandate was implemented at The University of Michigan Medical School to enhance diversity, inclusiveness, and greater equity throughout the campus. Mmeje and colleagues developed a comprehensive framework and model for their OB/GYN department through the engagement of their stakeholders (faculty, clinical and administrative staff, residents and fellows, and the local community).[20] A "bottom-up" approach that engaged employees in decision making—with leadership support and partnership of their Office of Health Equity and Inclusion. Their call to action provides a helpful model for meaningful engagement. A continued focus on the recruitment, selection, retention, and development of faculty and staff from underrepresented groups may result in sustained change and impact in the department.

Task Force on Diversity, Equity, and Inclusion in Obstetrics and Gynecology

The Association of Professors of Gynecology and Obstetrics prepared a call for action by all academic departments to achieve a future free from racism in OB/GYN education and health care.[21] As a result, a task force was created to support educators in their efforts to identify and create educational materials that augment antiracist educational goals and prepare, recruit, and retain a talented and diverse workforce. In their special report, the Task Force shared guidelines that describe best practices and set new standards to increase diversity, foster inclusivity, address systemic racism, and eliminate bias in OB/GYN. Their guidelines involved metrics for the learning environment (including inclusive language and antiracism education), pathway programs, recruitment, retention, and promotion in the health professions.

Pathway programs at all US medical schools are intended to enhance opportunities for URM students to enter careers in the health professions and health sciences and to increase the availability of science and technology education programs.[22] Continued mentorship by faculty has been identified as a mechanism to reduce the disparities associated with the small numbers of URM trainees and physicians. Guidelines by the Task Force are provided for recruitment, retention, and promotion of mentorship programs from college to completion of medical school.[21] Ensuring a welcoming workplace and learning environment and instilling a sense of belonging are similarly crucial to support, retain, and promote URM students, residents, and faculty.

Nontenure Faculty Appointments

Tenure, a category of indefinite academic appointment that can be terminated only for cause or extraordinary circumstances, has been a dominant influence in academia at nearly all medical schools.[23] However, the proportion of clinical physician faculty who were either tenured or tenure-eligible has declined by 26.7% during the past

25 years.[23,24] An observational study by Esters and colleagues, using data from the AAMC Faculty Roster, identified the remarkable increase in OB/GYN faculty from 1699 in 1978 to 6347 in 2017 and the finding that 4 in 5 new faculty were nontenured.[25] Those who were nontenured were predominantly female and URM faculty. These results were consistent with data from Walling and Nilson evaluating trends for all medical school faculty from 2006 to 2016.[26] These findings signal an essential need for examining career development and academic accomplishment for promoting nontenured faculty.

Language Barriers and Hispanic Faculty

The United States needs more Spanish-speaking and culturally competent physicians because 19% of the population is Hispanic and nearly 70% of the Hispanic community speak Spanish at home.[27] Barriers with language-discordant health-care providers can lead to misunderstandings and adverse events. Although OB/GYN had the highest percentage of Hispanic faculty compared with other clinical departments combined (4.5% vs 3.1% in 1990, respectively, and 7.2% vs 6.0% in 2021, respectively), it has not kept pace with the growth of the Hispanic community.[27] Despite a 2-fold increase in the US Hispanic population during the past 30 years, there was only a 60% increase in Hispanic OB/GYN faculty.[27,28] In contrast to other specialties, the percentages of Hispanic and non-Hispanic females in OB/GYN faculty increased more than males, which explains how the percentages of Hispanic and non-Hispanic men declined.[28]

FUTURE CONSIDERATIONS

Gender, racial, and ethnic diversity brings a variety of perspectives in health-care teams that improve group problem-solving, creativity, and accessibility to culturally sensitive care to underserved populations.[29,30] Increasing numbers of underrepresented minorities in medicine will lead to better learning environments in medical schools and improved patient access to more culturally appropriate care.[31,32] In a report of 12-year trends in academic OB/GYN, Wooding and colleagues indicate promising trends due to increasing proportions of URM physicians. However, the rate at which they are increasing is slow and will require many decades to reach population averages.[33] Therefore, continued efforts are imperative to increase the representation of minority groups in academic OB/GYN to better reflect the population it serves.

Research in policies and strategies may lead to positive changes in the workplace and shifting culture. A study designed to assess policies and institutions that display more favorable diversity profiles could identify which strategies are most effective. A practical, institution-based framework for advancing gender diversity and underrepresented minorities should be periodically and collaboratively reviewed and updated, including policies to create equal opportunities (such as stop the clock tenure track for childbirth), programs, and mentoring initiatives to equip underrepresented persons with leadership skills. There is also a need for increasing visibility of demographic data of those in leadership positions.[33,34]

Diversity studies often use long-standing terminology and lack certain data to help explain or control the underlying causes of these disparities (ie, academic productivity, age, experience, and medical school intake).[33] Past definitions of gender, such as assigned male or female at birth, did not include the full spectrum of contemporary gender identity (eg, transgender and nonbinary). In addition, the 4 most prevalent racial and ethnic groups (White, Black, Asian, and Hispanic) prompt challenges with obtaining and analyzing accurate data, as in multiethnic individuals, those who do not self-identify, or those from other minority groups aside from the ones included herein.[33] In addition, diversity data do not describe how intersectionality (eg, assessing the proportion of persons from racial or ethnic minorities) relates to the described metrics. Ethnicity is now rarely discussed alone, and diversity studies would benefit from demographic data that combined race and ethnic backgrounds (ie, Hispanic Black or non-Hispanic White) and perhaps country of origin (ie, Puerto Rican, Cuban, Mexican, and Brazilian).

Studies show that when the size of a minority group reaches a certain threshold or critical mass (around 15%), a qualitative change takes place among group interactions.[34] The literature suggests that this threshold may be even higher during the selection process. At such levels, the particular minority group can organize and reinforce itself. A critical mass in OB/GYN gender diversity has been recognized as a potential deterrent for female applicants in the past and male applicants currently, thus influencing recruitment demographics.[35–37]

Our examination of the data did not allow recruitment or retention of males or underrepresented minorities at separate institutions. Individual departments need to review their decisions on recruitment and selection criteria and identify those decisions that differ (or may be viewed differently) for gender, racially and ethnically diverse applicants.[34] Bowe and associates studied evidence of specialty-specific gender disparities.[17] Specialties that have not reached around 25% gender minority (ie, males in OB/GYN) have had a harder time improving gender diversity. Their findings in resident recruitment and selection would likely also apply to faculty. Intentional efforts to affect representation at various stages of the recruitment and selection process can help provide a level of critical mass that has been shown to reduce the impact of unconscious bias.[38]

Findings in this report support the ongoing calls for dedicated institutional and departmental programming and policy changes to increase the continued low Black and Hispanic representation. These calls involve many organizations, including the American Medical Association, National Medical Association, National Hispanic Medical Association, and National Centers of Excellence in Women's Health.[39–41] Attention should be paid at each successive stage from pathway and pipeline programs to encourage historically underrepresented students to medical school, OB/GYN residency training, and academic appointment.[42,43] Improved visibility of underrepresented OB/GYN physicians is necessary at all stages of faculty recruitment, selection, retention, and promotion. Institutional and department accountable strategies need to be in place to foster unbiased training for recruitment and academic advancement of more Black and Hispanic faculty, repetitive guidance about promotion and tenure criteria, increased mentorship, and reducing financial burden.

Despite more equity in residency and faculty diversity, progress has been much slower at leadership levels. Morahan and colleagues have offered 2 approaches to advancing women as leaders—the concept of a leadership continuum and a framework of practical approaches for moving equity at all ranks.[44] A commentary by Brubaker and colleagues synthesized available information about women holding academic leadership roles, as well as specific principles and leadership practices for promoting diversity and equity.[45] A core value in academic OB/GYN may be gender, race, and ethnic equity. A reflective dialog and departmental, institutional, and professional society efforts should explicitly prioritize and demonstrate a commitment to equity with tangible actions.

CLINICS CARE POINTS

- Diversity improves the morale and performance of health-care teams. The numbers and proportions of females, as well as racial and ethnic minorities, have increased in OB/GYN.
- OB/GYN has seen the most dramatic shift in gender composition with nearly all residents and most faculty being women.
- Increased representation of faculty who are historically excluded in medicine should improve team functioning, access to culturally appropriate care, and mentorship to other minorities.
- There remains a lower proportion of females and URM physicians in leadership positions, higher academic ranks, and tenure.
- Although racial and ethnic diversity of US medical students has improved over the years, similar changes will remain more gradual for OB/GYN residents and especially faculty.

DISCLOSURE

The author reports no conflict of interest.

REFERENCES

1. Xierali IM, Castillo-Page L, Zhang K, et al. AM last page: the urgency of physician workforce diversity. Acad Med 2014;89:1192.
2. Xierali I, Nivet M. The racial and ethnic composition and distribution of primary care physicians. J Health Care Poor Underserved 2018;29:556–70.
3. Bonifacino E, Ufomata E, Farkas A, et al. Mentorship of underrepresented physicians and trainees in academic medicine: a systematic review. J Gen Intern Med 2021;36:1023–34.
4. United States Census Bureau. 2018 American Community Survey 5-year Public Use Microdata Sample (PUMS) files. Available at: https://www.census.gov/programs-surveys/acs/microdata/. Accessed July 10, 2013.
5. Association of American Medical Colleges. Table B-3: Total U.S. medical school enrollment by race/ethnicity (alone) and sex, 2016-2017 through 2020-2021. Available at: https://FACTS_Table_B-s.pdf Published November 3, 2020. Accessed May 22, 2023.
6. Association of American Medical Colleges Table 8: U.S. medical school faculty by race/ethnicity, 2018. Available at : https://www.aamc.org/media/9711/download. Published December 31, 2019. Accessed June 13, 2023.
7. Henderson J, Weisman C. Physician gender effects on preventive screening and counseling: an analysis of male and female patients' health care experiences. Med Care 2001;39:1281–992.
8. Lindberg O. Gender, and role models in the education of medical doctors: a qualitative exploration of gendered ways of thinking. J Med Educ 2020;11:31–6.
9. Gonzalo J, Chuang C, Glod S, et al. General internists as change agents: opportunities and barriers to leadership in health systems and medical education transformation. J Gen Intern Med 2020;35:1865–9.
10. Umbach PD. The contribution of faculty of color to undergraduate education. Res High Educ 2006;47:317–45.
11. Nonnemaker L. Women physicians in academic medicine: new insights from cohort studies. N Engl J Med 2000;342:399–405.

12. Romero I, Tucker J, Phelan S, et al. The legacy and challenges of gender disparities in obstetrics and gynecology. Nashville, TN: Central Association of Obstetrics and Gynecology; 2023.
13. Rayburn WF. The obstetrician-gynecologist workforce in the United States: facts, figures, and implications. 2nd edition. Washington DC: American College of Obstetricians and Gynecologists; 2017.
14. Association of American Medical Colleges. Matriculants to US medical schools by sex, published academic years 1980-1981 through 2018-2019. Available at: https://www.aamc.org.system/files/reports/1/tactsdatachart3.pdf.   Accessed May 12, 2023.
15. Craig L, Smith C, Crow S, et al. Obstetrics and gynecology clerkship for males and females: similar curriculum, different outcomes? Med Educ Online 2013; 18:21506.
16. Rayburn W, Xierali I. Expanded fellowship training and residency graduates' availability for women's general health needs. Obstet Gynecol 2021;137: 1119–21.
17. Bowe S, Wang Z, Whipple M, et al. Evidence of specialty-specific gender disparities in resident recruitment and selection. J Grad Med Ed 2021;13:841–7.
18. Xierali IM, Nivet MA, Rayburn WF. Full-time faculty in clinical and basic science departments by sex and underrepresented in medicine status: a 40-year review. Acad Med 2021;96:568–75.
19. Rayburn W, Xierali I, McDade WA. Racial-ethnic diversity of obstetrics and gynecology faculty in the United States. Am J Obstet Gynecol 2022;226:862–4.
20. Mmeje O, Price EA, Johnson TR, et al. Galvanizing the future: a bottom approach to diversity, equity, and inclusion. Am J Obstet Gynecol 2020;223:715–20.
21. Buery-Joyner S, Baecher-Lind L, Clare C, et al. Educational guidelines for diversity and inclusion: addressing racism and eliminating biases in medical education. Am J Obstet Gynecol 2023;228:133–9.
22. Liaison Committee on Medical Education. LCME functions and structure of a Medical School: standards for accreditation of medical education programs leading to the MD degree 2021. Available at: https://lcme.org/publications/. Accessed June 11, 2023.
23. Walling A. Understanding tenure. Fam Med 2015;47:43–7.
24. Bunton S, Corrice A. Trends in tenure for clinical M.D. faculty in U.S. medical schools: a 25-year review. Anal Brief 2010;9:1–2.
25. Esters D, Xierali I, Nivet M, et al. The rise of nontenured faculty in obstetrics and gynecology by sex and underrepresented in medicine status. Obstet Gynecol 2019;134:34S–9S.
26. Walling A, Nilsen K. Tenure appointments for faculty of clinical departments at U.S. medical schools: does specialty designation make a difference? Accad Med 2018;93:1719–26.
27. Saxena MR, Ling AY, Carillo E, et al. Trends of academic faculty identifying as Hispanic at US medical schools, 1990-2021. J Grad Med 2023;15:175–9.
28. Xierali IM, Romero IL, Rayburn WF. Changes in the number and academic ranks of Hispanic Faculty in departments of obstetrics and gynecology. Am J Obstet Gynecol 2023;229(6):694–6.
29. Roth L, Markova T. Essentials for great teams: trust, diversity, communication and joy. Am Board Fam Med 2012;25:146–8.
30. Lanham H, McDaniel R, Crabtree B, et al. How improving practice relationships among clinicians and nonclinicians can improve quality in primary care. Joint Comm J Qual Patient Saf 2009;35:457–66.

31. Marrast L, Zallman L, Woolhandler S, et al. Minority physicians' role in the care of underserved patients: diversifying the physician workforce may be key in addressing health disparities. JAMA Intern Med 2014;174:289–91.

32. Komaromy M, Grumbach K, Drake M, et al. The role of black and Hispanic physicians in providing health care for underserved populations. N Engl J Med 1996; 334:1305–10.

33. Wooding DJ, Das P, Tiwana S, et al. Race, ethnicity, and gender in academic obstetrics and gynecology: 12-year trends. Am J Obstet Gynecol MFM 2020;2: 100178.

34. Etzkowitz H, Kemelgor C, Neuschatz M, et al. The paradox of critical mass for women in science. Science 1994;266:1389–91.

35. Chapman C, Hwang WT, Wan X, et al. Factors that predict for representation of women in physician graduate medical education. Med Edu Online 2019;24: 1624132.

36. Neumayer L, Kaiser S, Anderson K, et al. Perceptions of women medical students and their influence on career choice. Am J Surg 2002;183:146–50.

37. Rohde R, Wolf J, Adams J. Where are the women in orthopaedic surgery? Clin Orthop 2016;474:1950–6.

38. Isaac C, Lee B, Canes M. Interventions that affect gender bias in hiring: a systematic review. Acad Med 2009;84:1440–6.

39. AMA. AMA adopts new policy to increase diversity in physician workforce 2021. Available from: https://wwwama0assn.org.press-center/press-releases/ama-adopts-new-policiy-increase-diversity-physician workforce. Accessed February 5, 2023.

40. Fuentes-Afflick E, Dzau VJ. Inclusion, diversity, equity, and anti-racism in health and science professional: a call for action for membership and leadership organizations. NAM Perspec 2022;2022. https://doi.org/10.31478/202205b.

41. Morahan PS, Voytko M, Abbuhl S, et al. Ensuring the success of women faculty at AMCs: lessons learned from the National Centers of Excellence in Women's Health. Acad Med 2001;76:19–31.

42. Peek ME, Kim KE, Johnson JK, et al. "URM candidates are encouraged to apply": a national study to identify effective strategies to enhance racial and ethnic faculty diversity in academic departments of medicine. Acad Med 2013;88(3):405.

43. Ajayi AA, Rodriguez F, De Jesus Perez V. Prioritizing equity and diversity in academic medicine faculty recruitment and retention. JAMA Health Forum 2021;2: e212426.

44. Morahan PS, Rosen SE, Richman RC, et al. The leadership continuum: a framework for organizational and individual assessment relative to the advancement of women physicians and scientists. J Women's Health 2011;20:387–96.

45. Brubaker L, Marsh E, Cedars M, et al. Promotion of gender equity in obstetrics and gynecology: principles and practices for academic leaders. Am J Obstet Gynecol 2022;226:163–8.

Substance Use in Pregnancy and Its Impact on Communities of Color

Leah Habersham, MD[a], Joshua George, MD, MPH[b],
Courtney D. Townsel, MD, MSc[c],*

KEYWORDS

- Equity • Substance use • Pregnancy • Cannabis • Opioid • Cocaine
- Health disparities

KEY POINTS

- Several US legislative acts between 1914 and 1994 paved the way for disproportionate punitive actions and incarceration among people of color despite similar rates of substance use as other racial groups.
- Substance use in pregnancy increases maternal and neonatal morbidity and mortality—particularly in relation to placenta-mediated effects of cocaine exposure and morbidity associated with opioid overdose.
- Stigma and bias are exacerbated by the intersection of obstetric racism and substance use among birthing people of color.

INTRODUCTION

Substance use in pregnancy is a significant public health issue impacting the health of both the birthing person and the developing fetus. Over the past several decades, substance use in pregnancy has increased—impacting pregnancy outcomes and health trajectories of neonates. Between 2017 and 2020, drug overdose mortality increased approximately 81% among pregnant and postpartum people, mirroring trends among reproductive-aged people.[1] Compounding the negative health impacts of substance use in pregnancy are the stigma and bias perceived and experienced by these birthing individuals. Stigma toward pregnant and postpartum people who use drugs is common and seeks to define addiction as a moral weakness rather than a

[a] Department of Obstetrics, Gynecology and Reproductive Sciences, 22 South Greene Street, Suite P6H310, Baltimore, MD 21201, USA; [b] Department of Obstetrics and Gynecology, University of Michigan, 1500 East Medical Center Drive, Ann Arbor, MI 48109, USA; [c] Department of Obstetrics, Gynecology and Reproductive Sciences, University of Maryland Baltimore, 250 West Pratt Street, Suite 880, Baltimore, MD 21201, USA
* Corresponding author. Department of Obstetrics, Gynecology and Reproductive Sciences, 22 South Greene Street, Suite P6H310, Baltimore, MD 21201.
E-mail address: ctownsel@som.umaryland.edu

Obstet Gynecol Clin N Am 51 (2024) 193–210
https://doi.org/10.1016/j.ogc.2023.10.004
0889-8545/24/Published by Elsevier Inc.

obgyn.theclinics.com

chronic medical illness that requires resources and treatment. More concerning is the additive impact of substance use and racial discrimination, whose intersections present particularly challenging circumstances. In this article, the authors review the history of substance use in the United States and focus on 3 substances of abuse that illustrate the inequity faced by birthing people of color who use drugs.

History of Drug Use in the United States

Although drug use, especially opium and its derivatives, was common before the 1900s, the US federal government had little to no involvement in restriction or regulation of drugs for medical or recreational purposes. These matters were left to state jurisdictions.[2] This position changed in 1914 with the Harrison Narcotics Act, which ushered in federal involvement through registration and taxation.[3] Along with this bill came the inclusion of racism and racial disparities. Much of the context and impetus for this legislation were built on exaggerated accounts of crime committed by Black people under the influence of cocaine and threats from Chinese immigrants in opium dens.[4]

War on Drugs

No story of the US drug policy is complete without discussion of President Richard Nixon and the "War on Drugs"—a term famously popularized after a Special Message to Congress from the President in 1971.[5] This "war" led to passage of the Controlled Substances Act in 1971, formation of the Drug Enforcement Administration in 1973, passage of the Anti-Drug Abuse Act in 1986, and the Violent Crime Control and Law Enforcement Act in 1994. These policies resulted in an overall increase in incarceration, with a disproportionate burden experienced by individuals of color despite similar rates of substance use across racial groups.[6]

Punitive Implications

The legacy of this history for pregnant people—especially pregnant people of color—is impactful on several fronts. Incarceration and incarceration exposure directly impact adverse obstetric outcomes, such as preterm birth, low birth weight, and rates of infectious diseases and vertical infectious disease transmission. There are also indirect, generational impacts of incarceration on social determinants of health, such as poverty, education, and housing instability and safety.[7] Furthermore, there are downstream punitive policies surrounding substance use and pregnancy that have demonstrated clear evidence of bias, such as unequal mandatory reporting and involvement of child protective services.[8] Together, these impacts result in a vicious cycle of adverse outcomes and often prevent clinicians from addressing the barriers of systemic racism—instead driving "mother blame" narratives.

Obstetric Racism

Obstetric racism is a newly coined term that connects both obstetric violence and medical racism[9] to characterize the birthing experience of people of color. The World Health Organization defines obstetric violence as abuse, disrespect, and mistreatment in childbirth perpetrated by health professionals that results in violations of people's dignity and results in unnecessary pain and avoidable complications.[10] Medical racism involves discriminatory and directed medical practices driven by biases based on a patient's perceived race and ethnicity.[11] Obstetric racism has been strongly connected to the birthing experience of Black birthing people, in particular,[9] who continue to bear the brunt of significant obstetric-related health disparities, including higher ates of preterm birth, maternal morbidity, and maternal mortality compared with their white counterparts.[12,13]

When substance use is layered on top of racial identity, additional stigma and bias nsue—compounding and exacerbating the birthing experience for these individuals. Birthing people with substance use disorders have identified several barriers to engaging in care, including shame about using drugs while pregnant, fear of punitive action, and mistrust of health care professionals.[14]

Screening for Substance Use and Substance Use Disorders in Pregnancy

Substance use and substance use disorders have a significant impact on the prenatal period, with prevalence similar to many illnesses that are typically tested for during pregnancy.[15] For instance, in 2020, the National Survey on Drug Use and Health reported that 8.3% of pregnant people used illicit substances, with 10.6% using alcohol, .4% using tobacco products, and 0.4% using opioids.[16] Therefore, with substantial se of substances during pregnancy, it behooves practitioners to identify substance se ideally before, but at minimum during, pregnancy. There are several means of substance use identification, such as (1) biological testing (eg, urine toxicology testing); (2) questionnaire administration (eg, validated screening tool); and (3) patient interview.[17]

Screening is distinct from testing, as it involves the use of screening tools or questionnaires in the assessment of substance use. Testing refers to analysis of a biologic specimen, such as blood, saliva, urine, feces, or hair for the presence of specific substances. Screening tools and biologic tests are incapable of identifying a substance use disorder. Furthermore, biologic testing is only capable of determining the presence of a substance over a finite window of time—usually around 3 to 7 days[18] (Table 1). Therefore, relying on universal testing as the only means to identify substance use during pregnancy is an inherently flawed and potentially biased strategy. The American College of Obstetricians and Gynecologists (ACOG) recommends universal screening for substance use and substance use disorders during pregnancy using a validated screening tool[19] (Fig. 1). Despite these recommendations, there is still o universally held standard for the assessment of prenatal substance use during

Table 1
Substances and detection windows

Substance	Detection Window After Intake
Alcohol	7–12 h
Amphetamines	2–3 d
Benzodiazepines	
Short-acting	2 d
Long-acting	10–30 d
Cannabis	
Single to moderate use	3–7 d
Chronic heavy use	>30 d
Cocaine	2–3 d (up to 7 d at high doses)
Opioids	2–5 d
Phencyclidine	8 d

Screening Tools for the Pregnant Population

4Ps Plus: Four questions (Parents, Partner, Past, and Pregnancy) to assess substance use.

5Ps Plus: Expanded version of the 4Ps Plus and includes five questions (Parents, Partner, Past, Pregnancy, and Protection).

ASSIST-Pregnancy: Adapted version of the ASSIST (Alcohol, Smoking, and Substance Involvement Screening Test) to assess substance use disorders in pregnant individuals.

CRAFFT-Pregnancy: Adapted from the CRAFFT for adolescents—focuses on identifying substance use disorders in pregnant individuals ages 26 and under.

NIDA Quick Screen: Single question that asks about drug use in the past year: "How many times in the past year have you used an illegal drug or used a prescription medication for non-medical reasons?"

Substance Use Risk Profile-Pregnancy (SURP-P): A comprehensive screening tool that evaluates substance use, mental health, and psychosocial factors during pregnancy.

T-ACE: Four questions (Tolerance, Annoyance, Cut down, Eye-opener) to identify alcohol use disorders in pregnant women.

TWEAK-MS: Modified version of the TWEAK screening tool that focuses on identifying alcohol use disorders during pregnancy.

Fig. 1. Validated screening tools.

pregnancy; therefore, various strategies are used in prenatal clinics and hospitals across the United States, including biologic testing, screening tools, or both. Research has demonstrated that inequities abound in the realm of biologic testing and subsequent child protective services reporting. Despite historical evidence that substance use is nearly equal among Black and White pregnant people, Black birthing people are 10 times more likely to be reported to child protective services when positive toxicology testing is identified.[20]

Despite these facts, clinicians may still use biologic testing owing to concern that patient self-report of substance use may be unrevealing. In addition, a high percentage of pregnant people who report substance use are found to have gone untested for substance use via toxicology. Clinicians may then think that universal testing and universal screening are the answers, as they may increase the chance of identifying substance use during pregnancy while avoiding bias.[21–23] Despite these misconceptions, ACOG and the Society for Maternal-Fetal Medicine support screening questionnaires over biologic testing.[15,19,24]

DISCUSSION
The Tale of Three Epidemics

To illustrate the contemporary impact of substance use in birthing people of color, the authors review the history and existing impact of marijuana, cocaine, and opioid use in pregnancy.

Marijuana

History and legal status
Although products of the *Cannabis* plant have been used by humans for thousands of years, its pharmacologic and medicinal properties in the form of marijuana have only been realized in the United States since the 1800s.[25] Cannabis was widely used for its medicinal properties for a variety of conditions, including pain, cramping, appetite stimulation, and mental illness.[26] Toward the early 1900s, issues with dose variability and competition from other pharmaceutical agents initiated the trend toward legislation. The substance and its active ingredients, tetrahydrocannabinol (THC) and cannabidiol, were first regulated in 1937 with the passage of the Marihuana Tax Act, which

instituted the first tax on use, prescription, and distribution of marijuana.[27] This Act was spearheaded by the founding Commissioner of the Federal Bureau of Narcotics, Harry Anslinger, whose overtly racist rhetoric against Mexican immigrants and Black Americans was instrumental in fostering legislative support for the marijuana ban.[28] Attributing substance use and its associations with crime to minority communities was a trope initiated by Anslinger that has proven to be pervasive to this day.

A discussion of the impact of marijuana use on pregnancy in communities of color would be incomplete without mention of the impact of disproportionate drug-related incarceration. The mandatory sentencing policies for drug-related arrests that began with the passage of the Boggs Act of 1952 and the Narcotics Control Act of 1956 continued into the 1980s with the passage of the Anti-Drug Abuse Act, which grouped marijuana offenses into the same mandatory minimum punishments as substances such as cocaine.[29,30] This led to an exponential increase in the number of marijuana-related arrests over the next 2 decades, with Black people representing a disproportionate share of arrests despite similar rates of marijuana use between racial groups.[6,31] This increase is significant, as incarceration and incarceration exposure have been shown to result in a greater barrier to prenatal care as well as increased rates of preterm birth and low birth weight.[32,33] These adverse outcomes have also been shown to be increased even when paternal incarceration alone was present.[34]

Modern legal considerations and decriminalization

Alongside more stringent marijuana legislation in recent years have come many attempts at amendments and revisions of policy that mirror the US population's support for marijuana reform. However, this reform has proceeded at differing speeds between the federal and state levels.

Individual states began decriminalizing marijuana as early as 1973 by removing criminal penalties for low-level possession.[35] Although this trend stalled during the 1980s, the increase of medical and recreational policies—beginning with California's Compassionate Use Act in 1996—ushered in a new era of marijuana policies. As of 2023, 22 states have fully legalized marijuana for both medical and recreational purposes; 17 states have medical use—only policies; 5 states have low THC-only policies, and 6 states have no legal program (**Fig. 2**).[36] On the federal level, marijuana

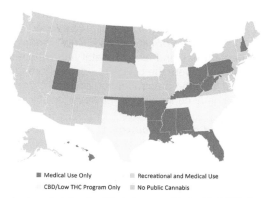

■ Medical Use Only ▫ Recreational and Medical Use
▫ CBD/Low THC Program Only ■ No Public Cannabis

Fig. 2. Cannabis use by legal status in US states as of July 15, 2023. Laws vary in the legal limit allowed for possession. (*Data from*: National Conference of State Legislatures. State Medical Cannabis Laws. Accessed August 11, 2023. https://www.ncsl.org/health/state-medical-cannabis-laws.)

is still classified as a Schedule 1 substance under the Controlled Substances Act, designating it as a substance with high potential for abuse and no current medical use for treatment in the United States.[37] However, recent legislation, such as the SAFE Banking Act of 2019 and the Marijuana Opportunity Reinvestment and Expungement Act of 2019 (MORE Act), which have been passed by the US House only, has challenged the integrity of federal marijuana criminalization policies.[35]

The increased rate of cannabis possession arrests for Black Americans compared with White Americans is well acknowledged. Both decriminalization and legalization policies hoped to address this gap, as well as the negative consequences of incarceration. Under current evaluation is the impact of drug policy liberalization on disparate outcomes in arrests between racial groups. Although most studies show a decrease in absolute arrests across racial groups, other analyses show that relative arrest disparities persist across multiple US cities.[38] This may be due to a variety of factors, including disproportionate enforcement of residual laws in place or nonstandard citation policies that regressively impact communities of color.[39]

Although cannabis use in the nonpregnant population has increased, the effect of decriminalization and legalization among pregnant people is still under further investigation. Several survey-based studies demonstrate that pregnant people would be more likely to use marijuana if it were legalized, but those who are aware of its potentially harmful effects are more likely to quit or cut down on their use.[40,41] This finding comes despite the recommendation from ACOG that people who are pregnant or contemplating pregnancy should be encouraged to discontinue marijuana use.[42] Legalization of marijuana may cause the public to misconstrue the substance as safe, which may not be true—especially in pregnancy and the postpartum period. As the national trend toward drug policy liberalization continues, it will be imperative for medical providers who care for pregnant people to be clear about current evidence and recommendations for marijuana use and cessation during pregnancy.

Epidemiology of marijuana use in pregnancy

Recent estimates of cannabis use show a prevalence of around 10% for the preconception period and 4% for the prenatal period.[43] Preconception use and postpartum use have also shown increasing trends in states that have legalized cannabis; prenatal use may also be increased but is subject to greater reporting and social desirability bias.[44] Data from the Pregnancy Risk Assessment Monitoring System (PRAMS) show that increased prenatal cannabis use is associated with single status, nulliparity, age younger than 24, lower socioeconomic status, unintended pregnancy, prior intimate partner violence, and tobacco or alcohol use. Non-Hispanic Black people self-reported more preconception use and less prenatal use, whereas Hispanic, Native American, and Pacific Islanders were the opposite—self-reporting increased use during the prenatal compared with the preconception period.[45] Whether race alone is a significant predictor of perinatal cannabis use, however, is still unclear.[46]

Pregnancy considerations and neonatal outcomes of marijuana use

Pregnancy risks. It is known that marijuana crosses the placenta and has been associated in some studies with adverse developmental effects for the fetus, such as low birth weight,[42,47] preterm birth, and stillbirth, as well as increased maternal risk for placentally mediated conditions, such as hypertensive disorders of pregnancy[48,49] **(Fig. 3)**. Data on these associations are mixed and confounded by concomitant tobacco use and poor capture of cannabis initiation and dosing. Counseling by obstetric providers on the risks of cannabis in pregnancy is often lacking, and when performed, often focuses on punitive implications—especially for individuals of color, who are

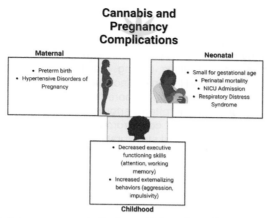

Fig. 3. Cannabis and pregnancy complications. Although evidence is often confounded by concomitant tobacco use and limited details of cannabis dose, studies have shown increased risk of adverse outcomes in all 3 domains. NICU, neonatal intensive care unit. Created with BioRender.com.

more likely to be asked about substance use in pregnancy. This inadequate counseling may be due in part to the lack of clear evidence from studies, which often are hampered by confounding from other exposures and limited by reporting and recall bias.[42]

Management and treatment. There is currently no Food and Drug Administration (FDA)-approved medical therapy for cannabis use disorder. The limited treatment options that exist fall into the realm of rehabilitation programs or psychosocial interventions. Integrated substance use disorder prenatal clinics may be beneficial in that they may provide access to comprehensive services (eg, mental health resources) and social services (eg, childcare, nutrition, and transportation), which have been shown to be beneficial in addressing additional identified risk factors for cannabis use in pregnancy that are more prevalent in communities of color.[50]

Although marijuana use has been associated with adverse pregnancy outcomes as described, there are no specific evidence-based recommendations regarding antepartum care for individuals who consume or use cannabis during pregnancy. There is insufficient evidence to recommend antenatal surveillance or growth ultrasounds to minimize risk of stillbirth or fetal growth restriction. There are also no specific modifications to decision making regarding delivery timing, modality, or standard obstetric intrapartum care. Obstetric anesthesia providers should be notified of cannabis use, as it may cause changes in vital signs. In addition, inhaled marijuana may cause airway irritation or edema, leading to an increased risk of anesthesia complications.[51]

Postpartum. The postpartum period is a vulnerable time, when increased rates of cannabis use are seen compared with the prenatal period.[52] Data from California and Maryland show decreased uptake of postpartum care among Hispanic and non-Hispanic Black birthing people.[53,54] This period is vital for engagement, as people who have quit or cut down on cannabis use owing to pregnancy are more likely to be receptive to continued cessation interventions. Various strategies, such as incentives and patient navigators, have demonstrated benefit in reducing disparities in postpartum care attendance and may also be beneficial in addressing postpartum substance use.[55]

The benefits of breastfeeding for infants are well-established by ACOG and the American Academy of Pediatrics. Both organizations recommend refraining from cannabis use during lactation owing to the limited clinical evidence on infant outcomes.[56] Although perhaps well-intentioned, these guidelines may in fact further exacerbate breastfeeding disparities among racial groups.[57] PRAMS data from 2017 to 2018 showed that non-Hispanic Black pregnant people who self-reported cannabis use in pregnancy were 4 times more likely to receive counseling against breastfeeding.[58] This counseling is often performed in a punitive manner and may further discourage birthing people of color from breastfeeding. Breastfeeding counseling should aim to reduce barriers of structural racism and bias to not only minimize infant risk but also optimize infant benefit.

Outcomes in neonates and children. The present evidence on neonatal outcomes after cannabis use in pregnancy includes those such as low birth weight, small for gestational age, preterm delivery, neonatal intensive care unit admission, decreased mean birth weight, APGAR score at 1 minute, and infant head circumference[59] (see **Fig. 3**). Data are complicated by multiple factors, including reporting bias, recall bias, and limited information on timing of administration, modality, and dosing. High rates of concomitant tobacco use also confound data interpretation. Several recent meta-analyses have shown differing results, but most studies show an increased risk of preterm birth and small for gestational age; other outcomes show increased risk but have a lower certainty of evidence.[60] Providers should be mindful of the limitations but recognize that cannabis use likely does come with increased neonatal risk without evidence of benefit for any maternal or neonatal indication.

Data on long-term outcomes have centered on neurodevelopmental outcomes, as cannabinoid type 1 receptors are expressed at early gestational ages and exposure has the potential to impact fetal brain development. Although childhood developmental studies are limited by multiple exposures, genetics, and environmental effects, evidence does suggest that cannabis may negatively impact neurobehavioral outcomes. This impact appears to be more significant in patients with earlier use and increased dose.[61] Counseling for cannabis cessation should include information about potential short- and long-term impacts.

Cocaine

The medical era

Originating from the leaves of the Erythroxylon coca plant, cocaine is a psychoactive alkaloid native to Bolivia, Colombia, and Peru. The substance was first used as a psychostimulant more than 5000 years ago. In the 1500s, Europeans traveling to South America discovered the benefits of coca leaves, including reduced fatigue and increased stamina. After coca leaf use, and likely overuse, in 1552, the Catholic church directed the world's first antidrug campaign banning its use.[62]

In the latter half of the nineteenth century, investigators began to research the therapeutic value of coca. Initially, these research efforts proved futile owing to variations in the quality of the coca product found in the United States. However, the chemist Albert Niemann was able to isolate cocaine from coca leaves and subsequently discovered its local anesthetic properties.[63] In 1884, physician Carl Koller decided to use cocaine to anesthetize the surface of the eye. Thereafter, cocaine began to be used as an alternative option to more dangerous general anesthetics, such as ether and chloroform.[62]

As the use of cocaine in surgery and other procedures became more common, its use began to extend to the fields of neurology and psychiatry. The substance was used to treat medical conditions, such as headaches, epilepsy, depression, and exhaustion. Cocaine even came to be used as a treatment for opioid addiction.[62] Cocaine's use was far-reaching and deep within the confines of early-modern medicine.

The popular era

As cocaine's medical use was increasingly exploited, new uses for the substance began to emerge. In the late 1890s, cocaine became a common pastime of young professional White men. The typical cocaine user was an overworked White male-identifying professional—stressed and seeking relief. However, by 1900, cocaine came to be known as the "hard drug" of choice, used by laborers and commercial sex workers. Employers introduced the drug to laborers, many of whom were Black, to optimize production.[64] Black Americans soon came to be associated with the use of cocaine, which came to be seen as a threat to the subservient social norms typically observed of Black Americans at that time. Beyond the use noted among laborers, cocaine began to extend to use among commercial sex workers—raising concern for its eventual use by people assigned female at birth and children more broadly. It was through these perceived negative associations that cocaine came to be seen as a substance used by those of social and moral failing.[62]

The crack era

The 1970s brought a rejuvenation of cocaine use among the young and elite. Cocaine once again was the substance of choice for the White professional to facilitate stress relief. By the 1980s, a new, more affordable and smokeable form of cocaine was introduced into major cities across the United States—coined "crack" owing to the sound it made during its formation. The popularity of this substance grew, and it became a favored choice among lower-income populations for production, sale, and use. It was out of cocaine's use in this environment that the war on drugs was born and propagated by politicians, such as Ronald Reagan and George H.W. Bush.

Epidemiology of crack cocaine use and pregnancy outcomes

In 2021, of people aged 12 years and older, 1.7% reported use of cocaine within the past 12 months, with cocaine use disorder reported by 0.5% of respondents. During this same year, more than 24,000 people died of an overdose that involved the use of cocaine.[65]

Cocaine is typically ingested orally, intranasally, intravenously, or through inhalation. The effect is most quickly experienced through inhalation, and next by injection. Because of the quick effect onset of inhaled "crack" cocaine, this form became favored by large numbers of people across the United States and worldwide. Cocaine use increases the risk of heart attacks, strokes, and seizures.[66] Cocaine use during pregnancy has been found to be associated with concurrent use of other substances, comorbid psychiatric disorders, poor nutrition, inadequate medical care, intimate partner violence, delays in prenatal care, and other confounding factors that lead to poor pregnancy outcomes.[67] Maternal use of cocaine is associated with placental abruption, preterm labor, cocaine overdose, and even death.[67]

Treating cocaine use disorder in pregnancy

There is no FDA-approved medication-assisted treatment option for cocaine use disorder. This leaves patients with limited choices to assist with recovery, including rehabilitation programs and psychosocial therapy. Often, patients who are pregnant are further limited owing to practical issues that tend to arise, including transportation, childcare, focus on partners, minimal focus on prenatal care, and limited focus on medical needs.[68]

One approach to managing these limitations in the care of pregnant people with cocaine use disorder sprouted in the 1990s—the introduction of integrated clinics.[69] The first was the MATER clinic in Philadelphia, which offered an opioid treatment program for people assigned female at birth where birthing people could receive treatment for opioid use disorder (OUD) and prenatal care concurrently.[70] This program served as a model for subsequent programs throughout the United States. Key components of this type of program's success include provision of health care and social needs, including prenatal and mental health care, vocational training and employment assistance, parenting skills, transportation support, onsite childcare, and colocation of other integral services.[69]

Barriers to cocaine use disorder treatment are further compounded by inequities of race and ethnicity, with marginalized and minoritized birthing people having higher referral rates to child protective services, facing rising rates in overdose death, and experiencing increased risks of untreated mental illness.[20,71–73]

Neonatal outcomes

First reported in the *New England Journal of Medicine*, which touted the burgeoning influx of "crack babies," researchers and clinicians alike have debunked this term, as it is not a supported finding in medical practice.[74] Among pregnant people, this substance has the potential of increasing risk of placental abnormalities, such as placental abruption, preterm labor and delivery, small for gestational age, low birth weight, and small head circumference.[67]

Opioids

Opioids are a class of drugs that includes illegal formulations such as heroin, synthetic forms such as fentanyl, and prescription forms such as hydromorphone. Opioids act by binding the opioid receptors (mu, delta, and kappa), which are responsible for mediating psychoactive and somatic effects. The central nervous system action of opioid drugs has led to its potential for misuse.

The crisis

In 2015, the US life expectancy declined for the first time in more than 100 years (2014: 78.8 years; 2015: 78.7 years; 2016: 78.5 years), which was directly connected to escalating deaths owing to opioid overdose. Between 1999 and 2021, opioid overdose deaths increased more than six-fold.[75] The "opioid epidemic" emerged as a result of the overprescribing of opioids by health care providers for pain and aggressive and fraudulent marketing by pharmaceutical manufacturers. In 1995, the American Pain Society launched a campaign that coined pain as the "fifth vital sign." Attention to pain and pain management increased, and physicians began to more liberally prescribe controlled substances without fear of prosecution. Even more concerning were reports from reputable journals insinuating that opioid addiction following receipt of an opioid prescription was rare. The *New England Journal of Medicine* published a study in 1980 that reported only 4 out of 11,882 patients became addicted to opioids after receiving a prescription.[76] Such studies contributed to the idea that opioids had low addiction potential. Alongside these occurrences were new opioid formulations, such as OxyContin, which was introduced in the mid-1990s as a treatment for chronic pain by Purdue Pharma, who claimed this medication was "less addictive" than other opioids. This false claim resulted in a $635 million fine in 2007,[77] but this truth did not reach doctors and patients until several years later.

The first wave of the epidemic occurred in the 1990s, with increased prescribing as mentioned earlier. The second wave began in 2010 as a result of escalating opioid overdose deaths related to heroin. The third wave began in 2013 with the increase in use of fentanyl, which led to even more overdose deaths. Today, illicitly manufactured fentanyl can be found in heroin, cocaine, and counterfeit pills.[75] An important aspect of this epidemic is the noted racial differences. Heroin use is highest among non-Hispanic White people.[78] In addition, after opioid use is detected, White patients receive treatment up to 80% more frequently than Black patients.[79] These racial disparities in addiction diagnosis and treatment persist into pregnancy. A recent study found that the majority (86.7%) of birthing people with OUD presenting to a northeastern urban substance use clinic were non-Hispanic White, 8.8% were Hispanic, and 4.5% were Black. Treatment was received by 69.9% of non-Hispanic White birthing people with OUD compared with only 49.4% of Hispanic patients and 46.2% of Black patients.[80]

The current epidemic

Between 1999 and 2021, almost 645,000 people died of an opioid overdose involving both prescription and illicit opioids.[81] Mirroring the US opioid epidemic, the rate of opioid use or dependence in pregnancy increased 131% between 2010 and 2017.[82] In addition, drug overdose mortality for birthing people increased 81% from 2017 to 2020.[1] Overdoses were lowest in the third trimester and highest 7 to 12 months after delivery. Birthing people with OUD who received pharmacotherapy treatment had reduced overdose rates in the postpartum period.[83]

Pregnancy and neonatal outcomes

Opioid use in pregnancy has been associated with numerous poor outcomes for the fetus and newborn infant. These conditions include, but are not limited to, preterm delivery, lack of prenatal care, placental abruption, fetal growth restriction, stillbirth, possible birth defects (eg, neural tube, cardiac, and gastroschisis), sudden infant death syndrome, and meconium passage before birth.[19,84] In addition, untreated OUD is associated with high-risk activities, such as commercial sex work and exchanging sex for drugs. These behaviors increase the risk of sexually transmitted infections, legal trouble, and violence. Birthing people with OUD often have cooccurring substance use disorders and mental health conditions. Tobacco use and marijuana use are the most common cooccurring substances, whereas cooccurring benzodiazepine use increases risk of mortality owing to overdose. Depression and posttraumatic stress disorder are common among this pregnant population.

Drug withdrawal in newborns caused by opioid exposure in utero is called neonatal opioid withdrawal syndrome (NOWS), which occurs in 30% to 80% of opioid-exposed neonates. NOWS is characterized by disturbances in the autonomic, gastrointestinal, and nervous systems resulting in poor feeding, irritability, and even seizure activity shortly after birth.[19] Treatment of NOWS ranges from supportive care through programs such as Eat-Sleep-Console (ESC) to pharmacotherapy agents. Of note, ESC was found to significantly reduce the length of stay compared with usual care for neonates prenatally exposed to opioids in a recent randomized controlled trial.[85] Long-term neonatal outcomes are less clear owing to cooccurring substance exposures that are frequently observed. In general, studies have not shown significant neurodevelopmental impairment at up to 5 years of age.[19]

Treatment: medication for opioid use disorder

Opioid agonist pharmacotherapy with either methadone (opioid receptor agonist) or buprenorphine (mixed opioid receptor agonist) is first-line therapy for patients with OUD. These agents are preferred to withdrawal and plan for abstinence because withdrawal and abstinence programs have been associated with higher rates of relapse.

Maternal medication for opioid use disorder (MOUD) dosages usually require up-titration in pregnancy, owing to the physiologic increased volume of distribution, to avoid withdrawal symptoms (eg, nausea, abdominal cramps, irritability, and anxiety). Clinicians should counsel pregnant people taking MOUD that dose and duration of MOUD do not predict severity of NOWS. Therefore, pregnant people on MOUD should be maintained on the dose of medication that controls their withdrawal symptoms. Although methadone is currently the most common pharmacotherapy agent in pregnancy, buprenorphine has been shown to result in lower rates of NOWS.[86] However, birthing people who enter pregnancy on methadone should not be switched to buprenorphine because of the potential for withdrawal owing to buprenorphine's partial agonist properties. Buprenorphine is available as a mono-product (Subutex) and in combination with naloxone (Suboxone), an opioid antagonist, to reduce diversion. Studies have found no adverse effects and similar outcomes when comparing buprenorphine alone with the combination of buprenorphine and naloxone.[87,88]

Naltrexone is a nonselective opioid receptor antagonist that blocks the effects of opioids. It is commonly used outside of pregnancy for OUD treatment but has limited data in pregnancy. One major downside is the need to abstain from opioids for 7 days before initiating naltrexone to reduce the risk of precipitated withdrawal. This transition period increases the risk of relapse. A recent study found favorable neonatal outcomes for pregnancies exposed to naltrexone, with lower rates of neonatal opioid

Table 2
Comparison of substances in pregnancy, associated complications, and interventions

Substance	Maternal Complications	Birth/Neonatal Complications	Recommended Therapies/ Interventions
Marijuana	• Hypertensive disorders of pregnancy	• Low birth weight • Preterm birth • Stillbirth • Long-term neurodevelopmental impact uncertain	• No FDA-approved pharmacotherapy • Supportive treatment for complications of cessations (eg, nausea and vomiting) • Integrated substance use prenatal clinics
Cocaine	• Heart attack • Stroke • Seizure • Placental abruption • Preterm labor • Cocaine overdose • Death	• Small for gestational age • Low birth weight • Small head circumference	• No FDA-approved treatment options • Consider psychosocial therapy and rehabilitation programs • Integrated substance use prenatal clinics
Opioids	• Placental abruption • Opioid overdose • Death	• Preterm delivery • Low birth weight • Stillbirth • Possible birth defects (eg, neural tube, cardiac, gastroschisis) • NOWS • Sudden infant death syndrome • Meconium passage before birth	• Medication for opioid use disorder (first line; eg, methadone, buprenorphine)

withdrawal (8.4%) compared with 75% in pregnancies with methadone or buprenorphine exposure.[89]

Juxtaposing Two Epidemics

Although both cocaine and OUD are thought to necessitate treatment, those with cocaine use and dependence are less likely than those with opioid use and dependence to receive treatment for their substance use disorders. Chronic use of heroin and other opioids has typically been viewed as an addiction, whereas cocaine has often been seen as a chosen vice within the control of its user. Similar to today, opioids hold the connotation of being the result of long-term use typically secondary to chronic ailments. Cocaine continues to be seen as a substance that is instead used for pleasure and associated with social deviance. These differences play out both along epidemics and also along racial and ethnic lines, as the cocaine epidemic has historically been seen as a "Black" issue, and the opioid epidemic has largely been seen as a "White" issue.[90]

SUMMARY

Substance use in pregnancy is prevalent and remains a critical public health issue. The histories of marijuana, cocaine, and opioid use in the United States serve as clear examples of stark differences in treatment received by communities of color. There remain several maternal and neonatal complications associated with use of these substances in pregnancy (**Table 2**). Clinicians should strive to implement universal screening practices to reduce bias. If substance use is identified, treatment and services should be offered to the individual, and punitive impacts should be minimized, when possible, to maintain the physician-patient relationship.

CLINICS CARE POINTS

- Provide universal screening and informed consent, with self-reporting practices preferred.
- Counsel on adverse maternal and fetal outcomes; recommend cessation or cutting down.
- Discuss recommendation to avoid breastfeeding with cannabis and cocaine use in the setting of limited evidence regarding risks; do not withdraw lactation support.
- Address nausea- and vomiting-related concerns early at the initial prenatal visit and treat based on standard guidelines to reduce and eliminate cannabis use in pregnancy.
- Screen for other substance use risk factors, including tobacco use, anxiety, depression, and intimate partner violence.
- Review safety of breastfeeding while taking prescribed opioids (eg, methadone, buprenorphine); individualize care as needed.
- The American College of Obstetricians and Gynecologists recommends universal screening for substance use and substance use disorders during pregnancy using a validated screening tool.
- Despite evidence that substance use is nearly equal among Black and White pregnant people, Black birthing people are 10 times more likely to be reported to child protective services when positive toxicology testing is identified.
- Marijuana crosses the placenta and is associated with low birth weight, preterm birth, and stillbirth, as well as increased hypertensive disorders of pregnancy.
- Opioid agonist pharmacotherapy with either methadone or buprenorphine is first-line therapy for patients with opioid use disorder and can be safely initiated in pregnancy.

DISCLOSURE

The authors report no conflicts of interest.

REFERENCES

1. Bruzelius E, Martins SS. US trends in drug overdose mortality among pregnant and postpartum persons 2017-2020. JAMA 2022;328(21):2159–61.
2. Sacco LN, Congressional Research Service. Drug enforcement in the United States: history, policy, and trends. Available at: https://sgp.fas.org/crs/misc/R43749.pdf. Accessed July 31, 2023.
3. SixtyThird Congress of the United States. Harrison Narcotics Tax Act, 1914. Available at: https://www.naabt.org/documents/Harrison_Narcotics_Tax_Act_1914.pdf. Accessed July 31, 2023.
4. Farahmand P, Arshed A, Bradley MV. Systemic Racism and Substance Use Disorders. Psychiatr Ann 2020;50(11):494–8.
5. The American Presidency Project. Special Message to the Congress on Drug Abuse Prevention and Control. Available at: https://www.presidency.ucsb.edu/node/240245. Accessed July 31, 2023.
6. King RS, Mauer M. The war on marijuana: the transformation of the war on drugs in the 1990s. Harm Reduct J 2006;3:6.
7. Sabol WJ, Minton TD, Harrison PM, et al. Prison and Jail Inmates at Midyear 2006. Available at: https://bjs.ojp.gov/library/publications/prison-and-jail-inmates-midyear-2006. Accessed August 11, 2023.
8. Roberts SCM, Thompson TA, Taylor KJ. Dismantling the legacy of failed policy approaches to pregnant people's use of alcohol and drugs. Int Rev Psychiatry 2021;33(6):502–13.
9. Davis DA. Obstetric Racism: The Racial Politics of Pregnancy, Labor, and Birthing. Med Anthropol 2019;38(7):560–73.
10. World Health Organization. The prevention and elimination of disrespect and abuse during facility-based childbirth. Available at: https://apps.who.int/iris/bitstream/handle/10665/134588/WHO_RHR_14.23_eng.pdf. Accessed August 11, 2023.
11. Nuriddin A, Mooney G, White AIR. Reckoning with histories of medical racism and violence in the USA. Lancet 2020;396(10256):949–51.
12. Martin JA, Hamilton BE, Osterman MJ, et al. Births: Final Data for 2015. Natl Vital Stat Rep 2017;66(1):1.
13. Hoyert DL. Maternal Mortality Rates in the United States, 2021. Available at: https://stacks.cdc.gov/view/cdc/124678. Accessed August 11, 2023.
14. Hilliard F, Goldstein E, Nervik K, et al. Voices of Women With Lived Experience of Substance Use During Pregnancy: A Qualitative Study of Motivators and Barriers to Recruitment and Retention in Research. Fam Community Health 2023;46(1):1–12.
15. Ecker J, Abuhamad A, Hill W, et al. Substance use disorders in pregnancy: clinical, ethical, and research imperatives of the opioid epidemic: a report of a joint workshop of the Society for Maternal-Fetal Medicine, American College of Obstetricians and Gynecologists, and American Society of Addiction Medicine. Am J Obstet Gynecol 2019;221(1):B5–28.
16. Center for Behavioral Health Statistics and Quality, Substance Abuse and Mental Health Services Administration. 2019 National Survey on Drug Use and Health: Final Analytic File Codebook. Available at: https://www.samhsa.gov/data/sites/default/files/2021-09/NSDUHAnalyticCodebookRDC2019.pdf. Accessed May 11, 2023.
17. Cook JL, Green CR, de la Ronde S, et al. Screening and Management of Substance Use in Pregnancy: A Review. J Obstet Gynaecol Can 2017;39(10):897–905.

18. Raouf M, Bettinger JJ, Fudin J. A Practical Guide to Urine Drug Monitoring. Fed Pract 2018;35(4):38–44.
19. American College of Obstetricians and Gynecologists. Committee Opinion No. 711. Opioid use and opioid use disorder in pregnancy. Obstet Gynecol 2017; 130(2):e81–94.
20. Chasnoff IJ, Landress HJ, Barrett ME. The prevalence of illicit-drug or alcohol use during pregnancy and discrepancies in mandatory reporting in Pinellas County, Florida. N Engl J Med 1990;322(17):1202–6.
21. Wexelblatt SL, Ward LP, Torok K, et al. Universal maternal drug testing in a high-prevalence region of prescription opiate abuse. J Pediatr 2015;166(3):582–6.
22. Klawans MR, Northrup TF, Villarreal YR, et al. A comparison of common practices for identifying substance use during pregnancy in obstetric clinics. Birth 2019;46(4):663–9.
23. Skelton KR, Donahue E, Benjamin-Neelon SE. Validity of self-report measures of cannabis use compared to biological samples among women of reproductive age: a scoping review. BMC Pregnancy Childbirth 2022;22(1):344.
24. American College of Obstetricians and Gynecologists Committee on Health Care for Underserved Women. AGOG Committee Opinion No. 473: substance abuse reporting and pregnancy: the role of the obstetrician-gynecologist. Obstet Gynecol 2011;117(1):200–1.
25. Malmo-Levine D. Recent history. In: Holland J, editor. The Pot Book: a complete Guide to cannabis. Rochester, VT, USA: Park Street Press; 2010.
26. Bridgeman MB, Abazia DT. Medicinal cannabis: history, pharmacology, and implications for the acute care setting. P & T. 2017;42(3):180–8.
27. Musto DF. The Marihuana Tax Act of 1937. Arch Gen Psychiatry 1972;26(2): 101–8.
28. Adams C, CBS News. The man behind the marijuana ban for all the wrong reasons. Available at: https://www.cbsnews.com/news/harry-anslinger-the-man-behind-the-marijuana-ban/. Accessed August 11, 2023.
29. PBS Frontline. Marijuana Timeline. Available at: https://www.pbs.org/wgbh/pages/frontline/shows/dope/etc/cron.html. Accessed August 11, 2023.
30. Vitiello M. Marijuana legalization, racial disparity, and the hope for reform. Lewis & Clark Law Review 2019;23(3):789–821.
31. Houston WT. The racial politics of marijuana. In: Houston WT, editor. Race and the Black male Subculture: the Lives of Toby Waller. New York, NY, USA: Palgrave Macmillan; 2016.
32. Testa A, Jackson DB. Incarceration exposure and barriers to prenatal care in the United States: findings from the pregnancy risk assessment monitoring system. Int J Environ Res Public Health 2020;17(19). https://doi.org/10.3390/ijerph17197331.
33. Lee RD, D'Angelo DV, Dieke A, et al. Recent incarceration exposure among parents of live-born infants and maternal and child health. Public Health Rep 2023; 138(2):292–301.
34. Yi Y, Kennedy J, Chazotte C, et al. Paternal jail incarceration and birth outcomes: evidence from New York City, 2010-2016. Matern Child Health J 2021;25(8):1221–41.
35. Hudak J. Marijuana: A short history. Washington, DC, USA: Brookings Institution Press; 2016.
36. Bort R, Garber-Paul E, Ward A, et al. The United States of Weed. Available at: https://www.rollingstone.com/feature/cannabis-legalization-states-map-831885/. Accessed August 11, 2023.
37. Department of Justice, Drug Enforcement Administration. Drug Fact Sheet: Marijuana/Cannabis. Available at: https://www.dea.gov/sites/default/files/2020-06/Marijuana-Cannabis-2020_0.pdf. Accessed August 11, 2023.

38. Joshi S, Doonan SM, Pamplin JR 2nd. A tale of two cities: Racialized arrests following decriminalization and recreational legalization of cannabis. Drug Alcohol Depend 2023;249:109911.
39. Gunadi C, Shi Y. Cannabis decriminalization and racial disparity in arrests for cannabis possession. Soc Sci Med 2022;293:114672.
40. Ng JH, Rice KK, Ananth CV, et al. Attitudes about marijuana use, potential risks, and legalization: a single-center survey of pregnant women. J Matern Fetal Neonatal Med 2022;35(24):4635–43.
41. Mark K, Gryczynski J, Axenfeld E, et al. Pregnant Women's Current and Intended Cannabis Use in Relation to Their Views Toward Legalization and Knowledge of Potential Harm. J Addict Med 2017;11(3):211–6.
42. American College of Obstetricians and Gynecologists Committee on Obstetric Practice. Committee Opinion No. 722: Marijuana Use During Pregnancy and Lactation. Obstet Gynecol 2017;130(4):e205–9.
43. Ko JY, Coy KC, Haight SC, et al. Characteristics of Marijuana Use During Pregnancy - Eight States, Pregnancy Risk Assessment Monitoring System, 2017. MMWR Morb Mortal Wkly Rep 2020;69(32):1058–63.
44. Skelton KR, Hecht AA, Benjamin-Neelon SE. Association of Recreational Cannabis Legalization With Maternal Cannabis Use in the Preconception, Prenatal, and Postpartum Periods. JAMA Netw Open 2021;4(2):e210138.
45. Sood S, Trasande L, Mehta-Lee SS, et al. Maternal Cannabis Use in the Perinatal Period: Data From the Pregnancy Risk Assessment Monitoring System Marijuana Supplement, 2016-2018. J Addict Med 2022;16(4):e225–33.
46. King KA, Vidourek RA, Yockey RA. Psychosocial Determinants to Prenatal Marijuana Use Among a National Sample of Pregnant Females: 2015–2018. J Drug Issues 2020;50(4):424–35.
47. Dodge P, Nadolski K, Kopkau H, et al. The impact of timing of in utero marijuana exposure on fetal growth. Front Pediatr 2023;11:1103749.
48. Prewitt KC, Hayer S, Garg B, et al. Impact of Prenatal Cannabis Use Disorder on Perinatal Outcomes. J Addict Med 2023;17(3):e192–8.
49. Metz TD, Stickrath EH. Marijuana use in pregnancy and lactation: a review of the evidence. Am J Obstet Gynecol 2015;213(6):761–78.
50. Bolnick JM, Rayburn WF. Substance use disorders in women: special considerations during pregnancy. Obstet Gynecol Clin North Am 2003;30(3):545–58, vii.
51. Hernandez M, Birnbach DJ, Van Zundert AA. Anesthetic management of the illicit-substance-using patient. Curr Opin Anaesthesiol 2005;18(3):315–24.
52. Skelton KR, Hecht AA, Benjamin-Neelon SE. Recreational Cannabis Legalization in the US and Maternal Use during the Preconception, Prenatal, and Postpartum Periods. Int J Environ Res Public Health 2020;17(3). https://doi.org/10.3390/ijerph17030909.
53. Thiel de Bocanegra H, Braughton M, Bradsberry M, et al. Racial and ethnic disparities in postpartum care and contraception in California's Medicaid program. Am J Obstet Gynecol 2017;217(1):47 e1–e47 e7.
54. Morgan I, Hughes ME, Belcher H, et al. Maternal Sociodemographic Characteristics, Experiences and Health Behaviors Associated with Postpartum Care Utilization: Evidence from Maryland PRAMS Dataset, 2012-2013. Matern Child Health J 2018;22(4):589–98.
55. Yee LM, Martinez NG, Nguyen AT, et al. Using a Patient Navigator to Improve Postpartum Care in an Urban Women's Health Clinic. Obstet Gynecol 2017;129(5):925–33.
56. Kilpatrick SJ, Papile L, Macones GA. Guidelines for perinatal care. 8th ed. Elk Grove Village, IL, USA: American Academy of Pediatrics/The American College of Obstetricians and Gynecologists; 2017.

57. Beauregard JL, Hamner HC, Chen J, et al. Racial Disparities in Breastfeeding Initiation and Duration Among U.S. Infants Born in 2015. MMWR Morb Mortal Wkly Rep 2019;68(34):745–8.

58. Nidey N, Hoyt-Austin A, Chen MJ, et al. Racial Inequities in Breastfeeding Counseling Among Pregnant People Who Use Cannabis. Obstet Gynecol 2022;140(5): 878–81.

59. Marchand G, Masoud AT, Govindan M, et al. Birth Outcomes of Neonates Exposed to Marijuana in Utero: A Systematic Review and Meta-analysis. JAMA Netw Open 2022;5(1):e2145653.

60. Lo JO, Shaw B, Robalino S, et al. Cannabis Use in Pregnancy and Neonatal Outcomes: A Systematic Review and Meta-Analysis. Cannabis Cannabinoid Res 2023;8(5). https://doi.org/10.1089/can.2022.0262.

61. Thompson M, Vila M, Wang L, et al. Prenatal cannabis use and its impact on offspring neuro-behavioural outcomes: A systematic review. Paediatr Child Health 2023;28(1):8–16.

62. Loue S. Diversity issues in substance abuse treatment and research. New York, NY, USA: Springer; 2003.

63. Ayres RU. Anesthesia, Surgery, and Modern Medicine. In: Ayres RU, editor. The history and future of Technology: can Technology Save Humanity from Extinction? New York, NY, USA: Springer; 2021. p. 223–50.

64. Spillane JF. Cocaine: from medical Marvel to modern Menace in the United States, 1884–1920. New York, NY, USA: The Johns Hopkins University Press; 2000.

65. National Institute on Drug Abuse. What is the scope of cocaine use in the United States? Available at: https://nida.nih.gov/publications/research-reports/cocaine/what-scope-cocaine-use-in-united-states. Accessed May 8, 2023.

66. National Institute on Drug Abuse. How is cocaine used? Available at: https://nida.nih.gov/publications/research-reports/cocaine/how-cocaine-used. Accessed May 8, 2023.

67. Dos Santos JF, de Melo Bastos Cavalcante C, Barbosa FT, et al. Maternal, fetal and neonatal consequences associated with the use of crack cocaine during the gestational period: a systematic review and meta-analysis. Arch Gynecol Obstet 2018;298(3):487–503.

68. Hull L, May J, Farrell-Moore D, et al. Treatment of cocaine abuse during pregnancy: translating research to clinical practice. Curr Psychiatry Rep 2010;12(5): 454–61.

69. Kandall SR. Women and drug addiction: a historical perspective. J Addict Dis 2010;29(2):117–26.

70. Gannon M, Population Health Matters (formerly Health Policy Newsletter). MATER: Innovative Programs for Maternal Addiction Education Treatment and Research. Available at: https://jdc.jefferson.edu/hpn/vol29/iss3/5/. Accessed May 11, 2023.

71. Thomas MMC, Waldfogel J, Williams OF. Inequities in Child Protective Services Contact Between Black and White Children. Child Maltreat 2023;28(1):42–54.

72. Han B, Einstein EB, Jones CM, et al. Racial and Ethnic Disparities in Drug Overdose Deaths in the US During the COVID-19 Pandemic. JAMA Netw Open 2022; 5(9):e2232314.

73. Snowden LR, Cordell K, Bui J. Racial and Ethnic Disparities in Health Status and Community Functioning Among Persons with Untreated Mental Illness. J Racial Ethn Health Disparities 2023;10(5):2175–84.

74. Glenn JE. The Birth of the Crack Baby and the History that "Myths" Make. Available at: https://citeseerx.ist.psu.edu/pdf/a46a9edbcd4e1d1675aa585cd8ec00aa05b a8066. Accessed May 11, 2023.
75. Centers for Disease Control and Prevention. Understanding the Opioid Epidemic. Available at: https://www.cdc.gov/opioids/basics/epidemic.html. Accessed August 11, 2023.
76. Porter J, Jick H. Addiction rare in patients treated with narcotics. N Engl J Med 1980;302(2):123.
77. Meier B, New York Times. In guilty plea, OxyContin maker to pay $600 million. Available at: http://www.nytimes.com/2007/05/10/business/11drug-web.html. Accessed August 11, 2023.
78. Schuler MS, Schell TL, Wong EC. Racial/ethnic differences in prescription opioid misuse and heroin use among a national sample, 1999-2018. Drug Alcohol Depend 2021;221:108588.
79. Barnett ML, Meara E, Lewinson T, et al. Racial Inequality in Receipt of Medications for Opioid Use Disorder. N Engl J Med 2023;388(19):1779–89.
80. Schiff DM, Nielsen T, Hoeppner BB, et al. Assessment of Racial and Ethnic Disparities in the Use of Medication to Treat Opioid Use Disorder Among Pregnant Women in Massachusetts. JAMA Netw Open 2020;3(5):e205734.
81. Centers for Disease Control and Prevention. CDC WONDER - Wide-ranging ONline Data for Epidemiologic Research. Available at: http://wonder.cdc.gov. Accessed August 11, 2023.
82. Centers for Disease Control and Prevention. About Opioid Use During Pregnancy. Available at: https://www.cdc.gov/pregnancy/opioids/basics.html. Accessed August 11, 2023.
83. Schiff DM, Nielsen T, Terplan M, et al. Fatal and Nonfatal Overdose Among Pregnant and Postpartum Women in Massachusetts. Obstet Gynecol 2018;132(2): 466–74.
84. Yazdy MM, Mitchell AA, Tinker SC, et al. Periconceptional use of opioids and the risk of neural tube defects. Obstet Gynecol 2013;122(4):838–44.
85. Young LW, Ounpraseuth ST, Merhar SL, et al. Eat, Sleep, Console Approach or Usual Care for Neonatal Opioid Withdrawal. N Engl J Med 2023;388(25):2326–37.
86. Minozzi S, Amato L, Bellisario C, et al. Maintenance agonist treatments for opiate-dependent pregnant women. Cochrane Database Syst Rev 2013;12:CD006318. https://doi.org/10.1002/14651858.CD006318.pub3.
87. Johnson RE, Jones HE, Fischer G. Use of buprenorphine in pregnancy: patient management and effects on the neonate. Drug Alcohol Depend 2003;70(2 Suppl):S87–101.
88. Debelak K, Morrone WR, O'Grady KE, et al. Buprenorphine + naloxone in the treatment of opioid dependence during pregnancy-initial patient care and outcome data. Am J Addict 2013;22(3):252–4.
89. Towers CV, Katz E, Weitz B, et al. Use of naltrexone in treating opioid use disorder in pregnancy. Am J Obstet Gynecol 2020;222(1):83 e1–e83 e8.
90. Canzater SL, O'Neill Institute for National & Global Health Law. A Thoughtful Comparison of the Government's Response to Crack Epidemic of the 1980s vs. the current Opioid Epidemic: A look at criminalization, race, and treatment. Available at: https:// oneill.law.georgetown.edu/a-thoughtful-comparison-of-the-governments-response-to-crack-epidemic-of-the-1980s-vs-the-current-opioid-epidemic-a-look-at-crimina lization-race-and-treatment/. Accessed August 11, 2023.

Achieving Reproductive Justice Within Family Planning

Rieham Owda, MD, Charisse Loder, MD, MSc*

KEYWORDS

- Reproductive health care • Reproductive justice • Abortion • Contraception

KEY POINTS

- Understanding the historical and present context to reproductive oppression is an essential component to provision of reproductive health care.
- The reproductive justice framework provides a structure for advocacy and clinical work that is centered on a person's desire to become pregnant, prevent pregnancy, and raise healthy families.
- Overlapping systems of inequity limit patient's access to comprehensive family planning services, such as contraceptive care and abortion care, in the United States and contribute to reproductive health disparities.
- Clinical care providers can advocate for dismantling injustice within reproductive health and family planning by leveraging power and privilege within health systems.

INTRODUCTION

Reproductive health care in the United States has a long and complex history. Contraception and abortion services continue to face a variety of limitations and are not always accessible to all people—especially those from marginalized communities. Owing to the long-standing history of oppression and inequality in reproductive health care, it is critical to approach the delivery of these services through a health justice lens. Using a reproductive justice (RJ) framework allows for a more holistic approach in addressing the multifaceted reproductive needs of both individuals and communities. To understand the reproductive experience within the United States, we must first acknowledge and unpack this complicated history so that we can better understand the present context and advocate for future changes in the reproductive health landscape.

Department of Obstetrics and Gynecology, University of Michigan, 1500 East Medical Center Drive, Ann Arbor, MI 48109, USA
* Corresponding author. 1500 East Medical Center Drive, SPC 5276, Ann Arbor, MI 48109-5276.
E-mail address: loder@med.umich.edu

Obstet Gynecol Clin N Am 51 (2024) 211–221
https://doi.org/10.1016/j.ogc.2023.11.006
0889-8545/24/© 2023 Elsevier Inc. All rights reserved.

obgyn.theclinics.com

Defining Reproductive Justice

Family planning services has historically included contraception care, abortion services, and general reproductive care. When providing these services, there are three distinct frameworks that can be used in a complementary manner to decrease reproductive oppression and advance reproductive human rights. The three frameworks—reproductive health, reproductive rights, and RJ—were first analyzed in the 2005 essay "A New Vision for Reproductive Justice" by Asian Communities for Reproductive Justice, which is now known as Forward Together.[1] The first framework, reproductive health, focuses on service delivery and addresses the reproductive health needs of individual people. This framework focuses on expanding health care services and improving access to care, as well as on improving health data that is available to help improve health care delivery. The second framework, reproductive rights, focuses on the legal right to reproductive health care and the advocacy needed to maintain and fight for this right. The third framework, RJ, on which we will focus most in this article, uses community advocates and organizing to understand how the differing intersections of identity, environment, and society all interact to cause reproductive oppression. It also combines the ideas of social justice and human rights to achieve full reproductive autonomy.

The RJ framework transcends the traditional boundaries of the reproductive health and reproductive rights frameworks. At its core, reproductive justice is ensuring that each individual—regardless of their race, class, gender, or ability—has the agency to make informed decisions about their reproductive life and are able to access the necessary resources to make that choice. This framework was created in 1994 by a group of Black female activists who felt that the frameworks present at the time did not address the needs of people of color and their reproductive autonomy.[2] The reproductive justice movement has played a crucial role in advocating for the empowerment of individuals in making informed choices about their bodies and their families.

To understand how the reproductive justice framework came to be, we must first examine other reproductive health movements and the history that led to their creation. In the early nineteenth century, abortion was legal within the United States until "quickening"—the time at which a pregnant individual perceived fetal movement. Around the middle of the century, a campaign to criminalize abortion was initiated based on concerns about its safety and the provision of abortion care by homeopaths and midwives. This campaign was supported by physicians, who wanted to curtail the provision of reproductive health care by nonphysicians through the backing and support of countless local and national medical societies. Local medical societies also used the Comstock Act, a federal law that criminalized the use of the United States Postal Service to distribute information regarding sexual health, abortion, and contraception. The goal was not only to stop the advertising of contraceptives but also to limit the distribution of abortion information and discontinue the mailing of abortifacients.[3,4] The antiabortion campaign was also fueled by White Protestant families, who were concerned that continued abortion access would lead to a decrease in the birth rates within their communities and, subsequently, an increase in overpopulation of minority communities.[5]

In response to decades of antiabortion campaigns, the feminist pro-choice movement to support abortion and reproductive rights was created.[6] This movement focused solely on the idea of choice—specifically the ways in which choosing not to continue a pregnancy could facilitate the liberation of women and allow them to have full autonomy. It gained significant momentum in the 1960s and 1970s. In 1965, the United States Supreme Court's decision in *Griswold v Connecticut* gave married couples the ability to buy and use contraceptives without government restriction, which overturned the prior Comstock Act.[7] Shortly thereafter, the Supreme Court ruled in the landmark decision of *Roe v Wade* in 1973, which legalized abortion in the United States. The time period after *Roe v Wade* highlighted the concept of reproductive choice, and the ability to decide what was best for an individual and their pregnancy. The pro-choice movement focused on reproductive decisions, but it did not account for the fact that choice alone is not enough in the fight for reproductive autonomy. During the 1970s and 1980s, women of color activists highlighted that people who come from historically marginalized communities do not have access to the same choices as those with privilege due to societal, environmental, and economic reasons.

Given the limitations of the pro-choice movement and recognizing that the idea of choice did not fully encompass the reproductive experiences of women of color, activists of color—many of whom are associated with SisterSong, an Atlanta-based reproductive justice organization—called for a different framework to achieve reproductive autonomy. They envisioned a movement that focused not only on the choice to prevent pregnancy but also on living in a healthy environment devoid of racism, where people have access to medical care and stable housing. As a result, the reproductive justice framework was built, addressing all the necessary aspects to achieve reproductive autonomy and freedom. Its aim was to merge reproductive rights and social justice to create a framework that meets those needs. Reproductive justice is made up of several primary principles defined as: "the human right to maintain personal bodily autonomy, have children, not have children, and parent the children we have in safe and sustainable communities."[2] SisterSong's executive director, Monica Simpson, recommends that in considering reproductive justice, "[we] consider the ways in which all social justice issues intersect and affect the way we are able to make decisions about our bodies and the creation of our futures."[8] In focusing on the greater structures and issues that lead to injustice, the reproductive justice movement widens the lens to encompass all reproductive issues, rather than focusing solely on abortion and contraception rights.

Historical Injustices

The reproductive ability and capacity of people of color has been governed for centuries by race, wealth, gender, and power hierarchies. Historically, reproductive health within the United States has been restricted by structural forces such as policies, health education, and health systems but also by societal discrimination such as racism and sexism that leads to injustice. Reproductive injustice can be pervasive and includes unequal access to reproductive health care, incomplete insurance coverage of services, and abuses within health care institutions such as provider bias, discrimination, and coercion. People of privilege and power, both inside and outside the medical establishment, have a history of exercising control over the reproductive freedoms of those with less power, leading to systematic marginalization of groups based on race, ethnicity, immigration status, ability, income, and education. To understand the history of reproductive rights in the United States, it is important to understand how reproductive freedoms were controlled since the colonization of North America. **Fig. 1** outlines some of the major reproductive justice legislation over time in the United States.

During colonization and in establishing an independent United States, Europeans acquired territory using not only military power but also reproductive control to establish dominance over indigenous and enslaved people. Colonizers used mass genocide to limit the growth of indigenous populations: "[Indigenous people] were hunted down

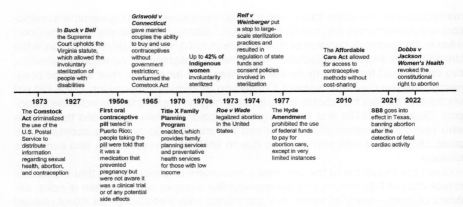

Fig. 1. Major legislative timeline of reproductive health care in the United States.

and slaughtered. [due to] the potential through childbirth to assure the continuance of the people."[9] In the eighteenth and nineteenth centuries, Indigenous American families were impacted by anti-native laws aimed at abolishing Indigenous American culture and the establishment of boarding schools to remove children from their families.[10] Not only were children discouraged from learning their native language, observing cultural practices, and maintaining contact with families, but they also suffered from atrocious physical and sexual abuses.

During this period, enslaved Black women also experienced dehumanization and reproductive control as White men, who claimed to own them, sought to restrict access to sexual partners, control birthing, and limit the ability to raise children throughout the trans-Atlantic slave trade and in the Antebellum South.[11] These practices were enacted through breeding programs, which became the only way for plantation owners to produce more enslaved people once the 1808 Ban on the importation of enslaved people was established.[12] As a result, thousands of Black enslaved women were subjected to violations of bodily autonomy including rape, assault, and forced reproduction.[13] With no rights and little power, enslaved women had few ways to regain bodily autonomy, but did so by seeking herbal remedies to attempt to prevent or end a pregnancy, often relying on the advice of elders or midwives within their communities.[12]

In the mid-1800s, medicine began to formalize with the increasing presence of organized medical societies and increasing physician credibility, along with the heightened importance on the reproduction of enslaved women in the United States for the perpetuation of slavery following the 1808 Ban. There evolved a shift in the provision of maternal and reproductive health care from midwifery care to physician-delivered care.[14] In fact, physicians sought to silence or repress midwifery expertise, claiming patients were "...exposed to the dangers of incompetence, ignorant, unclean midwives." Physicians began publishing new knowledge in periodicals and developed innovative treatments and surgical techniques aimed at improving reproductive function. The cost of formalizing gynecology, however, was borne by people of color who contributed to medicine, whereas they and their families simultaneously experienced reproductive oppression, racism, and enslavement.

Specifically, gynecology was built on experimentation on the bodies of enslaved Black women. J Marion Sims, known as the father of modern gynecology due to his contribution to the field, experimented on both Black and White women to develop new treatment options and surgical techniques for treating vesicovaginal fistulas. The purpose of these surgeries was twofold: to experiment with innovative surgical techniques, while also attempting to relieve these women of their symptoms. The desire to relieve enslaved women of their symptoms was so that they would be able to return to their enslavers and continue to labor without disruption. Surgical techniques were refined by White physicians, often without their own knowledge or concern of the risks and consequences to the patient, and without informed discussion or consent.[15] In identifying potential surgical subjects, Sims and other practicing physicians would in some instances lease Black women from their enslavers. None of these surgeries were performed under anesthesia, even when its use became more widespread. One concern among the medical community was that anesthetic use increased blood loss, which was later debunked. In addition, there were gross underestimates of the pain experienced by those undergoing vaginal surgery. Finally, there was a widespread belief that Black people experience pain differently than their White counterparts, a notion that continues to be perpetuated in current medical texts but holds no scientific merit.

The development of surgical techniques for treating vesicovaginal fistula, which was a key factor identifying Sims as a leader in gynecology, is one of many examples of how the bodies of Black women were not valued and were viewed as disposable, only to be used to accomplish certain social, political, or economic agendas.[15] Many of Sims' subjects were not known by name, and only three enslaved women were recognized in historical documents: Lucy, Anarcha, and Betsey. Although many physicians, like Sims, have been celebrated for the knowledge and skills that informed the contemporary practice of gynecology, the field has not traditionally acknowledged those who sacrificed their bodies without consent to the acquisition of this knowledge. It is only more recently that discussions about this history have occurred within medical societies and have been woven into medical education in a way that honors the contributions of Lucy, Anarcha, Betsey, and many others.[16] It has also taken over a century for the medical community to begin grappling with the legacy of Sims and other surgeons.

In the early 1900s, reproductive injustices continued as eugenics movements spread throughout the world and eugenics programs were established across the United States. Eugenics was a movement seeking to limit the fertility of those felt to be "unfit" or "feebleminded" while supporting the growth of privileged communities—often White communities with high socioeconomic status. Eugenics programs were fueled by racism, with the belief that some groups of people should not procreate and that allowing them to do so could dilute the population. Thousands of people—often selected based on race, ethnicity, disability, or immigration status—were sterilized through these eugenics programs.[17] Physicians were complicit in coercive sterilization practices, and sterilizations often occurred without patient knowledge or consent. One notable case, *Relf v Weinberger,* shed light on these practices by highlighting a case of two adolescents who were sterilized without parental knowledge. This case put a stop to large-scale sterilization practices and resulted in regulation of state funds and consent policies involved in sterilization. The legacy of the eugenics movement influences contemporary reproductive health care, as we continue to observe ways in which fertility is devalued and even controlled among those who have been marginalized in society.

In the 1950s, emerging hormonal contraceptive technologies introduced a new option for fertility control; however, the cost of being a research subject was again borne by marginalized communities. Unfortunately, contraceptive clinical trials were wrought with ethical concerns, from study recruitment to informed consent processes, which echoed coercive sterilization practices of the past. For example, contraceptive researchers first experimented with hormonal medications among institutionalized women with mental health disorders in Massachusetts. Large-scale birth control pill trials heavily recruited in communities of color and in Puerto Rico, where subjects were not compensated for participation[18] and trials were not subject to the same rules and regulations of the mainland United States. The first combined hormonal contraceptive pill was approved in 1960 and at first only available to married couples. However, unmarried people gained access to birth control methods in the following decades and benefited from the growth in contraceptive technologies that expanded options beyond the birth control pill. The progestin injectable, depot medroxyprogesterone acetate (DMPA), was widely used for contraception outside of the United States but struggled to achieve Food and Drug Administration (FDA) approval until 1992. Despite this, DMPA use was widespread among institutionalized populations and within the Indian Health Service[19,20] as a tool for menstrual control. Many who were treated with DMPA were not informed of its side effects—including its long-term contraceptive effect—or even notified of their participation in contraceptive trials. Ultimately, the full breadth of communities who unknowingly contributed to contraceptive science may never fully be known; consequently, there remains significant distrust of contraceptive technologies today due to these unethical practices.

As laws restricting contraception were relaxed and contraceptive use became more widespread, those holding power considered how to use it as a tool of reproductive control. Several politicians proposed to use birth control as a method of limiting family size to serve their own political agendas. For example, in the early 1990s, legislators in many states proposed dozens of bills that included financial or social incentives in exchange for utilization of Norplant,[21] a long-acting reversible contraceptive (LARC) device. Low-income communities were more likely to be targeted for these initiatives. Although these bills were ultimately not passed, they were problematic in that they devalued the fertility of those seeking social support programs, such as nutrition and housing assistance. Although these bills were not explicitly racist, they propagated an idea about who should and should not have children. Anthropologists first described this concept as stratified reproduction,[22] where the fertility of those with social and economic power is valued, whereas those without power are devalued. These disturbing patterns of reproductive injustices are pervasive and woven into the very fabric of US history.

Current Injustices in Family Planning and Their Impact

Given the nature of these injustices, it is hard to imagine that they could persist. Unfortunately, reproductive injustices continue to be perpetuated both inside and outside of the health care system. Although large-scale coercive sterilization programs were halted, more recent examples of sterilization without patient consent have been uncovered. One such example is the California State Auditor's report[23] of more than 100 sterilization procedures that were performed on incarcerated people in the early 2000s, which highlighted failures to document informed consent and/or to observe the 30-day waiting period. In addition, in 2022, a nurse whistleblower shed light on unindicated gynecologic procedures, such as hysterectomies being performed within an Immigration Detention Center. The resulting investigation revealed "female detainees appear to have undergone excessive, invasive, and often unnecessary gynecologic procedures"[24] and recommended against using the medical facility and physician for future detainee care. These examples highlight not only how the entire health care team may play a role in perpetuating injustice but also that health care systems and people within them can be instrumental in changing them.

Being able to control one's ability to become or not become pregnant is a core component of reproductive justice; however, access to affordable contraceptive care remains out of reach for many people in the United States. From a federal standpoint, there are multiple policies in place that have led to decreased access to essential reproductive health care. The passage of the Affordable Care Act in 2012 required states to expand Medicaid while also allowing for access to contraceptive methods without cost-sharing. Legal challenges resulted, with only 40 states expanding Medicaid coverage and leaving many without access to care.[25] In addition, religiously affiliated nonprofit and for-profit organizations upheld their right in court to refuse its provision. Limits on Title X funding, which funds a broad range of family planning services such as preconception health services, sexually transmitted disease testing, and contraceptive products,[26] have resulted in limited access to those in greatest need such as under- or uninsured communities. In addition, the Hyde amendment prohibits the use of federal funds to pay for abortion care, except in very limited instances (such as in situations where continuing the pregnancy would endanger a person's life). As unplanned pregnancy rates increase in the United States, along with increases in preterm birth and morbidity and mortality rates for pregnant and postpartum people, the lack of access to contraceptives and abortion care is particularly unjust.

As we consider the history of contraceptive care in the United States, it is no surprise that bias and pressure exist in care provision today.[27,28] LARC has been viewed as a powerful tool for preventing unplanned pregnancy; however, uptake has long been impeded by access to skilled providers and device cost. Several initiatives have used grant funding to expand access to LARC by providing free devices to low-income, uninsured patients (often referred to as the "LARC-first" approach). However, reproductive justice advocates and health care providers caution against this approach. It may not appropriately enable patient-centered, justice-informed care,[29] and does not acknowledge previous violations in reproductive autonomy and how bias can impact contraceptive recommendations and care. The "LARC -first" approach can also perpetuate the concept of stratified reproduction. Research shows that contraceptive providers do exhibit bias in making recommendations about intrauterine device (IUD) use depending on the patient's race, ethnicity, and perceived socioeconomic status.[28] In addition, studies have uncovered that patients experience undesired counseling approaches by their providers. In one study interviewing postpartum women about their experiences with contraceptive counseling, researchers found that women felt pressured to choose contraception. One subject described repeated attempts by her doctors to convince her to choose a method, stating, "They wanted to go with the IUD... they kept bringing it up over and over again." Others described being suspicious that providers were targeting patients based on race and/or ethnicity for LARC methods or potentially receiving financial incentives or "kickbacks" for placing them.[27,28] Other studies involving young women and Latinas accessing contraceptive care have revealed feelings of medical mistrust and perceived discrimination.[30] Given these findings, it is imperative that reproductive health care providers reflect on their own biases and develop approaches that mitigate these effects and prioritize a patient-centered and justice-informed approach.

In the last decade, abortion care has been significantly regulated and restricted, limiting access not only to abortion services but also to other types of reproductive health care. For example, 16 states have restricted the allocation of state funding for family planning services at private reproductive health clinics that counsel about abortion or offer abortion services.[31] There are also restrictions on funds typically used for sexually transmitted disease diagnosis and treatment. In addition, targeted regulation of abortion providers (known as targeted regulation of abortion providers [TRAP] laws) has led to an increase in state laws restricting abortion care and facilities that perform this care. Today, more than 20 states have regulations or policies that limit medical licensing, require physician admitting privileges, set building standards, or require transfer agreements.[32] Although the stated intention of these laws is to improve the safety of abortion care, there is no evidence that health outcomes have subsequently improved.[33] In fact, these regulations have resulted in the closing of reproductive health clinics, which leads to access issues and delays in patient care.

It is also hard to ignore the impact that the Dobbs decision has had on reproductive access. On June 24, 2022, the US Supreme Court ruled in *Dobbs v Jackson Women's Health*, overturning nearly 50 years of precedent that was set by *Roe v Wade* and revoked the constitutional right to abortion. This decision returned the right to abortion up to each individual state, meaning that laws and access vary from state to state. Texas is one of the most restricted states in the country, limiting access to pregnancy termination for pregnancies less than 6 weeks or in cases of pregnancy threatening maternal life, and invoked this law about 9 months before the *Dobbs* decision. Regulations around referral to abortion services or assisting a person in Texas to leave the state to obtain abortion care have created strains on the patient–physician relationship. Texas has therefore proven to be a case study for poor maternal health outcomes due to its severely restricted abortion care.[34] In fact, several studies demonstrate that abortion restrictions result in higher rates of maternal and infant morbidity and mortality.[35] At the time of this publication, 14 states have complete bans on abortion care and many others have significant restrictions that make it difficult for patients to access care. This lack of abortion access not only challenges the concept of reproductive justice but also represents a larger public health and women's rights issue.

Moving Forward Together

Although understanding the US history of reproductive health care is critical, many of these injustices continue to be perpetuated today. To achieve reproductive justice, systemic inequities must be addressed. There is a critical need for advocacy for policies and practices that ensure that all individuals not only have the resources and agency to make decisions about their reproductive lives, but they are also in safe environments to be able to do so. Below are some steps and considerations to achieving reproductive justice within family planning, which is represented in **Fig. 2**.

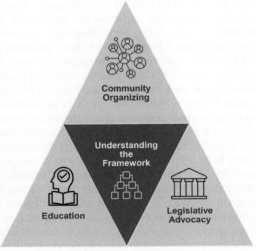

Achieving Reproductive Justice

Fig. 2. Strategy to addressing reproductive justice.

1. Understanding the Framework: It is imperative for people to familiarize themselves with the reproductive justice framework. This framework focuses on using an intersectional approach that considers race, class, gender, and other social determinants and the impact of those factors on a person's ability to achieve reproductive autonomy. It also focuses on the entire reproductive experience, not just abortion and contraception care.
2. Community Organizing: We must support grassroot movements and community organizations that are fighting for reproductive justice and recognize that community organizing is at the heart of this movement.
3. Education: We must continue to educate ourselves and others about the history of reproduction within the United States, especially that of marginalized individuals. Understanding the previous history allows us to understand the context under which we are providing care and to avoid perpetuating mistakes of the past.
4. Legislative Advocacy: It is critical, especially in this time, to advocate both on a state and national level for affordable and accessible health care services, including contraceptive care, abortion services, fertility treatments, prenatal care, and postpartum care regardless of an individual's income or geographic location.

Achieving reproductive justice and integrating this approach into reproductive care is an ongoing process that involves addressing both immediate and long-term societal issues. It requires collective action, advocacy, and a commitment to interrogating and dismantling the systems in which we work and live to ensure that everyone, regardless of what identities they hold, can achieve true reproductive autonomy.

SUMMARY

The state of reproductive health care continues to be challenging with many similarities to the past despite continuous fights to make this essential health care accessible to all moving forward. As restrictions on abortion and contraception access continue, it is imperative that we understand the historical context of reproduction in the United States. The historical legacy of injustice still has a lingering impact on how people access reproductive health care. It also informs what we must do to ensure that harms of the past are not perpetuated. By understanding the historical context that led to the development of reproductive justice and its core principles, health care providers can strive to deliver equitable and just care that recognizes and validates the experiences of marginalized communities. Using a reproductive justice lens when providing family planning services allows us to address an individual's right to have or not have children. It also reinforces the broader social justice issues that intersect with a person's reproductive health with the goal of achieving reproductive liberation.

CLINICS CARE POINTS

- Obstetrics and gynecology practitioners must understand the historical context of reproductive oppression and injustice in the United States.
- The reproductive justice framework is a lens which recognizes a person's autonomy and right to become pregnant, prevent pregnancy, and raise healthy families.
- Many marginalized communities have suffered injustices and may continue to be negatively impacted by reproductive legislation that limits access.
- Clinical providers must advocate for dismantling injustice in reproductive health.

DISCLOSURE

Dr C. Loder is a Principal Investigator for Contraceptive Clinical Trials for Merck & Co, Inc and Sebela Pharmaceuticals Inc and is an Educational Consultant for the American Medical Students' Association.

REFERENCES

1. Asian Communities for Reproductive Justice. A New Vision for advancing our movement for reproductive health, reproductive rights and reproductive justice. 2005; https://forwardtogether.org/wp-content/uploads/2017/12/ACRJ-A-New-Vision.pdf. Accessed October 24, 2023.
2. Ross LJ, Solinger R. Reproductive justice: an introduction. Oakland, CA: University of California Press; 2017.
3. Reagan LJ. When abortion was a crime: women, medicine, and law in the United States, 1867-1973. Berkeley, CA: University of California Press; 2022.
4. Burnette BR. Comstock Act of 1873. 2009; https://firstamendment.mtsu.edu/article/comstock-act-of-1873-1873/. Accessed October 24, 2023.
5. Pollitt K. Abortion in American History. 1997; https://www.theatlantic.com/magazine/archive/1997/05/abortion-in-american-history/376851/. Accessed October 24, 2023.
6. Nelson J. 6 women of color and the movement for reproductive justice: a human rights agenda. In: Nelson J, editor. More than medicine: a history of the feminist women's health movement. New York, NY: NYU Press; 2015.
7. Bollier D. Summary: Griswold v. Connecticut. https://www.jud.ct.gov/publications/Curriculum/Curriculum6.pdf. Accessed October 24, 2023.
8. Simpson M. To Be Pro-Choice, You Must Have the Privilege of Having Choices. 2022; https://www.nytimes.com/2022/04/11/opinion/abortion-black-brown-women.html. Accessed October 24, 2023.
9. Smith A, Ross L. Introduction: Native Women and State Violence. Soc Justice 2004;31(4):1–7.
10. National Native American Boarding School Healing Coalition. US Indian Boarding School History. https://boardingschoolhealing.org/education/us-indian-boarding-school-history/.
11. Franklin JH. From slavery to freedom. New York, NY: Alfred A. Knopf; 1947.
12. Roberts D. Killing the Black body. New York, NY: Vintage Books; 1997.
13. Townsend H. Second Middle Passage: How Anti-Abortion Laws Perpetuate Structures of Slavery and the Case for Reproductive Justice. Univ Pa J Const Law 2023;25(1):185–232.
14. Thompson JB, Varney H. A history of midwifery in the United States: the midwife said fear not. New York, NY: Springer Publishing; 2016.
15. Owens DC. Medical bondage: race, gender, and the origins of American gynecology. Athens, GA: University of Georgia Press; 2017.
16. American College of Obstetricians and Gynecologists. Betsey, Lucy, and Anarcha Days of Recognition. https://www.acog.org/about/diversity-equity-and-inclusive-excellence/betsey-lucy-and-anarcha-days-of-recognition. Accessed October 24, 2023.
17. Stern AM. Eugenics, sterilization, and historical memory in the United States. Hist Cienc Saude Manguinhos 2016;1(Suppl 1):195–212.
18. Pendergrass D.C., Raji M.Y., The Harvard Crimson. The Bitter Pill: Harvard and the Dark History of Birth Control. 2017. Available at: www.thecrimson.com/article/2017/9/28/the-bitter-pill/. Accessed October 24, 2023.

19. Stern AM. Eugenics, sterilization, and historical memory in the United States. Hist Cienc Saude Manguinhos 2016;23Suppl 1(Suppl 1):195–212.
20. Volscho TW. Racism and disparities in women's use of the depo-provera injection in the contemporary USA. Crit Sociol 2011;37(5):673–88.
21. American Civil Liberties Union. Norplant: A New Contraceptive with the Potential for Abuse. 1994; https://www.aclu.org/documents/norplant-new-contraceptive-potential-abuse#:~:text=In%201991%2C%201992%2C%20and%201993,induce%20them%20to%20use%20Norplant. Accessed October 24, 2023.
22. Ginsburg FD, Rapp R. Introduction: conceiving the new world order. In: Ginsburg FD, Rapp R, editors. Conceiving the new world order: the global politics of reproduction. Berkeley, CA: University of California Press; 1995.
23. California State Auditor. Sterilization of Female Inmates. 2014; https://www.auditor.ca.gov/pdfs/reports/2013-120.pdf. Accessed October 24, 2023.
24. Montoya-Galvez C, CBS News. Investigation finds women detained by ICE underwent "unnecessary gynecological procedures" at Georgia facility. 2022; https://www.cbsnews.com/news/women-detained-ice-unnecessary-gynecological-procedures-georgia-facility-investigation/. Accessed October 24, 2023.
25. The Commonwealth Fund. Impact of the Medicaid Coverage Gap: Comparing States That Have and Have Not Expanded Eligibility. September 11, 2023; https://www.commonwealthfund.org/publications/issue-briefs/2023/sep/impact-medicaid-coverage-gap-comparing-states-have-and-have-not. Accessed November 11, 2023.
26. Salganicoff A, Ranji U. A Focus on Contraception in the Wake of Dobbs. Wom Health Issues 2023;33(4):341–4.
27. Yee LM, Simon MA. Perceptions of coercion, discrimination and other negative experiences in postpartum contraceptive counseling for low-income minority women. J Health Care Poor Underserved 2011;22(4):1387–400.
28. Dehlendorf C, Ruskin R, Grumbach K, et al. Recommendations for intrauterine contraception: a randomized trial of the effects of patients' race/ethnicity and socioeconomic status. Am J Obstet Gynecol 2010;203(4):319.e1-8.
29. Gubrium AC, Mann ES, Borrero S, et al. Realizing reproductive health equity needs more than long-acting reversible contraception (LARC). Am J Publ Health 2016;106(1):18–9.
30. Higgins JA, Kramer RD, Ryder KM. Provider bias in long-acting reversible contraception (larc) promotion and removal: perceptions of young adult women. Am J Publ Health 2016;106(11):1932–7.
31. Guttmacher Institute. State Family Planning Funding Restrictions. 2023; https://www.guttmacher.org/state-policy/explore/state-family-planning-funding-restrictions. Accessed October 24, 2023.
32. Guttmacher Institute. Targeted Regulation of Abortion Providers. 2023; https://www.guttmacher.org/state-policy/explore/targeted-regulation-abortion-providers. Accessed October 24, 2023.
33. Austin N, Harper S. Assessing the impact of TRAP laws on abortion and women's health in the USA: a systematic review. BMJ Sex Reprod Health 2018;44(2):128–34.
34. Arey W, Lerma K, Beasley A, et al. A preview of the dangerous future of abortion bans - texas senate bill 8. N Engl J Med 2022;387(5):388–90.
35. Harper LM, Leach JM, Robbins L, et al. All-cause mortality in reproductive-aged females by state: an analysis of the effects of abortion legislation. Obstet Gynecol 2023;141(2):236–42.

Printed and bound by CPI Group (UK) Ltd, Croydon, CR0 4YY

08/05/2025

01864748-0004